THE CYTOKINE
FactsBook

Other books in the FactsBook Series:

A. Neil Barclay, Albertus D. Beyers, Marian L. Birkeland, Marion H. Brown,
Simon J. Davis, Chamorro Somoza, Alan F. Williams
The Leucocyte Antigen FactsBook

Rod Pigott and Christine Power
The Adhesion Molecule FactsBook

Ed Conley
The Ion Channel FactsBook

Shirley Ayad, Ray Boot-Handford, Martin J. Humphries, Karl E. Kadler and
Adrian Shuttleworth
The Extracellular Matrix FactsBook

Steve Watson and Steve Arkinstall
The G-Protein Linked Receptor Factsbook

Robin Hesketh
The Oncogene Factsbook

Graham D. Hardie and Steven Hanks
The Protein Kinase Factsbook

THE CYTOKINE
FactsBook

Robin E. Callard
Institute of Child Health,
University of London, London, UK

Andy J.H. Gearing
Neures Ltd,
Abingdon, UK

Academic Press
Harcourt Brace & Company, Publishers
LONDON   SAN DIEGO   NEW YORK   BOSTON
SYDNEY   TOKYO   TORONTO

ACADEMIC PRESS LIMITED
24–28 Oval Road
LONDON NW1 7DX

U.S. Edition Published by
ACADEMIC PRESS INC.
San Diego, CA 92101

This book is printed on acid-free paper

A catalogue record for this book is available from the British Library

ISBN 0–12–155143–1

Typeset by Columns Design and Production Services Ltd, Reading
Printed and bound in Great Britain by Mackays of Chatham PLC, Chatham, Kent

Contents

Section I   THE INTRODUCTORY CHAPTERS

Section II   THE CYTOKINES AND THEIR RECEPTORS

Interleukins

Other Cytokines (in alphabetical order)

Preface

The FactsBook series had its inception during a conversation between the authors and Susan King at Academic Press four years ago. The first of the series, The Leucocyte Antigen FactsBook, was published in 1993 and fully vindicates Susan's vision and hard work to get the series started. We hope that the present volume meets the same high standard set by the first FactsBook. There are many people who have helped with advice and information during the writing of this book. In particular, we would like to mention Luke O'Neill for advice on signal transduction, Julian Symons and Gordon Duff for information on IL-1, Mark Mercola for unpublished sequence data on murine PDGF, Tadimitsu Kishimoto for information on murine gp130, and Ken Grabstein for advance information on the latest cytokine IL-15. Robin Thorpe, Antony Meager and Tony Mire-Sluis helped frequently when we could not obtain some vital piece of information. Richard Armitage and David Gearing also supplied us with unpublished information on cytokine receptors. We are especially grateful to Neil Barclay for allowing us to use his carefully prepared diagrams of cytokine receptors which appeared in The Leucocyte Antigen FactsBook, and the many reviewers who were kind enough to comment on early drafts of the various chapters. We also wish to thank Susan King, and subsequently Tessa Picknett, Leona Daw and Claire Gilman for their hard work and patience in getting the manuscript into press.

One of us (R.E.C.) also wishes to acknowledge funding from Action Research, the Leukaemia Research Fund, the Medical Research Council, and the Wellcome Trust.

The other (A.J.H.G.) wishes to thank Kate Owen for cheery help, British Biotech for employment, Academic Press for very nearly understanding I had a day job (sorry Tessa!) and finally Frances, Jamie and Catherine.

There will undoubtedly be some omissions and errors in this volume although we hope they will be infrequent. We would greatly appreciate being informed of any inaccuracies by writing to the Editor, Cytokine FactsBook, Academic Press, 24-28 Oval Road, London NW1 7DX, UK, so that these can be rectified in future editions.

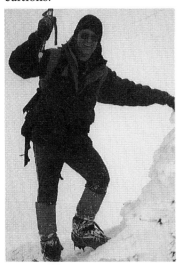 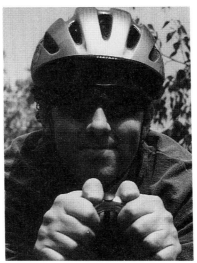

Left: *Robin Callard*, Right: *Andy Gearing*

Abbreviations

CCP-SF	Complement control protein superfamily
CKR-SF	Cytokine receptor superfamily
CSF	Colony stimulating factor
DAG	1,2-Diacylglycerol
EBV	Epstein–Barr virus
FNIII	Fibronectin type III domain
GAG	Glycosaminoglycan
GAP	GTPase activating protein
GF	Growth factor
GPI	Glycosyl-phosphatidylinositol
IFN	Interferon
IFNR-SF	Interferon receptor superfamily (also CKR-SF type II)
Ig-SF	Immunoglobulin superfamily
IL	Interleukin
IP_3	Inositol 1,4,5-trisphosphate
LAK	Lymphokine-activated killer
LPS	Lipopolysaccharide
LRR	Leucine-rich region
LTR	Long terminal repeat
M_r	Molecular ratio
NGFR-SF	Nerve growth factor receptor superfamily
NK	Natural killer
ORF	Open reading frame
PGE_2	Prostaglandin E_2
PHA	Phytohaemagglutinin
PI	Phosphatidylinositol
PIP_2	Phosphatidylinositol bisphosphate
PKC	Protein kinase C
PLC	Phospholipase C
PLD	Phospholipase D
PTK	Protein tyrosine kinase
PTKR-SF	Protein tyrosine kinase receptor superfamily
SF	Superfamily
STSR-SF	Seven transmembrane spanning receptor superfamily
TCR	T Cell receptor
4PS	I L-4 induced phosphotyrosine substrate

Abbreviations for all the cytokines are not included here as the abbreviation and full name appears at the beginning of each entry

THE INTRODUCTORY CHAPTERS

1 Introduction

AIMS OF THE BOOK

The main aim of this book is to provide a compendium of human and murine cytokines and their receptors. The information provided is confined largely to physicochemical properties, and includes amino acid sequences. The biological properties are not treated in detail but are described briefly. There are also introductory chapters on the nature of cytokines and cytokine families, the cytokine network, and cytokine receptor superfamilies.

WHAT IS A CYTOKINE?

Cytokines are soluble proteins or glycoproteins produced by leucocytes, and in many cases other cell types, which act as chemical communicators between cells, but not as effector molecules in their own right. Most are secreted, but some can be expressed on the cell membrane, and others are held in reservoirs in the extracellular matrix. Cytokines bind to specific receptors on the surface of target cells which are coupled to intracellular signal transduction and second messenger pathways. Most cytokines are growth and/or differentiation factors and they generally act on cells within the haematopoietic system.

Most of the molecules covered in this book fall easily within this definition of cytokines, but some do not. Erythropoietin (Epo) is not produced by leucocytes, but does act on haematopoietic precursors to generate red blood cells, and its receptor belongs to the cytokine receptor superfamily. Nerve growth factor (NGF), neurotrophin-3 (NT-3), and brain derived neurotrophic factor (BDNF) are all members of the same family of cytokines which are produced and act predominantly in the nervous system, but NGF also affects B cells, and its low affinity receptor is related to the tumour necrosis factor receptor (TNFR). Not all soluble peptide mediators are considered to be cytokines (e.g. insulin) and these exceptions have not been included. In the end, the decision whether to include a molecule as a cytokine or not must be somewhat arbitrary. If there are any omissions which offend, please let the Editor know and we will try to include them in the next edition. Information in this book is provided only for human and murine (or in some cases rat) cytokines which have been cloned, and for which there is a reasonable body of biological information. Where the receptors have been cloned, they are also included.

CYTOKINE FAMILIES

It should become clear from reading the entries in this book that cytokine nomenclature owes little to any systematic relationships between molecules. This is a reflection of the different historical approaches to naming new cytokines which were based either on cell of origin or initial defining bioassay. These systems have created anomalies such as tumour necrosis factor, originally defined as causing necrosis of solid tumours, but which is now thought to be primarily an immunomodulatory and pro-inflammatory cytokine, and which has proven ineffective as an anti-cancer agent in several clinical trials [1]. The interleukin nomenclature, which merely assigns a sequential number to new factors, is a rational system, but it has not been universally applied to new factors. This has created new anomalies such as IL-8 which is clearly a member of the chemokine cytokine family [2]. All of the molecules in this family share at least 25% amino acid homology, have similar structures and bind to seven transmembrane spanning receptors of the rhodopsin superfamily, but none of the other chemokines have been given interleukin numbers. The chemokines are further subdivided into the CXC or α-chemokines located on human chromosome 4, and the CC or β-chemokines located on chromosome 17. The CXC chemokines are neutrophil chemoattractants whereas the CC chemokines are predominantly monocyte chemoattractants. Other attempts to impose order on the cytokine field by grouping cytokines as lymphokines (lymphocyte-derived) or monokines (monocyte-derived) have usually proved misleading when sensitive detection systems are used [3].

With the availability of large quantities of recombinant cytokines, X-ray and NMR studies have generated accurate structures for many molecules, and these have been used to model the structures of related cytokines (see individual entries, and refs 4–6). Further homologies derived from studying gene organization, chromosomal location and receptor usage have allowed most cytokines to be placed into one of at least six different families [7,8]. Table 1.1 describes one scheme for these families, and Figure 1.1 shows solid models of representative members of each family. It seems unlikely that cytokine nomenclature will reflect these emerging family relations in the near future. However, information from these studies should at least help to establish general principles of the properties of the groups.

Table 1.1 *Structural families of cytokines*

Family	Members	Receptor type
Haematopoietins (4 α-helical bundles)	IL-2, IL-3, **IL-4**, IL-5, IL-6, IL-7, IL-9, IL-13, G-CSF, GM-CSF, CNTF, OSM, LIF, Epo	Cytokine receptor class I
	IL-10, IFNα, IFNβ, IFNγ	Cytokine receptor class II
	M-CSF	Tyrosine kinase
EGF (β-sheet)	**EGF**, TGFα	Tyrosine kinase
β-Trefoil	FGFα, FGFβ	Split tyrosine kinase
	IL-1α, **IL-1β**, IL-1Rα	IL-1 receptor
TNF (jelly roll motif)	**TNFα**, TNFβ, LTβ	NGF receptor
Cysteine knot	NGF	NGF receptor
	TGFβ1, **TGFβ2**, TGFβ3	Serine/threonine kinase
	PDGF, VEGF	Tyrosine kinase
Chemokines- (triple-stranded, anti parallel β-sheet in Greek key motif)	**IL-8**, MIP-1α, MIP-1β, MIP-2, PF-4, PBP, I-309/TCA-3, MCP-1, MCP-2, MCP-3, γIP-10	Rhodopsin superfamily

Cytokines in bold are illustrated in figure 1.

IL-4

EGF

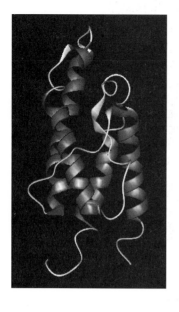

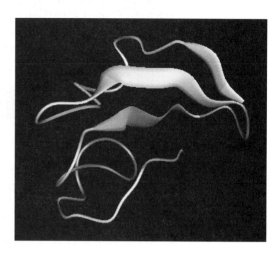

IL-1β

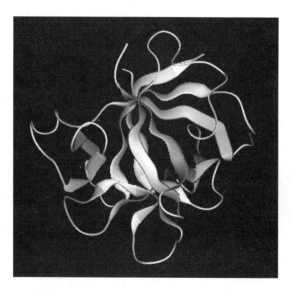

Figure 1.1. *Solid models not to scale of representative cytokines. These solid models of IL-4 (1BBN.PDB), EGF (1EGF.PDB), IL-1β (1I1B.PDB), TNFα trimer (1TNF.PDB), TGFβ 2 (2TGF.PDB) and IL-8 dimer (1IL8.PDB) were prepared with information from the Brookhaven database using the "Quanta" modelling package by Ed Hodgkin.*

TNFα trimer

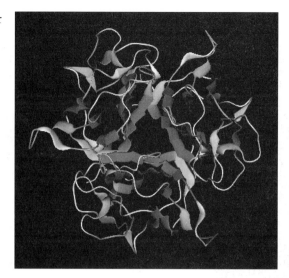

TGFβ2

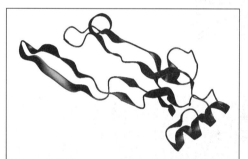

IL-8

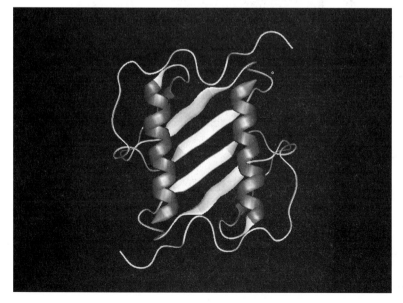

References

[1] Aggarwal, B.B. and Vilcek, J. (1991) Tumor Necrosis Factors: Structure, Function and Mechanism of Action, Dekker, New York.

[2] Oppenheim, J.J. et al. (1991) Ann. Rev. Immunol. 9, 617–648.

[3] Dumonde, D.C. et al. (1969) Nature 224, 38–42.

[4] DeVos, A.M. et al. (1992) Science 255, 306–312.

[5] Parry, D.A.D. et al. (1991) J. Mol. Recog. 4, 63–75.

[6] McDonald, M.Q. and Hendrickson, W.A. (1993) Cell 73, 421–424.

[7] Boulay, J.-L. and Paul, W.E. (1993) Curr. Biol. 3, 573–581.

[8] Bazan, J.F. (1990) Immunol. Today 11, 350–354.

2 Organization of the data

Each cytokine entry includes information under the following headings:

Other names

Most cytokines have more than one name. We have used the interleukin nomenclature whenever this has been assigned unequivocally. All other cytokines are entered under their most commonly accepted name. Alternative names are also listed.

THE MOLECULE

At the beginning of each entry is a brief description of the molecule and its main biological properties.

Crossreactivity

The degree of amino acid sequence homology between human and mouse cytokines is given when known together with cross species reactivity. In some cases, comparisons with other species are also given.

Sources

A list of cell types known to produce each cytokine is included.

Bioassays

Bioassays for each cytokine are described in brief. For the most part, these have been taken from methods used by the National Institute for Biological Standards, South Mimms, UK as described in refs 1 and 2.

Physicochemical properties of the cytokines

This table includes basic physicochemical information on human and mouse cytokines. The number of amino acids and predicted molecular weight for the mature proteins are calculated after removal of the signal peptide and propeptides where relevant. In some cases the cleavage point of the signal peptide has been determined by sequencing and in others from computer prediction. Potential N-linked glycosylation sites are identified by the consensus sequence Asn–X–Ser/Thr except when X is Pro or for the sequence Asn–X–Ser/Thr–Pro which is not usually glycosylated. The number of potential sites in the table is for the extracellular portion of the molecule only.

3-D structure

Information on the tertiary structure of each cytokine is taken from original papers or from Macromolecular Structures 1991–1993 published by Current Biology [3]. It includes data derived from X-ray or NMR structures, or predictions based on molecular models.

Gene structure and chromosomal localization

The chromosomal localization for the human cytokines is taken from original papers and/or the Human Gene Mapping (HGM 11)[4]. Mouse mapping data are taken from ref. 5. The exon–intron gene structure is drawn to scale from original papers with the number of amino acids shown for each exon.

Amino acid sequences

Human and mouse amino acid sequences are given for each cytokine and receptor where known. In some cases, the murine sequence is not available and the rat sequence is given instead. The sequences for most entries were taken directly from databases accessed through the VAX SEQNET computer at the Daresbury Laboratories using the Wisconsin GCG suite of programs. Where possible, amino acid sequences were obtained from the Swissprot database. Alternatively, cDNA nucleic acid sequences were obtained from EMBL and/or Genbank and translated. In each case, the accession number is listed with the sequence. Swissprot accession numbers begin with P. Recent submissions to EMBL and Genbank are assigned the same accession number, sometimes referred to as the Genembl accession number.

In all sequences, the single-letter amino acid code is used (Table 2.1). The numbering starts with the N-terminal amino acid after removal of the signal peptide. If the N-terminus has not been unequivocally assigned, the signal sequence is predicted according to consensus rules[6] and numbered to −1. Propeptides removed during post-translational modifications are shown in italics. The transmembrane portions of the sequences for cytokine receptors are underlined. The CNTF receptor is the only cytokine receptor so far which has been shown to have a GPI anchor and the proposed cleaved sequence is also shown in italics. Potential N-linked glycosylation sites marked by N in bold type are predicted by the presence of sequences Asn–X–Ser or Asn–X–Thr with the exceptions Asn–Pro–Ser/Thr which are not normally glycosylated and Asn–X–Ser/Thr–Pro which are often not glycosylated[7-9]. O-Linked glycosylation occurs at Ser or Thr residues. Although there is no clear-cut sequence motif that invariably indicates O-linked glycosylation, it usually occurs where there is a preponderance of Ser, Thr and Pro. When a high level of O-linked glycosylation on the receptors is expected, it is indicated on the receptor diagrams. Sequence motifs of particular interest are annotated under the sequence.

THE RECEPTORS

A brief description of the cytokine receptors with comments on important features is given in this section. A diagram of the receptor using the scheme described by Barclay et al.[10] is given for each receptor. In each case, the drawings are of the human receptors, and include protein domains, the mode of membrane attachment and degree of glycosylation. Orientation in the membrane is shown by labelling the intracellular terminus. The symbols used to represent the various domains, glycosylation and membrane attachment are taken directly from The Leucocyte Antigen FactsBook and are given in Figure 2.1.

The criteria used for defining cytokine receptor superfamilies are given in

Table 2.1 *Single-letter amino acid codes*

	Amino acid	Code	
Small hydrophilic	Serine	Ser	S
	Threonine	Thr	T
	Proline	Pro	P
	Alanine	Ala	A
	Glycine	Gly	G
Acid, acid amide	Asparagine	Asn	N
Hydrophillic	Aspartic	Asp	D
	Glutamine	Gln	Q
	Glutamic	Glu	E
Basic	Histidine	His	H
	Arginine	Arg	R
	Lysine	Lys	K
Small hydrophobic	Methionine	Met	M
	Isoleucine	Ile	I
	Leucine	Leu	L
	Valine	Val	V
Aromatic	Phenylalanine	Phe	F
	Tyrosine	Tyr	Y
	Tryptophan	Trp	W
Sulphydryl	Cysteine	Cys	C

Chapter 4. In those cases where no superfamily domain structure is known, the extracellular region is shown as a circle containing a question mark. The diameter of the circle is approximately proportional to the size of the extracellular region or domain. If a protein sequence contains a high proportion of Ser, Thr and Pro residues, it is probably heavily O-glycosylated, and is shown as an extended structure to distinguish it from regions likely to have a folded conformation. Only those disulphide bonds in the Ig superfamily (Ig-SF) domains are shown. The majority of cytoplasmic domains do not yet belong to well-defined superfamilies and are represented by wavy lines whose length is proportional to the number of amino acids.

Distribution

The tissue distribution of the receptors has been determined in some cases by ligand (cytokine) binding studies. Otherwise, it is assumed from mRNA expression or biological response.

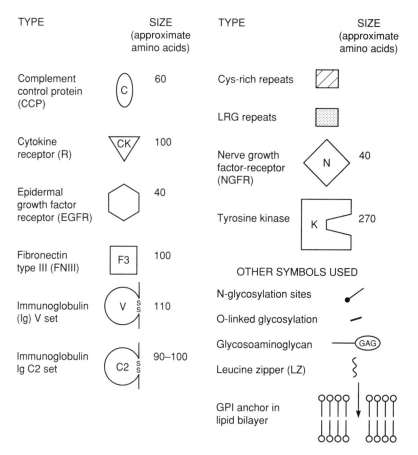

TYPE		SIZE (approximate amino acids)	TYPE		SIZE (approximate amino acids)
Complement control protein (CCP)	C	60	Cys-rich repeats		
			LRG repeats		
Cytokine receptor (R)	CK	100	Nerve growth factor-receptor (NGFR)	N	40
Epidermal growth factor receptor (EGFR)		40	Tyrosine kinase	K	270
Fibronectin type III (FNIII)	F3	100	OTHER SYMBOLS USED		
Immunoglobulin (Ig) V set	V	110	N-glycosylation sites		
			O-linked glycosylation		
Immunoglobulin Ig C2 set	C2	90–100	Glycosoaminoglycan	GAG	
			Leucine zipper (LZ)		
			GPI anchor in lipid bilayer		

Figure 2.1. *Models for domains and repeats found in leucocyte membrane proteins. These models are used in the diagrams drawn for the entries in Section II.*

Physicochemical properties of the receptors

This table includes the number of amino acids in both the precursor and the mature processed protein, predicted and expressed molecular ratio (M_r), and the number of N-linked glycosylation sites in the extracellular portion of the mature protein. The affinity of the receptor for its cytokine is also given. These data have been taken from binding studies with the natural receptor or the cloned receptor expressed on cells transfected with receptor cDNA.

Signal transduction

This section describes what is known about the intracellular signal transduction pathways coupled to the cytokine receptors.

Chromosomal location

The chromosomal location of the receptors is taken from original papers and/or HGM 11 [4,5].

Amino acid sequences of cytokine receptors

Sequence data for human and mouse receptors are given as described above for the cytokines. Transmembrane domains are underlined and short sequences of particular interest such as the WSXWS motif in fibronectin type III (FNIII) domains are annotated under the sequence.

References

[1] Thorpe, R. et al. (1992) Blood Rev. 6, 133–148.
[2] Wadhwa, M. et al. (1992) In Cytokines: A Practical Approach, Balkwill, F.R., ed., IRL Press, Oxford, pp. 309–330.
[3] Macromolecular Structures (1991, 1992, 1993) Hendrickson, W.A. and Wuthrich, K., ed., Current Biology Ltd., London.
[4] Human Gene Mapping 11 (HGM 11) (1991) Cytogenet. Cell Genet. 58, 1–2200.
[5] Copeland N.G. et al. (1993) Science 262, 57–66.
[6] von Heijne, G. (1983) Eur. J. Biochem. 133, 17–21.
[7] Bause, E. and Hettkamp, H. (1979) FEBS Lett. 108, 341–344.
[8] Kornfeld, R. and Kornfeld, S. (1985) Annu. Rev. Biochem. 54, 631–664.
[9] Gavel, Y. and von Heijne, G. (1990) Protein Engineering 3, 433–442.
[10] Barclay, N.A. et al. (1993) The Leucocyte Antigen FactsBook, Academic Press, London.

3 The cytokine network

INTERACTIONS BETWEEN CYTOKINES

Individually, cytokines are potent molecules which, *in vitro*, can cause changes in cell proliferation, differentiation and movement at nanomolar to picomolar concentrations. Injection of cytokines into animals and humans either systemically or locally can also have profound effects on leucocyte migration and function, haematopoietic cell numbers, temperature regulation, acute phase responses, tissue remodelling and cell survival. The individual chapters in this book describe the specific properties of each cytokine, but delineation of the mechanisms by which cytokines cause these effects is complicated by the tendency of cytokines to affect the expression of other cytokines and/or their receptors. In addition, it is clear that there are no circumstances *in vivo* in which cytokines are produced individually. Rather they are produced together with other cytokines in patterns characteristic of the particular stimulus or disease. The potency of cytokines, and the potential for amplification and damage which excessive cytokine production carries, has resulted in elaborate controls on cytokine production and action. The current view of cytokine biology reflecting these concepts is of a network of positive and negative cytokines, and cytokine inhibitors and inducers, which combine to give an overall biological or clinical response [1-5].

From experiments using cytokine proteins as agonists, or by blocking cytokine production or action with drugs or monoclonal antibodies, the contributions which many individual cytokines can make to particular aspects of immunity, inflammation and haematopoiesis are now beginning to be delineated. Where simple *in vitro* sytems have been studied, it has been possible to demonstrate roles for particular cytokines. A good example is the regulation of antibody responses where several cytokines are known to control B lymphocyte growth and differentiation [reviewed in ref 6]. From a wealth of experimentation over the past ten years it is known that IL-2 promotes growth and differentiation of B lymphocytes, IL-4 stimulates IgE and IgG4 secretion, IL-6 promotes plasma cell formation, IL-7 stimulates the growth and development of pre-B cells, IL-10 promotes B cell growth and antibody formation, IL-11 is a plasma cell stimulant, IL-13 promotes IgM, IgE and IgG4, IL-14 promotes B lymphocyte proliferation but inhibits Ig synthesis, nerve growth factor is a B lymphocyte growth factor, interferon-γ promotes IgG2α, and TGFβ promotes IgA secretion but inhibits cell proliferation. Any attempt to catalogue all of the possible combination effects of this partial list of cytokines would be a Herculean task (and likely to be extremely dull). It is possible, however, to ask questions such as what are the minimal cytokines needed to make a population of lymph node cells secrete IgE as opposed to IgG2a, or what cytokines are capable of suppressing an ongoing antibody response? Evidence from such experiments can allow predictions to be made which can be tested in animal models or in the clinic. An example of this type of work has been the description of TH1/TH2 cytokine patterns [7].

Work by Mossman and colleagues identified two groups of cytokines produced by different T helper (TH) lymphocytes which favour either cell mediated and inflammatory immunity (TH1) or antibody-mediated humoral immunity (TH2) [7-9]. The TH2 cytokines such as IL-4, IL-5, IL-6, IL-10 and IL-13 generally promote B cell function, specifically favouring IgE and IgA responses. The TH1 cytokines such as IFNγ and IL-2 can also have some antibody promoting effects but favour an IgG2a response. These two cytokine groups are also antagonistic in that IFNγ inhibits TH2 cytokine production, whereas IL-10, IL-4 and IL-13 inhibit TH1 cytokine production, probably via effects on antigen presenting cells. The initiating factors which predispose towards TH1 or TH2 responses are not fully understood; however, IL-12 is thought to be a key mediator in stimulating a TH1 response to antigenic challenge [10]. The *in vitro* properties of TH1 or TH2 cytokines have implicated these two groups either in DTH/CMI (delayed type hypersensitivity/cell mediated immunity) diseases (TH1) or in allergic/parasitic/humoral diseases (TH2). In pre-clinical models, IL-4 knockout mice have low levels of IgE, whereas IL-4 transgenic mice have hyper-IgE [11,12]. In addition, anti-IL-4 strategies are effective in allergic and parasitic disease causing marked reduction in IgE levels [13]. The *in vitro* observation that TH1 cytokines antagonize the TH2 response has also been tested *in vivo* where IFNγ inhibits the murine IgE response, and reduces IgE levels in patients with atopic dermatitis or hyper IgE syndrome [reviewed in ref 14]. It is a major triumph of cytokine biology that diseases such as asthma with an allergic pathology are now regarded as "TH2 diseases" [15–17], and considerable effort is being put into finding ways to suppress the TH2 phenotype.

Although the contributory cytokines in processes such as haematopoiesis, wound repair and inflammation seem to have been largely identified, information on the operation of the cytokine network even in simple experimental systems is far from complete. It is well beyond the scope of this book to review the literature on cytokine interactions in physiology and pathology. For more extensive information, the reader is referred to the General Bibliography on page 259 which covers the biology and clinical use of cytokines. This chapter gives a simple review of the regulatory components of cytokine networks.

REGULATION OF CYTOKINE PRODUCTION AND ACTION
Gene Expression

There is some evidence for the constitutive expression of haematopoietic cytokines such as M-CSF, G-CSF, SCF, IL-6 and Epo which are necessary to maintain steady state haematopoiesis. Moreover, several cytokines are pre-synthesized, and stored either in cytoplasmic granules, e.g. GM-CSF, TGFβ, PF-4, PDGF [18]; as membrane proteins, e.g. TNFα, IL-1β, EGF, TGFα [19]; or complexed with cell surface binding proteins or extracellular matrix, e.g. TGFβ, MIP-1β, IL-8 [20,21]. These pools of cytokine protein are available for rapid release in response to stimulation. Most cytokines, however, are not constitutively expressed in adult animals, but are rapidly produced in response to stimulation. The stimuli for gene expression are well characterized, particularly for the haematopoietic cells. In general, infectious agents such as bacteria, viruses, fungi and parasites, as well as mechanical injury and toxic stimuli are potent cytokine inducers. In addition to classical antigens, infectious agents also express many non-specific cytokine-inducing molecules, e.g. endotoxins [22]. Inflammatory mediators such as complement components, and lipid mediators such as PAF which are generated in response to infection can also stimulate cytokine production [23]. For many cells, cytokines are themselves potent cytokine inducers. Some, such as IL-1, TNF and IFNγ, are particularly potent inducers of cytokine gene expression, and are referred to as pro-inflammatory cytokines [24]. Others, like IL-1 and TNF, are even capable of stimulating their own production [25].

For most cytokines, the nature and extent of the transcription factors which regulate gene expression are not fully characterized. The specific consensus nucleotide recognition sequences for known transcription factors can be identified in genomic DNA, and simple experiments using reporter genes linked to the 5'sequences can support a role for particular transcription factors [26]. However, the biochemistry of the regulation imposed even by the known transcription factors is complex. For example, to induce IL-2 gene transcription requires both constitutive (NFAT-1 and NFIL-2A) and inducible factors (AP-1 and NFkB). The importance of other regulatory sequences outside the 5' regions is largely unknown. One particular feature common to many cytokine genes is a consensus sequence in the 3' end of the mRNA which promotes message instability [27]. This TTATTTAT sequence is responsible for limiting the extent of protein production characteristic of many cytokines.

In addition to the many positive stimuli, several mediators act to limit or prevent cytokine gene expression, or to limit cytokine action. The classical inhibitors of cytokine gene expression are the glucocorticoid hormones and the synthetic steroids which are widely used as immunosuppressants and anti-inflammatory drugs [28]. They are thought to act as part of an intracellular glucocorticoid receptor complex which binds to glucocorticoid response elements present in the IL-1, IL-2, IL-3, IL-6, IL-8 and IFNγ genes. The mode of action of this complex is unknown. Newer agents such as cyclosporin A, FK506 and rapamycin also act via cytokine pathways [29–31]. Prostaglandins are also known to inhibit the production of cytokines. As described above, many cytokines act to inhibit cytokine production. The antagonistic TH1 and TH2 cytokines are the best studied examples of this. Other examples include TGFβ, which is a broad spectrum inhibitor of cytokine production, and IL-10 which is a potent inhibitor of TNF and IL-1 production by monocytes [32,33].

Processing

Control of cytokine function can also be achieved by regulating the processing of precursor forms. Many cytokines are initially produced as biologically active integral membrane proteins which need to be proteolytically cleaved to release the active molecule. Examples in this category include EGF, TGFα, IL-1β, IL-1α, TNFα [19]. Alternatively, cytokines such as TGFβ are produced as secreted, but biologically inactive precursors, which are enzymatically processed to the active forms [34]. The identity of most of the processing enzymes is unknown, although the cysteine protease which mediates the processing of IL-1β, known as ICE, has recently been cloned [35,36].

Sequestration

Some growth factors such as TGFβ, FGF, LIF and IL-1 are sequestered on extracellular matrix in connective tissues, skin and bone [20]. This serves as a sink of active cytokine which can be rapidly released when the matrix is broken down during injury or tissue repair. Other cytokines, such as GM-CSF, IL-3 and SCF are localized to stromal cell layers in bone marrow where they stimulate haematopoiesis [37]. Others, including MIP-1β, and IL-8, bind to endothelial cells at sites of inflammation where they promote leucocyte extravasation [21]. In general, these cytokines are sequestered onto glycosaminoglycans such as heparin, decorin or CD44-like molecules .

Soluble binding proteins

Several binding proteins for cytokines are found in blood and tissue fluids. Some of these are secreted forms of the specific cell membrane receptors such as for TNF, IL-1, IL-2 and IL-6, whereas others are less specific such as α-2-macroglobulin [38–40]. These binding proteins may serve as passive carriers of the cytokines, either extending their half-lives or promoting their excretion, or they may act as circulating inhibitors limiting systemic effects of the cytokines. The soluble form of the IL-6 receptor is unusual in that it complexes with IL-6 to form a biologically active molecule which binds directly to the IL-6 receptor signalling chain [41].

Receptor antagonists

To date the only naturally occurring cytokine receptor antagonist that has been identified is IL-1Ra. It is structurally related to IL-1α and IL-1β and binds to the IL-1 receptors, but does not cause signal transduction, thereby acting as a specific receptor antagonist [42–44].

Receptor modulation

Control of cytokine function can also be achieved by modulating receptor number through controlling gene expression, internalization or receptor shedding. Modulation of receptor affinity or function can also occur by control of receptor phosphorylation, or by competition for shared receptor chains or signal transduction molecules [38,45].

Virokines

Recent papers have demonstrated that pathogenic organisms, particularly pox viruses, have subverted the cytokine network to their own ends. For example, vaccinia and cowpox viruses encode a secreted IL-1β binding protein, Shope fibroma virus encodes a secreted TNF binding protein, myxoma virus contains a secreted protein related to the IFNγ receptor, cowpox virus contains an inhibitor of the IL-1β converting enzyme, and vaccinia virus contains an analogue of epidermal growth factor called vaccinia growth factor [46–50]. Similarly, Epstein–Barr virus contains a homologue of IL-10, and cytomegalovirus a homologue of the MIP-1α receptor [51,52]. The expression of these genes is thought to confer an immunological advantage to the viruses.

References
1 Balkwill, F. and Burke, F. (1989) Immunol. Today 10, 299–304.
2 Wong, G.C. and Clark, S.C. (1988) Immunol. Today 9, 137.
3 Paul, W.E. (1989) Cell 57, 521–524.

4 Chatenoud, L. (1992) Eur. Cyt. Network 3, 509–513.

5 Aria, K. et al. (1992) J. Dermatol. 19, 575–583.

6 Callard, R.E. (1990) Cytokines and B-Lymphocytes, Academic Press, London.

7 Mosmann, T.R. and Coffman, R.L. (1989) Annu. Rev. Immunol. 7, 145–173.

8 Mosmann, T.R. et al. (1986) J. Immunol. 136, 2348–2357.

9 Moller, G. (1991) Immunol. Rev. 123, 2–229.

10 Trinchieri, G. et al. (1993) Prog. Growth Factor Res. 4, 355–368.

11 Kuhn, R. et al. (1991) Science 254, 707–710.

12 Tepper, R.I. et al. (1990) Cell 62 ,457–467.

13 Finkelman, F.D. et al. (1991) Annu. Rev. Immunol. 8, 303–333.

14 Banchereau, J. and Miossec, P. (1993) In Clinical Applications of Cytokines, Oppenheim, J.J. et al., eds, Oxford University Press, Oxford.

15 Ricci, M. and Romagnani, S. (1991) Ann. Ital. Med. Interna. 6, 183–191.

16 Robinson, D.S. et al. (1992) N. Engl. J. Med. 326, 298–304.

17 Kapsenberg, M.L. et al. (1992) Curr. Biol. 4, 788–793.

18 Jyung, R.W. and Mustoe, T.A. (1993) In Clinical Applications of Cytokines, Oppenheim, J.J. et al., eds, Oxford University Press, Oxford.

19 Massague, J. and Pandiella, A. (1993) Annu. Rev. Biochem. 62, 515–541.

20 Noble, N.A. et al. (1992) Prog. Growth Factor Res. 4, 369–382.

21 Tanaka, Y. et al. (1993) Immunol. Today 14, 111–115.

22 Sturk, A. et al., eds (1991) Bacterial Endotoxins: Cytokine Mediators and New Therapies for Sepsis, Wiley-Liss, New York.

23 Rola-Pleszcynski, M. (1991) Adv. Exp. Med. Biol. 314, 205–221.

24 Aria, K. et al. (1990) Annu. Rev. Biochem. 59, 783–836.

25 Spriggs, D.R. et al. (1990) Cancer Res. 50, 7101–7107.

26 Muegge, K. and Durum, S. (1990) Cytokine 2, 1–8.

27 Cosman, D. (1987) Immunol. Today 8, 16–17.

28 Almalwi, W.Y. et al. (1990) Prog. Leuk. Biol. 10A, 321–326.

29 Elliot, J.F. et al. (1984) Science 226, 1439–1441.

30 Bierer, B.E. et al. (1990) Proc. Natl. Acad. Sci. USA 87, 9231–9235.

31 Henderson, D.J. et al. (1992) Immunology 73, 316–321.

32 Sporn, M.B. and Roberts, A.B. (1990) Peptide Growth Factors and Their Receptors, Springer-Verlag, Berlin.

33 Howard, M. et al. (1993) J. Exp. Med. 177, 1205–1208.

34 Harper, J.G. et al. (1993) Prog. Growth Factor Res. 4, 321–335.

35 Cerretti, D.P. et al. (1992) Science 256, 97–100.

36 Thornberry, N.A. et al. (1992) Nature 356, 37–41.

37 Gordon, M.Y. et al. (1987) Nature 326, 403–405.

38 Cosman, D. (1993) Cytokine 5, 95–106.

39 Van Zee, K.J. et al. (1992) Proc. Natl. Acad. Sci. USA 89, 4845–4849.

40 James, K. (1990) Immunol. Today 11, 163–166

41 Taga, T. et al. (1989) Cell 58, 573–581

42 Carter, D.B. et al. (1990) Nature 344, 633–638.

43 Hannum, C.H. et al. (1990) Nature 343, 336–340.

44 Eisenberg, S.P. et al (1990) Nature 343, 341–346

45 Ullrich, A. and Schlessinger, J. (1990) Cell 61, 203–212.

46 Blomquist, M.C. et al. (1984) Proc. Natl. Acad. Sci. USA 81, 7363–7367.

47 Upton, C. et al (1991) Virology 184, 370–382.

48 Ray, C.A. et al. (1992) Cell 69, 597–604.

49 Spriggs, M.K. et al. (1992) Cell 71, 145–152.
50 Upton, C. et al. (1992) Science 258, 1369–1372.
51 Moore, K.W. et al. (1990) Science 248, 1230–1234.
52 Neote, K. et al. (1993) Cell 72, 415–425.

4 Cytokine receptor superfamilies

INTRODUCTION

The receptors for many cytokines have now been cloned and analysis of their primary structures has enabled many of them to be grouped into superfamilies based on common homology regions. There is no agreed nomenclature for most of the superfamilies. In order to achieve conformity within the FactsBook series, we have used the same nomenclature as Barclay et al [1] based on the most commonly used names. The abbreviation "R" is used for receptor and "SF" for superfamily. The main superfamilies recognized today are the cytokine receptor superfamily (CKR-SF) sometimes known as the haematopoietic receptor superfamily, the immunoglobulin superfamily (Ig-SF), the protein tyrosine kinase receptor superfamily (PTKR-SF), the nerve growth factor receptor superfamily (NGFR-SF), the interferon receptor superfamily (IFNR-SF), also known as the cytokine receptor superfamily type II, the G-protein-coupled seven transmembrane spanning receptor superfamily (STSR-SF), and the complement control protein superfamily (CCP-SF). The term "superfamily" was first used by Dayhoff et al. [2] for proteins with amino acid sequence homology of 50% or less and "family" for those with homology of more than 50%. In fact, homologies within superfamilies are often 15–25% and it can be difficult to establish an evolutionary relationship rather than a chance similarity until structural information is obtained. Conserved amino acids in superfamilies are often clustered in domains or repeats, but even then the homology may be low with the conserved amino acids clustered in small sequences throughout the 40–110 residues that make up superfamily domains and repeats. It is also important to note that many cytokine receptors have combinations of different domains or repeats. For example, both the IL-6 binding α-chain and the gp130 β-chain of the IL-6 receptor contain cytokine receptor (CK) and fibronectin type III (FNIII) domains characteristic of the cytokine receptor superfamily, and a Ig-SF C2 set domain.

A domain is a sequence or segment of a protein which is likely to form a discrete structural unit. Three criteria are used to identify a domain. First, tertiary structure. Domains established by their tertiary structure include Ig (C1 and C2), complement control protein (CCP), fibronectin type III (FNIII) and the cytokine receptor (CK). Secondly, superfamily segments that exist as the sole extracellular sequence, or as a sequence contiguous with hinge-like regions containing a high content of Ala, Gly, Pro, Ser and Thr residues may be considered as domains. Thirdly, superfamily segments coded for by single exons which can be readily spliced to form a new gene with an open reading frame may also be considered as domains.

Superfamily segments may not always be independent structural units (domains), in which case the term "repeat" may be used. For example, in the NGFR-SF, blocks of three or four repeats are found without intervening sequences between the repeats. The pattern of exons does not correspond to the repeats, and in this superfamily it seems that a precursor structure evolved by gene duplication of a primordial repeat. Additional members of the superfamily have evolved by duplication and divergence of this repeat.

The term motif describes a smaller sequence pattern which probably does not form a folded structural unit. An example is the Trp–Ser–X–Trp–Ser (WSXWS) motif in the FNIII domain found in most members of the CKR-SF.

THE CYTOKINE RECEPTOR SUPERFAMILY (CKR-SF)

Also known as the haematopoietic receptor superfamily, this is the largest receptor superfamily and includes IL-2R β- and γ-chains, IL-4R, IL-3R α- and β-chains, IL-5R α- and β-chains, IL-6R, gp130, IL-9R, IL-12R, G-CSFR, GM-CSFR, CNTFR, LIFR, EpoR, PRLR and GHR. The IL-7R is also usually included in this family but the case for its inclusion is weak. It has a very low ALIGN score[2] and few of the conserved amino acids in the CK domain [1].

Domain structure of the CKR-SF

The extracellular regions of the CKR-SF all contain combinations of CK, FNIII and in some cases C2 Ig domains. Initially, the CK and FNIII domains were not distinguished, and the term haematopoietic receptor superfamily was commonly used. The CK domain has a length of about 100 amino acids with a characteristic Cys–X–Trp motif and three other conserved Cys residues. The FNIII domain was first identified in an extracellular matrix protein, but it is also common in membrane molecules in the nervous system which often have a characteristic Ig-SF domain [3]. It includes the Trp–Ser–X–Trp–Ser (WSXWS) motif required for ligand binding and signal transduction [4]. The extracellular binding domain of the growth hormone receptor has been co-crystallized with its ligand (GH) and the three-dimensional structure solved at a resolution of 2.8 Å by X-ray crystallography [5,6] and NMR [7]. The receptor has two domains (CK and FNIII) of about 100 residues each, consisting of two antiparallel β-sheets of four and three strands with a similar folding pattern to the Ig-SF C2 set domain, and the domains of the PapD chaperone protein (Figure 1). Interestingly, the WSXWS motif is located away from the binding surfaces. However, this motif is highly conserved and is essential for ligand binding and receptor-mediated signal transduction [4]. Two GHR molecules crystallized with a single GH ligand had identical surfaces of the two GHR subunits binding to non-identical surfaces on the GH ligand. The areas of contact between the two GHR molecules and GH were of unequal size (1230 Å^2 and 900 Å^2) and the area of contact between the two GHR chains was 500Å^2. This structure is compatible with ligand induced receptor dimerisation.

Structures of the CKR complexes

For some members of the cytokine receptor superfamily, transfection of receptor cDNA results in high affinity ligand binding similar to that observed with responsive cells (e.g. EpoR, G-CSFR and GHR), suggesting that only one receptor subunit is required for high affinity binding. Ligand-induced receptor homodimerization has been shown for GH/GHR and G-CSF/G-CSFR interactions, and may occur with other members of this group. For example, a mutation in the extracellular domain of the EpoR has been shown to result in homodimerization and signal transduction without ligand binding.

In contrast to this group, receptor binding studies have revealed the existence of more than one binding affinity for several members of the cytokine receptor superfamily. Typically, these are high (10–100pM) and low (1–10nM) affinity binding sites. For these receptors, additional subunits have been identified which are required for high affinity receptor expression. These additional subunits are

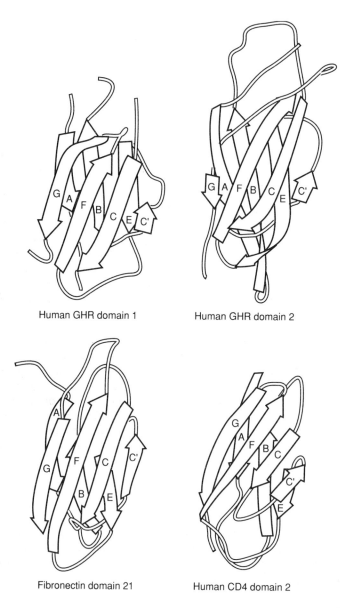

Human GHR domain 1

Human GHR domain 2

Fibronectin domain 21

Human CD4 domain 2

Figure 1. *The folding patterns of the cytokine receptor superfamily and fibronection type III superfamily domains. Ribbon diagrams are shown for the CK and FNIII domains from human growth hormone receptor, the FNIII domain 21 from human fibronection and (for comparison) the IgSF C2 set domain from human CD4 domain 2. The β-strands are shown as broad arrows pointing from the N- to C-direction and the connecting loops are shown as thinner lines. Some gaps are present in the loops of the growth hormone receptor where the structure has not been fully resolved. Each β-strand is labelled using the same nomenclature as in the IgSF.*

sometimes referred to as affinity converters or converter chains. Moreover, some of these subunits are shared by more than one cytokine receptor giving rise to heterodimeric and in some cases heterotrimeric structures. The elucidation of these complex multisubunit receptors is now beginning to allow an understanding of the functional crossreactivity and redundancy of some cytokines. These are grouped in the following discussion according to the identity of the shared subunit(s).

GM-CSFR β-chain users

IL-3, IL-5 and GM-CSF all have unique and specific low affinity receptors with similar structures including short intracytoplasmic segments which are unable to transduce a signal. In humans, a second β chain (KH97) common to all three receptors converts the low affinity receptors to high affinity receptors but does not itself bind ligand [8,9]. The KH97 β-subunit has a much longer intracytoplasmic portion, and is able to transduce a signal. In the mouse, there are two β subunits, AIC2A and AIC2B [10–13]. Of these, AIC2B is similar to the human KH97 and associates with all three low affinity receptors to form high affinity receptors, but does not itself bind ligand. On the other hand, AIC2A binds IL-3 with low affinity and can associate with the IL-3 receptor α-chain to form a high affinity IL-3 receptor, but it does not associate with either the GM-CSF or IL-5 receptor α-chains [9,13,14].

IL-6R β-chain (gp130) users

Another group of receptors (IL-6R, CNTFR, LIFR and OSMR) share a common signalling subunit known as gp130 which has some structural homology with the G-CSFR. The IL-6R binds IL-6 with low affinity but is itself unable to signal. This IL-6/IL-6R complex binds two gp130 molecules to form a gp130 disulphide-linked homodimer [15]. Dimerization results in tyrosine phosphorylation of gp130 and is required for signal transduction. The high affinity CNTFR complex has a similar structure [16]. Binding of CNTF to the CNTFR results in association with gp130 and the low affinity receptor for LIF (LIFR) to form a gp130/LIFR heterodimeric structure. Like the gp130 homodimer, formation of the gp130/LIFR heterodimer results in tyrosine phosphorylation and is required for signal transduction. The LIFR/gp130 heterodimer is also a high affinity receptor for both LIF and OSM. LIF binds to the LIFR with low affinity but does not bind to gp130 whereas OSM binds to gp130 with low affinity, but not to the LIFR. The LIFR/gp130 heterodimer is required for high affinity binding to both ligands, and for signal transduction. There is, however, some evidence for different signalling pathways activated by LIF and OSM [17], and there may be another component to the OSMR complex [18,19]. gp130 may also form part of the IL-11 receptor [20].

IL-2Rγ-chain users

The IL-2 receptor is also a complex of three chains [21]. The IL-2R α-chain (Tac, CD25 or p55) is not a member of the CKR-SF, but has two domains with homology to the complement control protein (CCP). It binds IL-2 with low affinity (K_d 1.4×10^{-8}M), but does not signal. The other two components are the IL-2R β-chain (p75), and the IL-2R γ-chain (p64), both of which are members of the CKR-SF [22,23]. The IL-2R β-chain binds IL-2 with intermediate affinity (K_d 1.2×10^{-7}M), but the γ-chain (p64) does not bind IL-2. Receptor complexes consisting of α/γ or β/γ heterodimers bind IL-2 with an affinity of about 10^{-9}M. The high affinity receptor complex is an α/β/γ heterotrimer. It has an equilibrium K_d of 1.3×10^{-11}M and a dissociation half-life of

50 min [23]. Both β/γ and α/β/γ complexes are able to mediate signal transduction. The β-chain is also a component of the IL-15 receptor. At least two distinct cytoplasmic regions of the IL-2 β-chain are involved in IL-2-mediated cellular signalling. A serine-rich region is critical for induction of c-*myc* and cell proliferation (signal 1), whereas an acidic region is required for physical association with *src*-like protein tyrosine kinase (PTK) p56[lck], activation of p21[ras], and induction of c-*fos* and c-*jun* (signal 2) [21]. The IL-2R γ-chain has an SH2-like homology domain which may be involved in binding to phosphotyrosine residues on other signalling proteins. Recently, mutations in the IL-2R γ-chain have been shown to cause X-linked severe combined immunodeficiency (X-SCID) in humans [24]. This is a lethal disease characterized by absent or greatly reduced T cells and severely depressed cell-mediated and humoral immunity. The IL-2R γ-chain is also a functional component of the IL-4R [25,26] the IL-7R [27], and the IL-15 receptor, and there is some evidence that it is also part of the IL-9 and IL-13 receptor complexes.

Signal transduction by CKRs

There are no consensus sequence motifs in the intracytoplasmic portions of CKR molecules associated with known enzymic activity, and other membrane enzymes such as tyrosine kinases or phosphatases must associate with the ligand–receptor complex for signal transduction.

Two functional intracytoplasmic domains have been identified on some of the CKR members by mutational analysis. A region of 55–60 amino acids proximal to the transmembrane domain has two highly conserved sequence motifs [28]. This domain is necessary and sufficient for proliferative signals delivered by G-CSFR, gp130 and IL-2R β-chains. A second less well-defined and more distal domain is also important for signalling. Downstream events after ligand binding are not well defined for the CKR-SF although tyrosine phosphorylation of several cellular proteins has been described in response to IL-2, IL-3, IL-4, IL-5, IL-6, IL-7, G-CSF, GM-CSF, Epo, LIF and CNTF. The substrates include PI 3-kinase [29,30], p120[GAP] [31], and Raf-1 kinase [32]. Activation of p21[ras] has also been described for IL-2, IL-3 and GM-CSF, but not IL-4 [33]. The JAK kinases are also phosphorylated and activated in response to many cytokines including IL-3 [34], IFN [35], GH [36] and Epo [37] (reviewed [39b]). They are also associated with gp130 in receptor complexes for IL-6 [38], CNTF, LIF and OSM [39]. Phosphorylation of receptor chains has been described for IL-2Rβ, IL-3R, gp130 and EpoR. As the CK receptors do not have intrinsic protein tyrosine kinase (PTK) activity, they must associate with or indirectly activate other PTKs. The IL-2R β-chain associates with p56[lck] and other *src*-like kinases [40], and the GHR associates with an unidentified PTK [41]. Signal transduction by IL-2, IL-3 and GM-CSF involves Ras [33], and IL-4 has been shown to induce phosphorylation of the IL-4 induced phosphotyrosine substrate (4PS) which is associated with the p85 subunit of PI 3-kinase after cytokine stimulation [30-42]. IL-4 also stimulates PIP_2 hydrolysis, yielding IP_3 and subsequent calcium flux followed after a 10 min lag period by increased intracellular cAMP [43].

Soluble CKRs

Alternatively spliced mRNA giving rise to secreted receptors lacking the transmembrane region and the cytoplasmic proximal charged residues that anchor the protein in the membrane have been described for the IL-4R [44], IL-5R [45], IL-7R [46], IL-9R [47], GM-CSFR [48], G-CSFR [49], GHR [50] and LIFR [51]. Soluble CK receptors can also be generated by proteolysis of cell surface receptors, e.g. GHR, and by phospholipase action on the GPI-linked CNTFR. The *in vivo* function of soluble CKR molecules is not established. They may act as antagonists by competitive ligand binding, but the affinity of cytokines for soluble receptors is generally low. sIL-4R has been shown to inhibit IL-4-mediated responses [52]. Alternatively, soluble receptors could act as transport proteins to carry cytokines to sites where they are required for biological activity or even to sites where they would have no biological activity for removal from the body. More interestingly, soluble receptors complexed with cytokine may act as agonists. Such a role has been described for IL-6R/IL-6 complexes which bind to gp130 and transduce a signal [53]. Similarly CNTF/CNTFR complexes bind to LIFR/gp130 heterodimers [54], and the IL-12 p35/p340 complex binds to the IL-12 receptor [55,56].

THE INTERFERON RECEPTOR SUPERFAMILY (IFNR-SF)

The interferon receptor superfamily, otherwise known as the cytokine receptor type II superfamily, includes the IFNα/β receptor, IFNγ receptor, IL-10 receptor and tissue factor [57–60]. The members of this family are single spanning transmembrane glycoproteins characterized by either one (IFNγR and IL-10R) or two (IFNα/βR) homologous extracellular regions of about 200 amino acids, each of which has two FNIII domains. The first of these FNIII domains has two conserved tryptophans and a pair of conserved cysteines, whereas the second has a unique disulphide loop formed from the second pair of conserved cysteines, but no WSXWS motif characteristic of type I cytokine receptors. Signal transduction by the IFN receptors involves phosphorylation and activation of JAK and TYK2 protein tyrosine kinases [35,61–63]. The mechanism for signal transduction by the IL-10R is not yet known.

THE IMMUNOGLOBULIN SUPERFAMILY (IG-SF)

The immunoglobulin superfamily is the largest known superfamily with about 40% of known leucocyte membrane polypeptides containing one or more Ig-SF domains. Cytokine receptors with Ig-SF domains in their extracellular sequences include the IL-1R, IL-6R, FGFR, PDGFR, M-CSFR and SCFR (c-kit). The Ig-SF domains are characterized by a structural unit of about 100 amino acids with a distinct folding pattern known as the Ig fold [64], consisting of a sandwich of two β-sheets, each made up from antiparallel β-strands of about 5-10 amino acids with a conserved disulphide bond between the two sheets in most but not all domains. The tertiary structure has been solved by X-ray crystallography for Ig V and Ig C domains, β2-microglobulin, the α3 domain of MHC class I, CD4 domains 1 and 2, and CD8. Ig and TCR V regions have common sequence patterns and are known as the V set. The Ig, TCR and MHC antigen C type domains all share the same sequence patterns and are known as the C1 set. A third set of domains with similar structure to C domains but with some sequence homology with the V set are known as the C2 set. The CD4 domain 2 is a C2 set sequence as are most of the Ig domains in the cytokine receptors. For a detailed description of the Ig-SF domain sets see ref. 1.

THE PROTEIN TYROSINE KINASE RECEPTOR SUPERFAMILY (PTKR-SF)

Receptor tyrosine kinases all have a large glycosylated extracellular ligand binding domain, a single transmembrane domain and an intracellular tyrosine kinase catalytic domain. [65,66]. This superfamily of receptors can be divided into four subclasses. Subclass I receptors are monomeric with two extracellular cysteine-rich repeat sequences and includes the EGFR. Disulphide-linked heterotetrameric ($\alpha2\beta2$) structures with similar cysteine-rich sequences are found in subclass II receptors such as insulin-R and insulin growth factor 1 receptor (IGF-1R). Subclass III (PDGFR, CSF-1R, SCFR) and IV (FGFR, flg, bek) receptors have five and three extracellular Ig-SF domains respectively. The tyrosine kinase domain of these two subclasses is interrupted by a hydrophilic insertion sequence of varying length. Another group is the trkA, trkB and trkC receptors for the NGF family of neurotrophins including NGF, BDNF, NT-3 and NT-4 [67,68]. Signal transduction by these receptors is mediated by ligand-induced oligomerization [69]. Oligomerization may be induced by monovalent ligands such as EGF, inducing conformational changes in the receptor, or bivalent ligands such as PDGF and CSF-1 that mediate oligomerization of nearby receptors. A significant feature of signal transduction by these receptors is ligand-induced autophosphorylation. The resultant phospho-tyrosine residues on the cytoplasmic domains of these receptors bind to SH2 domains of other proteins involved in the signalling cascade. The signal cascade for EGFR has recently been elucidated [70]. EGF binds to its receptor, inducing oligomerization and autophosphorylation of tyrosine residues. The receptor then binds a GRB2–Sos complex which in turn activates Ras. The activated Ras then activates Raf-1 kinase which is responsible for activating MAP kinases which induce c-*myc*, c-*fos* and c-*jun*.

The tyrosine kinase domain contains 11 highly conserved subdomains [65]. One of these contains the Gly–X–Gly–X–X–Gly–X(15–20)–Lys consensus sequence which forms part of the binding site for ATP. Another subdomain contains an invariant Lys which appears to be involved in the phosphotransfer reaction, and a third contains the Pro–Ile/Val–Lys/Arg–Trp–Thr/Met–Ala–Pro–Glu sequence character-istic of tyrosine kinases.

THE NERVE GROWTH FACTOR RECEPTOR SUPERFAMILY (NGFR-SF)

The NGFR-SF includes both cytokine receptors (NGFR, TNFR-I (p55) and TNFR-II (p75)) and several other leucocyte surface glycoproteins including CD27, CD30, CD40, OX40, 4-1BB and Fas antigen. The members of this superfamily are characterized by three or four cysteine-rich repeats of about 40 amino acids in the extracellular part of the molecule [71]. These repeats contain four or six conserved cysteine residues in a pattern characteristic of the NGFR-SF, but distinct from cysteine-rich repeats in other molecules such as low density lipoprotein. Several members of this superfamily including the NGFR and TNFR-II (p75) also have a hinge-like region characterized by a lack of cysteine residues and a high proportion of Ser, Thr and Pro, suggesting that it may be glycosylated with O-linked sugars. The gene structure shows that the repeats do not correspond to particular exons, suggesting that the receptors did not arise by duplication of exons encoding single repeats. A primordial gene encoding four repeats may have arisen by unequal crossing-over. Other members of the NGFR-SF would then have evolved by gene duplication and divergence.

One unusual feature of the NGFR-SF is that some of the receptors bind more than one ligand. Moreover, unlike most other cytokines, the ligands are dimeric or trimeric. Both TNFα and TNFβ bind TNFR-I and TNFR-II with high affinity even though these two cytokines are only 31% identical in amino acid sequence (see section on TNF). Similarly, NGF, NT-3 and BDNF all bind the NGFR.

The mode of signal transduction by the NGFR-SF has not been elucidated. The cytoplasmic portions of this family of receptors have little homology with each other or any other receptors. However, CD40 is phosphorylated in response to ligand binding, and recently the transmembrane tyrosine kinase trk has been shown to be a component of the NGFR.

G-PROTEIN-COUPLED SEVEN TRANSMEMBRANE SPANNING RECEPTOR SUPERFAMILY (STSR-SF)

The STSR-SF is a very large family of receptors related to rhodopsin. It includes receptors for C5a, IL-8 (and the many related chemokines) as well as platelet activating factor and formyl peptide [72]. The family also includes viral chemokine receptors US 28 from cytomegalovirus and ECRF3 from *Herpes saimari* virus which may bind specific chemokines and activate signal transduction pathways [73]. The Duffy blood group antigen is similarly related to this family, and binds IL-8 and related chemokines [74].

The receptors have a characteristic structure of a relatively short acidic extracellular N-terminal sequence followed by seven transmembrane spanning domains with three extracellular and three intracellular loops. There are conserved cysteine residues in the N-terminal sequence and in the third extracellular loop which form a disulphide bond required for ligand binding. A second disulphide bond is probably formed between conserved cysteine residues in the first and second extracellular loop. The receptor ligands are highly cationic (pI>8.5) proteins which are as large or larger than the projected extracellular domains of their receptors and it is likely that contact points of ligand and receptor includes membrane or intracellular portions [reviewed in ref. 72].

The receptors are coupled to heterotrimeric GTP binding proteins which induce PIP_2 hydrolysis and activate kinases, phosphatases and ion channels. The α-subunit is pertussis toxin sensitive (presumably $Gi\alpha2$ or $Gi\alpha3$) but the identity of the β- and γ-subunits is not known.

THE COMPLEMENT CONTROL PROTEIN SUPERFAMILY (CCP-SF)

The α-chain (p55) of the IL-2R has two domains belonging to the complement control protein superfamily (CCP-SF) which are involved in protein binding [75]. The CCP-SF domain is also called the short consensus repeat, and is found in proteins which control the complement cascade including factor H, which consists solely of 20 CCP-SF domains, factors B and C2 with 3 CCP-SF domains, CD35 with 30 domains, and L-selectin with two domains. The structure of the CCP-SF domain in factor H has been solved by NMR and shown to consist of two antiparallel β-sheets and a short triple-stranded β-sheet with no α-helical structure [76,77].

References
1 Barclay, A.N. et al. (1993) Academic Press, London.
2 Dayhoff, M.O. et al. (1983) Meth. Enzymol. 91, 524–545.
3 Patthy, L. (1990) Cell 61, 13-14.
4 Miyazaki, T. et al. (1991) EMBO. J. 10, 3191–3197.
5 de Vos, A.M. et al. (1992) Science. 255, 306–312.
6 Cunningham, B.C. et al. (1991) Science. 254, 821–825.
7 Baron, M. et al. (1992) Biochemistry. 31, 2068–2073 .
8 Hayashida, K. et al. (1990) Proc. Natl Acad. Sci. USA 87, 9655–9659.
9 Gearing, D.P. and Ziegler, S. F. (1994) Curr. Opin. Haematol. (in press).
10 Kitamura, T. et al. (1991) Proc. Natl Acad. Sci. USA 88, 5082–5086.
11 Gorman, D.M. et al. (1990) Proc. Natl Acad. Sci. USA 87, 5459–5463.
12 Takaki, S. et al. (1991) EMBO J. 10, 2833–2838.
13 Hara, T. and Miyajima, A. (1992) EMBO J. 11, 1875–1884.
14 Cosman, D. (1993) Cytokine 5,95–106.
15 Murakami, M. et al. (1993) Science 260, 1808–1810.
16 Davis, S. et al. (1993) Science 260, 1805–1808.
17 Gearing, D.P. (1993) Adv. Immunol. 53, 31-58.
18 Gearing, D.P. et al. (1992) Science 255, 1434–1437.
19 Gearing, D.P. and Bruce, A. G. (1992) New Biol. 4, 61–65 .
20 Yin, T. et al. (1993) J. Immunol. 151, 2555–2561.
21 Minami, Y. et al. (1993) Annu. Rev. Immunol. 11, 245–267.
22 Takeshita, T. et al. (1992) Science 257, 379–382.
23 Taniguchi, T. and Minami, Y. (1993) Cell 73, 5–8.
24 Noguchi, M. et al. (1993) Cell 73, 147–157.
25 Russell, S.M. et al. (1993) Science 262, 1880–1883.
26 Kondo, M. et al. (1993) Science 262, 1874–1877.
27 Noguchi, M. et al. (1993) Science 262, 1877–1880.
28 Murakami, M. et al. (1991) Proc. Natl Acad. Sci. USA 88, 11349–11353.
29 Remillard, B. et al. (1991) J. Biol. Chem. 266, 14167–14170.
30 Wang, L.-M. et al. (1992) EMBO J. 11, 4899–4908.
31 Torti, M. et al. (1992) J. Biol. Chem. 267, 8293–8298.
32 Miyajima, A. et al. (1992) Annu. Rev. Immunol. 10, 295–331.
33 Satoh, T. et al. (1991) Proc. Natl Acad. Sci. USA. 88, 3314–3318.
34 Silvennoinen, O. et al. (1993) Proc. Natl Acad. Sci. USA 90, 8429–8433.
35 Muller, M. et al. (1993) Nature 366, 129–135.
36 Argetsinger, L. S. et al. (1993) Cell 74, 237–244.
37 Witthuhn, B.A. et al. (1993) Cell 74, 227–236.
38 Lutticken, C. et al. (1994) Science 263, 89–92.
39 Stahl, N. et al. (1994) Science 263, 92–95.
39b Ihle, J.N. et al. (1994) Trends Biochem. Sci. 19, 222–227.
40 Hatakeyama, M. et al. (1991) Science. 252, 1523–1528.
41 Carter Su, C. et al. (1989) J. Biol. Chem. 264, 18654–18661.
42 Wang, L.-M. et al. (1993) Proc. Natl Acad. Sci. USA 90, 4032–4036.
43 Finney, M. et al. (1990) Eur. J. Immunol. 20, 151–156.
44 Mosley, B. et al. (1989) Cell 59, 335–348.

45 Murata, Y. et al. (1992) J. Exp. Med. 175, 341–351.
46 Goodwin, R.G. et al. (1990) Cell 60, 941–951.
47 Renauld, J.C. et al. (1992) Proc. Natl Acad. Sci. USA 89, 5690–5694.
48 Raines, M.A. et al. (1991) Proc. Natl Acad. Sci. USA 88, 8203–8207.
49 Fukunaga, R. et al. (1990) Proc. Natl Acad. Sci. USA 87, 8702–8706.
50 Sadeghi, H. et al. (1990) Mol. Endocrinol. 4, 1799–1805.
51 Gearing, D.P. et al. (1991) EMBO J. 10, 2839–2848.
52 Fanslow, W.C. et al. (1991) J. Immunol. 147, 535–540.
53 Taga, T. et al. (1989) Cell 58, 573–581.
54 Davis, S. et al. (1993) Science 259, 1736–1739.
55 Gearing, D.P. and Cosman, D. (1991) Cell. 66, 9–10.
56 Chizzonite, R. et al. (1992) J. Immunol. 148, 3117–3124.
57 Aguet, M. et al. (1988) Cell 55, 273–280.
58 Bazan, J.F. (1990) Proc. Natl Acad. Sci. USA 87, 6934–6938.
59 Lutfalla, G. et al. (1992) J. Biol. Chem. 267, 2802–2809.
60 Ho, A.S.Y. et al. (1993) Proc. Natl Acad. Sci. USA 90, 11267–11271.
61 Hunter, T. (1993) Nature 366, 114–116.
62 Watling, D. et al. (1993) Nature 366, 166–170.
63 Velazquez, L. et al. (1992) Cell 70, 313–322.
64 Amzel, L.M. and Poljak, R. J. (1979) Annu. Rev. Biochem. 48, 961–967 .
65 Hanks, S.K. et al. (1988) Science 241, 42–52.
66 Ullrich, A. and Schlessinger, J. (1990) Cell 61, 203–212.
67 Bradshaw, R.A. et al. (1993) Trends Biochem. Sci. 18, 48–52.
68 Schneider, R. and Schweiger, M. (1991) Oncogene 6, 1807–1811.
69 Schlessinger, J. (1988) Trends Biochem. Sci. 13, 443–447.
70 Marx, J. (1993) Science 260, 1588-1590.
71 Mallett, S. and Barclay, A. N. (1991) Immunol. Today 12, 220–223.
72 Gerard, C. and Gerard, N. P. (1994) Curr. Opin. Immunol. 6, 140–145.
73 Ahuja, S.K. and Murphy, P. M. (1993) J. Biol. Chem. 268, 20691–20694.
74 Neote, K. et al. (1993) J. Biol. Chem. 268, 12247–12249.
75 Reid, K.B. and Day, A.J. (1989) Immunol. Today. 10, 177–180.
76 Norman, D.G. et al. (1991) J. Mol. Biol. 219, 717–725.
77 Barlow, P.N. et al. (1991) Biochemistry. 30, 997–1004.

THE CYTOKINES
AND
THEIR
RECEPTORS

IL-1

Other names
Lymphocyte activating factor (LAF), endogenous pyrogen (EP), leucocyte endogenous mediator (LEM), mononuclear cell factor (MCF), catabolin.

THE MOLECULES

Interleukin 1 has a very wide range of biological activities on many different target cell types including B cells, T cells, monocytes [1-3]. *In vivo,* it induces hypotension, fever, weight loss, neutrophilia and acute phase response. There are two distinct molecular forms of IL-1 (IL-1α and IL-1β) derived from two different genes. Amino acid sequence homology between human IL-1α and IL-1β is only 20% and that between murine IL-1α and IL-1β is 23%. Despite the low sequence homology, these molecules bind to the same receptor and have very similar if not identical biological properties. IL-1α is mostly cell associated and IL-1β is mostly released. In addition, an IL-1 receptor antagonist (IL-1Ra) has been described which is structurally related to IL-1β and binds to the IL-1 receptor [4]. An intracellular form of human IL-1Ra has also been identified [5]. The antagonist is made by the same cells that secrete IL-1 and may be an important physiological regulator. A cysteine protease (converting enzyme) which releases mature IL-1β has also been cloned [6,7]. A cowpox virus inhibitor (CRMA) of the IL-1 converting enzyme has been described which inhibits the host inflammatory response [8].

Crossreactivity
There is 62% amino acid sequence homology between human and mouse IL-1α and 68% for IL-1β. Both forms crossreact between humans and mice. There is 77% sequence homology between human and mouse IL-1Ra.

Sources
A wide variety of cells secrete IL-1, including monocytes, tissue macrophages, Langerhans cells, dendritic cells, T lymphocytes, B lymphocytes, natural killer (NK) cells, large granular lymphocytes (LGL), vascular endothelium and smooth muscle, fibroblasts, thymic epithelia, astrocytes, microglia, glioma cells, keratinocytes, and chondrocytes.

Bioassays
Activation of murine thymocytes or murine T cell lines. PGE_2 induction in fibroblasts using an IL-1 neutralizing antibody as control. *In vivo* (rabbit) pyrogen assay.

Physicochemical properties of IL-1α and IL-1β

Property	IL-1α		IL-1β	
	Human	Mouse	Human	Mouse
pI	5	5	7	7
Amino acids – precursor	271	270	269	269
– mature[a]	159	156	153	159
M_r (K) – predicted	18.0	18.0	17.4	17.4
– expressed	17.5	17.4	17.3	17.5
Potential N-linked glycosylation sites[b]	2	3	1	2
Disulphide bonds	0	0	0	0

[a] After proteolytic removal of propeptide
[b] IL1 is not normally glycosylated

3-D structure

The structure of IL-1α has been determined at a resolution of 2.7 Å by X-ray crystallography and IL-1β at lower resolution by NMR spectroscopy. [9,10] Both forms of IL-1 are stable tetrahedral globular proteins formed by an antiparallel six-stranded barrel closed at one end by a six-stranded β-sheet to form a bowl-like structure.

Gene structure [11–14]

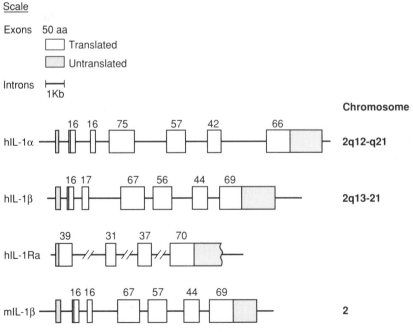

Mouse IL-1α, IL-1β and IL-1Ra genes are all on chromosome 2, and have a very similar structure to the human genes.

Amino acid sequence for human IL-1α [15]

Accession code: Swissprot P01583

```
  1  MAKVPDMFED LKNCYSENEE DSSSIDHLSL NQKSFYHVSY GPLHEGCMDQ
 51  SVSLSISETS KTSKLTFKES MVVVATNGKV LKKRRLSLSQ SITDDDLEAI
101  ANDSEEEIIK PRSAPFSFLS NVKYNFMRII KYEFILNDAL NQSIIRANDQ
151  YLTAAALHNL DEAVKFDMGA YKSSKDDAKI TVILRISKTQ LYVTAQDEDQ
201  PVLLKEMPEI PKTITGSETN LLFFWETHGT KNYFTSVAHP NLFIATKQDY
251  WVCLAGGPPS ITDFQILENQ A
```

Propeptide 1–112 (in italics) is removed to form the mature protein. Conflicting sequence A->S at position 114.

Amino acid sequence for human IL-1β [15]

Accession code: Swissprot P01584

```
  1  MAEVPKLASE MMAYYSGNED DLFFEADGPK QMKCSFQDLD LCPLDGGIQL
 51  RISDHHYSKG FRQAASVVVA MDKLRKMLVP CPQTFQENDL STFFPFIFEE
101  EPIFFDTWDN EAYVHDAPVR SLNCTLRDSQ QKSLVMSGPY ELKALHLQGQ
151  DMEQQVVFSM SFVQGEESND KIPVALGLKE KNLYLSCVLK DDKPTLQLES
201  VDPKNYPKKK MEKRFVFNKI EINNKLEFES AQFPNWYIST SQAENMPVFL
251  GGTKGGQDIT DFTMQFVSS
```

Propeptide 1–116 (in italics) is removed to form the mature protein. Conflicting sequence K->E at position 6, D->H at position 20, E->Q at position 111, G->A at position 177, and R->P at position 214.

Amino acid sequence for human IL-1 receptor antagonist (IL-1Ra) [4,16]

Accession code: Swissprot P18510

```
 -7                  MA LETIC
-25  MEICRGLRSH LITLLLFLFH SETIC
  1  RPSGRKSSKM QAFRIWDVNQ KTFYLRNNQL VAGYLQGPNV NLEEKIDVVP
 51  IEPHALFLGI HGGKMCLSCV KSGDETRLQL EAVNITDLSE NRKQDKRFAF
101  IRSDSGPTTS FESAACPGWF LCTAMEADQP VSLTNMPDEG VMVTKFYFQE
151  DE
```

A second intracellular form of the IL-1 receptor antagonist has been reported [5] with a short seven amino acid N-terminal sequence MALETIC instead of the longer signal sequence of the secreted form.

Amino acid sequence for mouse IL-1α [17]

Accession code: Swissprot P01582

```
  1  MAKVPDLFED LKNCYSENED YSSAIDHLSL NQKSFYDASY GSLHETCTDQ
 51  FVSLRTSETS KMSNFTFKES RVTVSATSSN GKILKKRRLS FSETFTEDDL
101  QSITHDLEET IQPRSAPTYT QSDLRYKLMK LVRQKFVMND SLNQTIYQDV
151  DKHYLSTTWL NDLQQEVKFD MYAYSSGGDD SKYPVTLKIS DSQLFVSAQG
201  EDQPVLLKEL PETPKLITGS ETDLIFFWKS INSKNYFTSA AYPELFIATK
251  EQSRVHLARG LPSMTDFQIS
```

Propeptide 1–114 (in italics) is removed to form the mature protein

Amino acid sequence for mouse IL-1β [18]

Accession code: Swissprot: P10749

```
  1   MATVPELNCE  MPPFDSDEND  LFFEVDGPQK  MKGCFQTFDL  GCPDESIQLQ
 51   ISQQHINKSF  RQAVSLIVAV  EKLWQLPVSF  PWTFQDEDMS  TFFSFIFEEE
101   PILCDSWDDD  DNLLVCDVPI  RQLHYRLRDE  QQKSLVLSDP  YELKALHLNG
151   QNINQQVIFS  MSFVQGEPSN  DKIPVALGLK  GKNLYLSCVM  KDGTPTLQLE
201   SVDPKQYPKK  KMEKRFVFNK  IEVKSKVEFE  SAEFPNWYIS  TSQAEHKPVF
251   LGNNSGQDII  DFTMESVSS
```

Propeptide 1–117 (in italics) is removed to form the mature protein.

Amino acid sequence for mouse IL-1 receptor antagonist (IL-1Ra) [19,20]

Accession code: Swissprot P25085

```
-26   MEICWGPYSH  LISLLLILLF  HSEAAC
  1   RPSGKRPCKM  QAFRIWDTNQ  KTFYLRNNQL  IAGYLQGPNI  KLEEKIDMVP
 51   IDLHSVFLGI  HGGKLCLSCA  KSGDDIKLQL  EEVNITDLSK  NKEEDKRFTF
101   IRSEKGPTTS  FESAACPGWF  LCTTLEADRP  VSLTNTPEEP  LIVTKFYFQE
151   DQ
```

THE IL-1 RECEPTORS

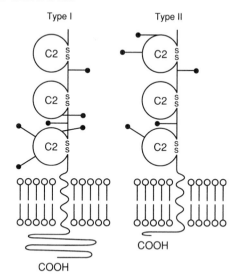

There are two IL-1 receptors. The type I receptor (CDw121a) is a transmembrane glycoprotein with an M_r of 80 000. It is a member of the Ig superfamily with three Ig-SF C2 set domains. The cytoplasmic domain is highly conserved between human and mouse with 78% sequence identity and it is essential for signal transduction. The receptor binds IL-1α, IL-1β and IL-1Ra mature proteins. In transfection experiments, human IL-1 receptor cDNA resulted in expression of low and high affinity receptors with dissociation constants similar to those found on the original T cell clone ($K_d \sim 10^{-9}$ and $\sim 10^{-11}$M). The type II receptor (CDw121b) is a glycoprotein with an M_r of 60 000 with three Ig-SF C2 set domains in its extracellular region, a single transmembrane segment, and a short (29 amino acid) cytoplasmic domain. The type II receptor can bind IL-1α, IL-1β and IL-1Ra. An open reading frame in the Vaccinia virus genome has significant homology with the type II IL-1R [21]. There is also significant homology between the transmembrane region of type II IL-1R and the membrane spanning segment of the Epstein–Barr virus protein BHRF1 [21]. This suggests an interaction with a common second subunit. A soluble receptor found in normal human serum and secreted by the human B cell line RAJI which binds preferentially to IL-1β has also been described [22].

Distribution

The type I IL-1 receptor is widely distributed on many cell types including T cells, B cells, monocytes, NK cells, basophils, neutrophils, eosinophils, dendritic cells, fibroblasts, endothelial cells, vascular endothelial cells and neural cells. The type II receptor is also expressed on a number of different tissues including T cells, B cells, monocytes and keratinocytes.

Physicochemical properties of the IL-1 receptors

Property	Type I		Type II	
	Human	Mouse	Human	Mouse
Amino acids – precursor	569	576	398	410
– mature[a]	552	557	385	397
M_r (K) – predicted	63.5	64.6	44.0	44.3
– expressed	80	80–90	60–68	60
Potential N-linked glycosylation sites[b]	6	7	5	4
Affinity K_d (M)[c]	$\sim 10^{-9}$	$\sim 10^{-9}$	$\sim 10^{-9}$	$\sim 10^{-9}$

[a] After removal of predicted signal peptide.
[b] There are five conserved N-linked glycosylation sites in human and murine IL-1 receptors.
[c] The affinity of IL-1α, IL-1β and IL-1Ra binding to type I and type II receptors is described in detail in ref. 21.

Signal transduction

IL-1 has been reported to induce hydrolysis of phosphatidylethanolamine (but not other phospholipids) which will release DAG and activate PKC without releasing calcium. It has also been reported to stimulate pertussis toxin-sensitive elevation of cAMP, suggesting it activates a G-protein-regulated adenyl cyclase [reviewed in ref. 23]. The IL-1 receptor has an intracellular sequence moiety resembling sequences that are conserved in many nucleotide binding proteins, suggesting that the receptor might act as its own G-protein [24]. Translocation of IL-1 receptor complexes from the cell surface to the nucleus has also been observed [25]. There is evidence that IL-1 signalling occurs only through the type I receptor [26].

Chromosomal location
Human type I IL-1R maps to 2q12 and the type II IL-1R to 2q12–q22. The mouse type I and type II receptors both map to the centromere-proximal region of chromosome 1 [27].

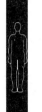

Amino acid sequence for human type I IL-1 receptor [24]

Accession code: Swissprot P14778

```
 -17  MKVLLRLICF  IALLISS
   1  LEADKCKERE  EKIILVSSAN  EIDVRPCPLN  PNEHKGTITW  YKDDSKTPVS
  51  TEQASRIHQH  KEKLWFVPAK  VEDSGHYYCV  VRNSSYCLRI  KISAKFVENE
 101  PNLCYNAQAI  FKQKLPVAGD  GGLVCPYMEF  FKNENNELPK  LQWYKDCKPL
 151  LLDNIHFSGV  KDRLIVMNVA  EKHRGNYTCH  ASYTYLGKQY  PITRVIEFIT
 201  LEENKPTRPV  IVSPANETME  VDLGSQIQLI  CNVTGQLSDI  AYWKWNGSVI
 251  DEDDPVLGED  YYSVENPANK  RRSTLITVLN  ISEIESRFYK  HPFTCFAKNT
 301  HGIDAAYIQL  IYPVTNFQKH  MIGICVTLTV  IIVCSVFIYK  IFKIDIVLWY
 351  RDSCYDFLPI  KASDGKTYDA  YILYPKTVGE  GSTSDCDIFV  FKVLPEVLEK
 401  QCGYKLFIYG  RDDYVGEDIV  EVINENVKKS  RRLIIILVRE  TSGFSWLGGS
 451  SEEQIAMYNA  LVQDGIKVVL  LELEKIQDYE  KMPESIKFIK  QKHGAIRWSG
 501  DFTQGPQSAK  TRFWKNVRYH  MPVQRRSPSS  KHQLLSPATK  EKLQREAHVP
 551  LG
```

Ig-SF C2 set domains at residues 20–86, 118–186 and 224–302. Disulphide bonds between Cys27–79, 125–179 and 231–295.

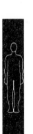

Amino acid sequence for human type II IL-1 receptor [21]

Accession code: Swissprot P27930

```
 -13  MLRLYVLVMG  VSA
   1  FTLQPAAHTG  AARSCRFRGR  HYKREFRLEG  EPVALRCPQV  PYWLWASVSP
  51  RINLTWHKND  SARTVPGEEE  TRMWAQDGAL  WLLPALQEDS  GTYVCTTRNA
 101  SYCDKMSIEL  RVFENTDAFL  PFISYPQILT  LSTSGVLVCP  DLSEFTRDKT
 151  DVKIQWYKDS  LLLDKDNEKF  LSVRGTTHLL  VHDVALEDAG  YYRCVLTFAH
 201  EGQQYNITRS  IELRIKKKKE  ETIPVIISPL  KTISASLGSR  LTIPCKVFLG
 251  TGTPLTTMLW  WTANDTHIES  AYPGGRVTEG  PRQEYSENNE  NYIEVPLIFD
 301  PVTREDLHMD  FKCVVHNTLS  FQTLRTTVKE  ASSTFSWGIV  LAPLSLAFLV
 351  LGGIWMHRRC  KHRTGKADGL  TVLWPHHQDF  QSYPK
```

Ig-SF C2 set domains at residues 30–102, 132–201 and 238–320. Disulphide bonds between Cys37–95, 139–194 and 245–313.

Amino acid sequence for mouse type I IL-1 receptor [28]

Accession code: Swissprot P13504

```
-19  MENMKVLLGL ICLMVPLLS
  1  LEIDVCTEYP NQIVLFLSVN EIDIRKCPLT PNKMHGDTII WYKNDSKTPI
 51  SADRDSRIHQ QNEHLWFVPA KVEDSGYYYC IVRNSTYCLK TKVTVTVLEN
101  DPGLCYSTQA TFPQRLHIAG DGSLVCPYVS YFKDENNELP EVQWYKNCKP
151  LLLDNVSFFG VKDKLLVRNV AEEHRGDYIC RMSYTFRGKQ YPVTRVIQFI
201  TIDENKRDRP VILSPRNETI EADPGSMIQL ICNVTGQFSD LVYWKWNGSE
251  IEWNDPFLAE DYQFVEHPST KRKYTLITTL NISEVKSQFY RYPFICVVKN
301  TNIFESAHVQ LIYPVPDFKN YLIGGFIILT ATIVCCVCIY KVFKVDIVLW
351  YRDSCSGFLP SKASDGKTYD AYILYPKTLG EGSFSDLDTF VFKLLPEVLE
401  GQFGYKLFIY GRDDYVGEDT IEVTNENVKK SRRLIIILVR DMGGFSWLGQ
451  SSEEQIAIYN ALIQEGIKIV LLELEKIQDY EKMPDSIQFI KQKHGVICWS
501  GDFQERPQSA KTRFWKNLRY QMPAQRRSPL SKHRLLTLDP VRDTKEKLPA
551  ATHLPLG
```

Ig-SF C2 set domains at residues 20–87, 119–187 and 225–303. Disulphide bonds between Cys27–80, 126–180 and 232–296. Thr 537 is phosphorylated by PKC.

Amino acid sequence for mouse type II IL-1 receptor [21]

Accession code: Swissprot P27931

```
-13  MFILLVLVTG VSA
  1  FTTPTVVHTG KVSESPITSE KPTVHGDNCQ FRGREFKSEL RLEGEPVVLR
 51  CPLAPHSDIS SSSHSFLTWS KLDSSQLIPR DEPRMWVKGN ILWILPAVQQ
101  DSGTYICTFR NASHCEQMSV ELKVFKNTEA SLPHVSYLQI SALSTTGLLV
151  CPDLKEFISS NADGKIQWYK GAILLDKGNK EFLSAGDPTR LLISNTSMDD
201  AGYYRCVMTF TYNGQEYNIT RNIELRVKGT TTEPIPVIIS PLETIPASLG
251  SRLIVPCKVF LGTGTSSNTI VWWLANSTFI SAAYPRGRVT EGLHHQYSEN
301  DENYVEVSLI FDPVTREDLH TDFKCVASNP RSSQSLHTTV KEVSSTFSWS
351  IALAPLSLII LVVGAIWMRR RCKRRAGKTY GLTKLRTDNQ DFPSSPN
```

Ig-SF C2 set domains at residues 44–114, 144–213 and 250–332. Disulphide bonds between Cys51–107, 151–206 and 257-325.

References

[1] Dinarello, C.A. (1989) Adv. Immunol. 44, 153–205.
[2] Fuhlbrigge, R.C. et al. (1989) In The Year in Immunology 1988: Immunoregulatory Cytokines and Cell Growth, Vol. 5, Cruse, J.M. and Lewis, R.E. ed, Karger, Basle, pp.21–37.
[3] di Giovine, F.S. and Duff, G. W. (1990) Immunol. Today 11, 13–20.
[4] Eisenberg, S.P. et al. (1990) Nature 343, 341–346.
[5] Haskill, S. et al. (1991) Proc. Natl Acad. Sci. USA 88, 3681–3685.
[6] Cerretti, D.P. et al. (1992) Science 256, 97–100.
[7] Thornberry, N.A. et al. (1992) Nature 356, 768–774
[8] Ray, C.A. et al. (1992) Cell 69, 597–604.
[9] Graves, B.J. et al. (1990) Biochem. 29, 2679–2684.

10 Priestle, J.P. et al. (1988) Embo. J. 7, 339–349.
11 Lennard, A. et al. (1992) Cytokine 4, 83–89.
12 Bensi, G. et al. (1987) Gene 52, 95–101.
13 Telford, J.L. et al. (1986) Nucl. Acids Res. 14, 9955–9963.
14 Furutani, Y. et al. (1986) Nucl. Acids Res. 14, 3167–3179.
15 March, C.J. et al. (1985) Nature 315, 641–647.
16 Carter, D.B. et al. (1990) Nature 344, 633–638.
17 Lomedico, P.T. et al. (1984) Nature 312, 458–462.
18 Gray, P.W. et al. (1986) J. Immunol. 137, 3644–3648.
19 Matsushime, H. et al. (1991) Blood 78, 616–623.
20 Zahedi, K. et al. (1991) J. Immunol. 146, 4228–4233.
21 McMahan, C.J. et al. (1991) EMBO J. 10, 2821–2832.
22 Symons, J.A. et al. (1991) J. Exp. Med. 174, 1251–1254.
23 Rigley, K.P. and Harnett, M. (1990) In Cytokines and B Lymphocytes, Callard, R. ed., Academic Press , London, pp.39–63.
24 Sims, J.E. et al. (1989) Proc. Natl Acad. Sci. USA 86, 8946–8950.
25 Curtis, B.M. et al. (1990) J. Immunol. 144, 1295–1303.
26 Sims, J.E. et al. (1993) Proc. Natl Acad. Sci. USA 90, 6155–6159.
27 Copeland, N.G. et al. (1991) Genomics 9, 44–50.
28 Sims, J.E. et al. (1988) Science 241, 585–589.

Other names

T Cell growth factor (TCGF).

THE MOLECULE

Interleukin 2 is a T cell-derived cytokine which was first described as a T cell growth factor (TCGF). It is now known to stimulate growth and differentiation of T cells, B cells, NK cells, LAK cells, monocytes, macrophages and oligodendrocytes [1-3].

Crossreactivity

There is about 60% homology between human and mouse IL-2. Human IL-2 is active on mouse lymphocytes, but mouse IL-2 is not active on human lymphocytes.

Sources

T Cells.

Bioassays

Proliferation of activated T cells or IL-2-dependent T cell lines. Proliferation of B cells co-stimulated with anti-IgM.

Physicochemical properties of IL-2

Property	Human	Mouse
pI	8.2	?
Amino acids – precursor	153	169
– mature[a]	133	149
M_r (K) – predicted	15.4	17.2
– expressed	15–20	15–30
Potential N-linked Glycosylation sites[b]	0	0
Disulphide bonds[c]	1	1

[a] After removal of signal peptide.

[b] O-Linked glycosylation of the threonine residue at position 3 in human and mouse IL-2 is responsible for size and charge heterogeneity of the mature protein. Glycosylation is not required for biological activity.

[c] Disulphide bonds between Cys 58 and 105 (human) and 72 and 120 (mouse).

3-D structure

The IL-2 structure has been determined at a resolution of 3 Å [4]. It is a globular protein composed of six α-helical regions (A–E) with a disulphide bridge between Cys58 and Cys105 (human) following a bent loop between α-helixes A and B. α-Helixes C, D, E and F form an apparent antiparallel α-helical bundle. An alternative folding based on the structures of GM-CSF and IL-4 has been proposed [5]. A site on the B α-helix is thought to bind to the p55 chain of the receptor [6].

Gene structure [7–9]

Scale

Exons   50 aa

☐ Translated

▨ Untranslated

Introns ⊢—⊣
         1Kb

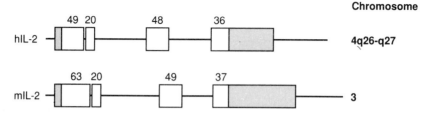

Chromosome

hIL-2   49 20   48   36   4q26-q27

mIL-2   63 20   49   37   3

Amino acid sequence for human IL-2 [10–12]

Accession code: Swissprot P01585

```
-20  MYRMQLLSCI ALSLALVTNS
  1  APTSSSTKKT QLQLEHLLLD LQMILNGINN YKNPKLTRML TFKFYMPKKA
 51  TELKHLQCLE EELKPLEEVL NLAQSKNFHL RPRDLISNIN VIVLELKGSE
101  TTFMCEYADE TATIVEFLNR WITFCQSIIS TLT
```

Amino acid sequence for mouse IL-2 [13,14]

Accession code: Swissprot P04351

```
-20  MYSMQLASCV TLTLVLLVNS
  1  APTSSSTSSS TAEAQQQQQQ QQQQQQHLEQ LLMDLQELLS RMENYRNLKL
 51  PRMLTFKFYL PKQATELKDL QCLEDELGPL RHVLDLTQSK SFQLEDAENF
101  ISNIRVTVVK LKGSDNTFEC QFDDESATVV DFLRRWIAFC QSIISTSPQ
```

Mouse IL-2 has an insertion of 12 repeat glutamine residues (15–26) which is not found in human IL-2.

THE IL-2 RECEPTOR

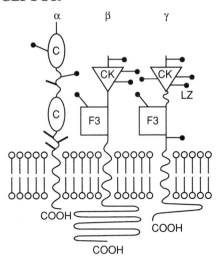

The IL-2 receptor is a complex of three distinct polypeptide chains [15]. The α-chain (Tac, p55 or CD25) binds IL-2 with low affinity (K_d 1.4×10⁻⁸M) and a short dissociation half-life of 1.7 s. A longer p75 subunit (β-chain) CD122 binds IL-2 with an affinity of 1.2×10⁻⁷M (K_d). The third p64 subunit (γ-chain) does not bind IL-2. Intermediate affinity (K_d 10⁻⁹M) IL-2R complexes are formed from α/γ or β/γ heterodimers. The high affinity receptor complex is an α/β/γ heterotrimer. It has an equilibrium K_d of 1.3×10⁻¹¹M and a half-life of 50 min [16]. The IL-2R β- and γ-chains are both members of the cytokine receptor superfamily. In addition, the γ-chain has a leucine zipper motif between the CK and FNIII domains, and an SH2-like domain at the proximal end of the cytoplasmic region. The α-chain is not a member of the CKR-SF, but it has two domains in its extracellular region with homology to the complement control protein (CCP). The γ-chain is also a functional component of the IL-4R, IL-7R and IL-15R, and possibly IL-9R and IL-13R and is now known as the common γ(γc) chain. Mutations in the IL-2R γ-chain are responsible for X-linked severe combined immunodeficiency (X-SCID) in humans [17]. This is a lethal disease characterized by absent or greatly reduced T cells, and severely depressed cell-mediated and humoral immunity.

Distribution

T Cells, B cells, NK cells, monocytes and macrophages.

Physicochemical properties of the IL-2 receptor

Property	α-Chain		β-Chain		γ-Chain	
	Human	Mouse	Human	Mouse	Human	Mouse
Amino acids – precursor	272	268	551	539	369	369
– mature[a]	251	247	525	513	347	348
M_r (K) – predicted	28.4	28.4	59.4	57.7	39.9	39.8
– expressed	55	50–60	70–75	70–75	64	?
Potential N-linked glycosylation sites	2	4	4	6	6	7
Affinity K_d (M)b	10^{-8}	10^{-8}	10^{-7}	10^{-7}	none	none

[a] After removal of predicted signal peptide.

[b] The high affinity receptor (K_d 10^{-11}M) is a complex of the p55 (α), p75 (β) and p64 (γ) chains. α/β and β/γ receptor complexes have intermediate affinities of 10^{-10}M and 10^{-9}M respectively [15].

Signal transduction

At least two distinct cytoplasmic regions of the IL-2R β-chain are involved in IL-2-mediated cellular signalling. A serine-rich region is critical for induction of c-*myc* and cell proliferation (signal 1) whereas an acidic region is required for physical association with *src*-like protein tyrosine kinase (PTK) p56*lck*, for activation of p21*ras*, and induction of c-*fos* and c-*jun* (signal 2) [15]. Binding of IL-2 to its receptor induces tyrosine phosphorylation of the β-chain [18]. The IL-2R γ-chain has an SH2-like homology domain which may be involved in binding to phosphotyrosine residues on other signalling proteins. There is conflicting evidence for phosphatidylinositol hydrolysis and elevation of cAMP [19,20].

Chromosomal location

The human IL-2R α-chain is located on 10p15–p14, the β-chain on 22q11.2–q12 (a region associated with some lymphoid tumours), and the γ-chain on Xq13. The mouse β-chain is on chromosome 15, and the γ-chain is on the X chromosome.

Amino acid sequence for human IL-2 receptor p55 (α-chain) [21–23]

Accession code: Swissprot P01589

```
-21   MDSYLLMWGL LTFIMVPGCQ A
  1   ELCDDDPPEI PHATFKAMAY KEGTMLNCEC KRGFRRIKSG SLYMLCTGNS
 51   SHSSWDNQCQ CTSSATRNTT KQVTPQPEEQ KERKTTEMQS PMQPVDQASL
101   PGHCREPPPW ENEATERIYH FVVGQMVYYQ CVQGYRALHR GPAESVCKMT
151   HGKTRWTQPQ LICTGEMETS QFPGEEKPQA SPEGRPESET SCLVTTTDFQ
201   IQTEMAATME TSIFTTEYQV AVAGCVFLLI SVLLLSGLTW QRRQRKSRRT
251   I
```

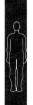

Amino acid sequence for human IL-2 receptor p75 (β-chain) [24]

Accession code: Swissprot P14784

```
-26   MAAPALSWRL  PLLILLLPLA  TSWASA
  1   AVNGTSQFTC  FYNSRANISC  VWSQDGALQD  TSCQVHAWPD  RRRWNQTCEL
 51   LPVSQASWAC  NLILGAPDSQ  KLTTVDIVTL  RVLCREGVRW  RVMAIQDFKP
101   FENLRLMAPI  SLQVVHVETH  RCNISWEISQ  ASHYFERHLE  FEARTLSPGH
151   TWEEAPLLTL  KQKQEWICLE  TLTPDTQYEF  QVRVKPLQGE  FTTWSPWSQP
201   LAFRTKPAAL  GKDTIPWLGH  LLVGLSGAFG  FIILVYLLIN  CRNTGPWLKK
251   VLKCNTPDPS  KFFSQLSSEH  GGDVQKWLSS  PFPSSSFSPG  GLAPEISPLE
301   VLERDKVTQL  LLQQDKVPEP  ASLSSNHSLT  SCFTNQGYFF  FHLPDALEIE
351   ACQVYFTYDP  YSEEDPDEGV  AGAPTGSSPQ  PLQPLSGEDD  AYCTFPSRDD
401   LLLFSPSLLG  GPSPPSTAPG  GSGAGEERMP  PSLQERVPRD  WDPQPLGPPT
451   PGVPDLVDFQ  PPPELVLREA  GEEVPDAGPR  EGVSFPWSRP  PGQGEFRALN
501   ARLPLNTDAY  LSLQELQGQD  PTHLV
```

Amino acid sequence for human IL-2 receptor p64 (γ-chain) [25]

Accession code: GenEMBL D11086

```
-22   MLKPSLPFTS  LLFLQLPLLG  VG
  1   LNTTILTPNG  NEDTTADFFL  TTMPTDSLSV  STLPLPEVQC  FVFNVEYMNC
 51   TWNSSSEPQP  TNLTLHYWYK  NSDNDKVQKC  SHYLFSEEIT  SGCQLQKKEI
101   HLYQTFVVQL  QDPREPRRQA  TQMLKLQNLV  IPWAPENLTL  HKLSESQLEL
151   NWNNRFLNHC  LEHLVQYRTD  WDHSWTEQSV  DYRHKFSLPS  VDGQKRYTFR
201   VRSRFNPLCG  SAQHWSEWSH  PIHWGSNTSK  ENPFLFALEA  VVISVGSMGL
251   IISLLCVYFW  LERTMPRIPT  LKNLEDLVTE  YHGNFSAWSG  VSKGLAESLQ
301   PDYSERLCLV  SEIPPKGGAL  GEGPGASPCN  QHSPYWAPPC  YTLKPET
```

Leucine zipper motif between residues 143 and 164. SH2-like domain between residues 266 and 299.

Amino acid sequence for mouse IL-2 receptor p55 (α-chain) [26,27]

Accession code: Swissprot P01590

```
-21   MEPRLLMLGF  LSLTIVPSCR  A
  1   ELCLYDPPEV  PNATFKALSY  KNGTILNCEC  KRGFRRLKEL  VYMRCLGNSW
 51   SSNCQCTSNS  HDKSRKQVTA  QLEHQKEQQT  TTDMQKPTQS  MHQENLTGHC
101   REPPPWKHED  SKRIYHFVEG  QSVHYECIPG  YKALQRGPAI  SICKMKCGKT
151   GWTQPQLTCV  DEREHHRFLA  SEESQGSRNS  SPESETSCPI  TTTDFPQPTE
201   TTAMTETFVL  TMEYKVAVAS  CLFLLISILL  LSGLTWQHRW  RKSRRTI
```

Conflicting sequence [27] M->T at position –15, T->A at position 97, E->V at position 119, F->L at position 195, and E->V at position 206.

Amino acid sequence for mouse IL-2 receptor p75 (β-chain) [28]

Accession code: Swissprot P16297

```
 -26  MATIALPWSL  SLYVFLLLLA  TPWASA
   1  AVKNCSHLEC  FYNSRANVSC  MWSHEEALNV  TTCHVHAKSN  LRHWNKTCEL
  51  TLVRQASWAC  NLILGSFPES  QSLTSVDLLD  INVVCWEEKG  WRRVKTCDFH
 101  PFDNLRLVAP  HSLQVLHIDT  QRCNISWKVS  QVSHYIEPYL  EFEARRRLLG
 151  HSWEDASVLS  LKQRQQWLFL  EMLIPSTSYE  VQVRVKAQRN  NTGTWSPWSQ
 201  PLTFRTRPAD  PMKEILPMSW  LRYLLLVLGC  FSGFFSCVYI  LVKCRYLGPW
 251  LKTVLKCHIP  DPSEFFSQLS  SQHGGDLQKW  LSSPVPLSFF  SPSGPAPEIS
 301  PLEVLDGDSK  AVQLLLLQKD  SAPLPSPSGH  SQASCFTNQG  YFFFHLPNAL
 351  EIESCQVYFT  YDPCVEEEVE  EDGSRLPEGS  PHPPLLPLAG  EQDDYCAFPP
 401  RDDLLLFSPS  LSTPNTAYGG  SRAPEERSPL  SLHEGLPSLA  SRDLMGLQRP
 451  LERMPEGDGE  GLSANSSGEQ  ASVPEGNLHG  QDQDRGQGPI  LTLNTDAYLS
 501  LQELQAQDSV  HLI
```

Amino acid sequence for mouse IL-2 receptor p64 (γ-chain) [29]

Accession code: GenEMBL L20048

```
 -21  MLKLLLSPRS  FLVLQLLLLR  A
   1  GWSSKVLMSS  ANEDIKADLI  LTSTAPEHLS  APTLPLPEVQ  CFVFNIEYMN
  51  CTWNSSSEPQ  ATNLTLHYRY  KVSDNNTFQE  CSHYLFSKEI  TSGCQIQKED
 101  IQLYQTFVVQ  LQDPQKPQRR  AVQKLNLQNL  VIPRAPENLT  LSNLSESQLE
 151  LRWKSRHIKE  RCLQYLVQYR  SNRDRSWTEL  IVNHEPRFSL  PSVDELKRYT
 201  FRVRSRYNPI  CGSSQQWSKW  SQPVHWGSHT  VEENPSLFAL  EAVLIPVGTM
 251  GLIITLIFVY  CWLERMPPIP  PIKNLEDLVT  EYQGNFSAWS  GVSKGLTESL
 301  QPDYSERFCH  VSEIPPKGGA  LGEGPGGSPC  SLHSPYWPPP  CYSLKPEA
```

References

1 Smith, K.A. (1984) Ann. Rev. Immunol. 2, 319–333.
2 Smith, K.A. (1988) Science 240, 1169–1176.
3 Kuziel, W.A. and Greene, W. C. (1991) In The Cytokine Handbook, Thomson, A., ed., Academic Press, London, pp.83–102.
4 Brandhuber, B.J. et al. (1987) Science 238, 1707–1709.
5 Bazan, J.F. (1992) Science 257, 410-413.
6 Sauve, K. et al. (1991) Proc. Natl. Acad. Sci. USA 88, 4636–4640.
7 Holbrook, N.J. et al. (1984) Proc. Natl Acad. Sci. USA 81, 1634–1638.
8 Fujita, T. et al. (1983) Proc. Natl. Acad. Sci. USA 80, 7437–7441.
9 Fuse, A. et al. (1984) Nucl. Acids Res. 12, 9323–9331.
10 Taniguchi, T. et al. (1983) Nature 302, 305–310.
11 Maeda, S. et al. (1983) Biochem. Biophys. Res. Comm. 115, 1040–1047.
12 Devos, R. et al. (1983) Nucl. Acids Res. 11, 4307–4323.
13 Yokota, T. et al. (1985) Proc. Natl Acad. Sci. USA 82, 68–72.
14 Kashima, N. et al. (1985) Nature 313, 402–404.
15 Minami, Y. et al. (1993) Ann. Rev. Immunol. 11, 245–267.
16 Taniguchi, T. and Minami, Y. (1993) Cell 73, 5–8.
17 Noguchi, M. et al. (1993) Cell 73, 147–157.
18 Asao, H. et al. (1990) J. Exp. Med. 171, 637–644.

19 Rigley, K. P. and Harnett, M. (1990) In Cytokines and B lymphocytes, Callard, R., ed., Academic Press , London, pp. 39–63.
20 Tigges, M.A. et al. (1989) Science 243, 781–786.
21 Leonard, W. J. et al. (1984) Nature 311, 626–631.
22 Cosman, D. et al. (1984) Nature 312, 768–771.
23 Nikaido, T. et al. (1984) Nature 311, 631–635.
24 Hatakeyama, M. et al. (1989) Science 244, 551–556.
25 Takeshita, T. et al. (1992) Science 257, 379–382.
26 Miller, J. et al. (1985) J. Immunol. 134, 4212–4217.
27 Shimuzu, A. et al. (1985) Nucl. Acids Res. 13, 1505–1516.
28 Kono, T. et al. (1990) Proc. Natl Acad. Sci. USA 87, 1806–1810.
29 Cao, X. et al. (1993) Proc. Natl Acad. Sci., USA 90, 8464–8468.

Other names

Mast cell growth factor (MCGF), multi-colony stimulating factor (multi-CSF), eosinophil-CSF (E-CSF), haematopoietic cell growth factor (HCGF), burst-promoting activity (BPA), P-cell stimulating factor activity, thy-1 inducing factor, WEHI-3 growth factor.

THE MOLECULE

Interleukin 3 is a haematopoietic growth factor which stimulates colony formation of erythroid, megakaryocyte, neutrophil, eosinophil, basophil, mast cell and monocytic lineages [1]. IL-3 may also stimulate multipotent progenitor cells, but it is more likely to be important in committing progenitor cells to a differentiation pathway rather than self-renewal of primitive stem cells. Many of the activities of IL-3 are enhanced or depend upon co-stimulation with other cytokines. IL-3 does not stimulate lymphocyte colony formation, but it is a growth factor for B lymphocytes and it activates monocytes, suggesting that it may have an additional immunoregulatory role. IL-3 has been used clinically to expand haematopoietic precursors after bone marrow transplantation, aplastic anaemia and chemotherapy [2].

Crossreactivity

Amino acid sequence homology between mouse and human IL-3 is only 29% and there is no cross-species reactivity.

Sources

Activated T cells, mast cells, eosinophils.

Bioassays

Proliferation of TF-1 (human erythroleukaemia), MO7e (human megakaryoblastic leukaemia) or AML-193 (acute myeloid leukaemia) cell lines. Stimulation of erythroid, granulocyte and macrophage colony formation in bone marrow colony assay.

Physicochemical properties of IL-3

Property	Human	Mouse
pI	4–8	4–8
Amino acids – precursor	152	166
– mature[a]	133	140
M_r (K) – predicted	15.1	15.7
– expressed	14–30	28
Potential N-linked glycosylation sites	2	4[b]
Disulphide bonds	1	2

[a] After removal of predicted signal peptide.

[b] Glycosylation only at positions 16 and 86 (see sequence). Glycosylation is not required for biological activity.

3-D structure

Similar to IL-4, GM-CSF and M-CSF.

Gene structure [3]

Scale

Exons   50 aa
         ☐ Translated
         ▨ Untranslated

Introns ⊢—⊣
         1Kb

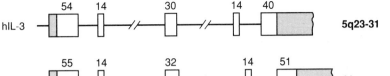

Chromosome

5q23-31

11

Amino acid sequence for human IL-3 [4,5]

Accession code: Swissprot P08700

```
-19   MSRLPVLLLL QLLVRPGLQ
  1   APMTQTTPLK TSWVNCSNMI DEIITHLKQP PLPLLDFNNL NGEDQDILME
 51   NNLRRPNLEA FNRAVKSLQN ASAIESILKN LLPCLPLATA APTRHPIHIK
101   DGDWNEFRRK LTFYLKTLEN AQAQQTTLSL AIF
```

Conflicting sequence [5] P->S at position 8. Disulphide bonds between
Cysteines 16-84.

Amino acid sequence for mouse IL-3 [6,7]

Accession code: Swissprot P01586

```
-26   MVLASSTTSI HTMLLLLLML FHLGLQ
  1   ASISGRDTHR LTRTLNCSSI VKEIIGKLPE PELKTDDEGP SLRNKSFRRV
 51   NLSKFVESQG EVDPEDRYVI KSNLQKLNCC LPTSANDSAL PGVFIRDLDD
101   FRKKLRFYMV HLNDLETVLT SRPPQPASGS VSPNRGTVEC
```

Disulphide bonds between Cysteines 17–80 and 79–140.

THE IL-3 RECEPTOR

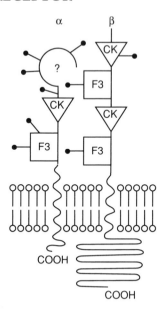

The high affinity IL-3 receptor is formed by association of a low affinity IL-3 binding α-subunit (IL-3Rα) (CD123) with a second β-subunit [8]. In humans, the β-subunit (KH97) is common to the IL-3, IL-5 and GM-CSF receptors, but does not itself bind any of these cytokines [9]. In mice, there are two β-subunits, AIC2A and AIC2B [10]. Of these, AIC2B is similar to KH97 and is shared with IL-5 and GM-CSF receptors, but does not itself bind cytokine [11,12]. In contrast, AIC2A binds IL-3 and associates only with the IL-3Rα chain. The IL-3R α-subunit is a member of the CKR-SF. It has an N-terminal region of about 100 amino acids with homology to a similar sequence in the α-subunits of the IL-5 and GM-CSF receptors, followed by a CKR domain and an FNIII domain that contains the WSXWS motif. It has a short cytoplasmic domain, and is unable to signal. The β-subunit has two homologous segments in the extracellular region, each with a CKR domain followed by an FNIII domain (see diagram). It has a much longer cytoplasmic domain with a Ser/Pro-rich region in common with the IL-2R β-chain, the IL-4R and the EpoR.

Distribution

Haematopoietic progenitor cells derived from pluripotent stem cells, monocytes, pre-B cells and B cells [13].

Physicochemical properties of the IL-3 receptor

Property	α-Chain		β-Chain		
	Human	Mouse	Human KH97	Mouse AIC2A	Mouse AIC2B
Amino acids – precursor	378	396	897	878	896
– mature[a]	360	380	881	856	874
M_r (K) – predicted	41.3	41.5	95.7	94.7	96.6
– expressed	70	60–70	120	110–120	120–140
Potential N-linked glycosylation sites	6	5	3	2	3
Affinity K_d (M)[b]	10^{-7}	5×10^{-8}	none	10^{-8}	none

[a] After removal of predicted signal peptide

[b] High affinity receptor is a complex of α- and β-chains. Human IL-3R α/β (KH97) K_d 10^{-10}M [14], mouse α/β (AIC2A) K_d 3×10^{-10}M, mouse α/β (AIC2B) K_d 4×10^{-10}M [15]. KH97 and AIC2B also associate with IL-5Rα and GM-CSFRα subunits.

Signal transduction

IL-3 binding to its receptor results in rapid tyrosine and serine/threonine phosphorylation of a number of cellular proteins [16-18], including the IL-3R β-subunit itself [19]. The cloned IL-3 receptor has no consensus sequence for tyrosine kinase, indicating that the receptor and associated tyrosine kinase, are separate molecules. There is also some evidence for PKC translocation. Signal transduction requires the presence of the β-subunit.

Chromosomal location
The human IL-3 receptor α-chain is located in the pseudo-autosomal region of the sex chromosomes at Yp13.3 and Xp22.3. The β-chain is on chromosome 22. AIC2A and AIC2B are both on mouse chromosome 15.

Amino acid sequence for the human IL-3 receptor α-chain [14]

Accession code: GenEMBL M74782

```
-18   MVLLWLTLLL IALPCLLQ
  1   TKEDPNPPIT NLRMKAKAQQ LTWDLNRNVT DIECVKDADY SMPAVNNSYC
 51   QFGAISLCEV TNYTVRVANP PFSTWILFPE NSGKPWAGAE NLTCWIHDVD
101   FLSCSWAVGP GAPADVQYDL YLNVANRRQQ YECLHYKTDA QGTRIGCRFD
151   DISRLSSGSQ SSHILVRGRS AAFGIPCTDK FVVFSQIEIL TPPNMTAKCN
201   KTHSFMHWKM RSHFNRKFRY ELQIQKRMQP VITEQVRDRT SFQLLNPGTY
251   TVQIRARERV YEFLSAWSTP QRFECDQEEG ANTRAWRTSL LIALGTLLAL
301   VCVFVICRRY LVMQRLFPRI PHMKDPIGDS FQNDKLVVWE AGKAGLEECL
351   VTEVQVVQKT
```

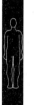

Amino acid sequence for the human IL-3 receptor β-chain (KH97) [9]

Accession code: GenEMBL M59941, M38275

```
-16     MVLAQGLLSM ALLALC
  1     WERSLAGAEE TIPLQTLRCY NDYTSHITCR WADTQDAQRL VNVTLIRRVN
 51     EDLLEPVSCD LSDDMPWSAC PHPRCVPRRC VIPCQSFVVT DVDYFSFQPD
101     RPLGTRLTVT LTQHVQPPEP RDLQISTDQD HFLLTWSVAL GSPQSHWLSP
151     GDLEFEVVYK RLQDSWEDAA ILLSNTSQAT LGPEHLMPSS TYVARVRTRL
201     APGSRLSGRP SKWSPEVCWD SQPGDEAQPQ NLECFFDGAA VLSCSWEVRK
251     EVASSVSFGL FYKPSPDAGE EECSPVLREG LGSLHTRHHC QIPVPDPATH
301     GQYIVSVQPR RAEKHIKSSV NIQMAPPSLN VTKDGDSYSL RWETMKMRYE
351     HIDHTFEIQY RKDTATWKDS KTETLQNAHS MALPALEPST RYWARVRVRT
401     SRTGYNGIWS EWSEARSWDT ESVLPMWVLA LIVIFLTTAV LLALRFCGIY
451     GYRLRRKWEE KIPNPSKSHL FQNGSAELWP PGSMSAFTSG SPPHQGPWGS
501     RFPELEGVFP VGFGDSEVSP LTIEDPKHVC DPPSGPDTTP AASDLPTEQP
551     PSPQPGPPAA SHTPEKQASS FDFNGPYLGP PHSRSLPDIL GQPEPPQEGG
601     SQKSPPPGSL EYLCLPAGGQ VQLVPLAQAM GPGQAVEVER RPSQGAAGSP
651     SLESGGGPAP PALGPRVGGQ DQKDSPVAIP MSSGDTEDPG VASGYVSSAD
701     LVFTPNSGAS SVSLVPSLGL PSDQTPSLCP GLASGPPGAP GPVKSGFEGY
751     VELPPIEGRS PRSPRNNPVP PEAKSPVLNP GERPADVSPT SPQPEGLLVL
801     QQVGDYCFLP GLGPGPLSLR SKPSSPGPGP EIKNLDQAFQ VKKPPGQAVP
851     QVPVIQLFKA LKQQDYLSLP PWEVNKPGEV C
```

Amino acid sequence for the mouse IL-3 receptor α-chain [15]

Accession code: GenEMBL X64534

```
-16     MAANLWLILG LLASHS
  1     SDLAAVREAP PTAVTTPIQN LHIDPAHYTL SWDPAPGADI TTGAFCRKGR
 51     DIFVWADPGL ARCSFQSLSL CHVTNFTVFL GKDRAVAGSI QFPPDDDGDH
101     EAAAQDLRCW VHEGQLSCQW ERGPKATGDV HYRMFWRDVR LGPAHNRECP
151     HYHSLDVNTA GPAPHGGHEG CTLDLDTVLG STPNSPDLVP QVTITVNGSG
201     RAGPVPCMDN TVDLQRAEVL APPTLTVECN GSEAHARWVA RNRFHHGLLG
251     YTLQVNQSSR SEPQEYNVSI PHFWVPNAGA ISFRVKSRSE VYPRKLSSWS
301     EAWGLVCPPE VMPVKTALVT SVATVLGAGL VAAGLLLWWR KSLLYRLCPP
351     IPRLRLPLAG EMVVWEPALE DCEVTPVTDA
```

Amino acid sequence for the mouse IL-3 receptor AIC2A β-chain [20]

Accession code: GenEMBL M29855

```
-22     MDQQMALTWG LCYMALVALC WG
  1     HEVTEEEETV PLKTLECYND YTNRIICSWA DTEDAQGLIN MTLLYHQLDK
 51     IQSVSCELSE KLMWSECPSS HRCVPRRCVI PYTRFSNGDN DYYSFQPDRD
101     LGIQLMVPLA QHVQPPPPKD IHISPSGDHF LLEWSVSLGD SQVSWLSSKD
151     IEFEVAYKRL QDSWEDASSL HTSNFQVNLE PKLFLPNSIY AARVRTRLSA
201     GSSLSGRPSR WSPEVHWDSQ PGDKAQPQNL QCFFDGIQSL HCSWEVWTQT
251     TGSVSFGLFY RPSPAAPEEK CSPVVKEPQA SVYTRYRCSL PVPEPSAHSQ
```

```
301  YTVSVKHLEQ  GKFIMSYYHI  QMEPPILNQT  KNRDSYSLHW  ETQKIPKYID
351  HTFQVQYKKK  SESWKDSKTE  NLGRVNSMDL  PQLEPDTSYC  ARVRVKPISD
401  YDGIWSEWSN  EYTWTTDWVM  PTLWIVLILV  FLIFTLLLAL  HFGRVYGYRT
451  YRKWKEKIPN  PSKSLLFQDG  GKGLWPPGSM  AAFATKNPAL  QGPQSRLLAE
501  QQGVSYEHLE  DNNVSPLTIE  DPNIIRDPPS  RPDTTPAASS  ESTEQLPNVQ
551  VEGPIPSSRP  RKQLPSFDFN  GPYLGPPQSH  SLPDLPGQLG  SPQVGGSLKP
601  ALPGSLEYMC  LPPGGQVQLV  PLSQVMGQGQ  AMDVQCGSSL  ETTGSPSVEP
651  KENPPVELSV  EKQEARDNPM  TLPISSGGPE  GSMMASDYVT  PGDPVLTLPT
701  GPLSTSLGPS  LGLPSAQSPS  LCLKLPRVPS  GSPALGPPGF  EDYVELPPSV
751  SQAATSPPGH  PAPPVASSPT  VIPGEPREEV  GPASPHPEGL  LVLQQVGDYC
801  FLPGLGPGSL  SPHSKPPSPS  LCSETEDLDQ  DLSVKKFPYQ  PLPQAPAIQF
851  FKSLKY
```

Amino acid sequence for the mouse IL-3 receptor AIC2B β-chain [10]

Accession code: GenEMBL M34397

```
-22  MDQQMALTWG  LCYMALVALC  WG
  1  HGVTEAEETV  PLKTLQCYND  YTNHIICSWA  DTEDAQGLIN  MTLYHQLEKK
 51  QPVSCELSEK  LMWSECPSSH  RCVPRRCVIP  YTRFSITNED  YYSFRPDSDL
101  GIQLMVPLAQ  NVQPPLPKNV  SISSSEDRFL  LEWSVSLGDA  QVSWLSSKDI
151  EFEVAYKRLQ  DSWEDAYSLH  TSKFQVNFEP  KLFLPNSIYA  PRVRTRLYPG
201  SSLSGRPSRW  SPEAHWDSQP  GDKAQPQNLQ  CFFDGIQSLH  CSWEVWTQTT
251  GSVSFGLFYR  PSPVAPEEKC  SPVVKEPPGA  SVYTRYHCSL  PVPEPSAHSQ
301  YTVSVKHLEQ  GKFIMSYNHI  QMEPPTLNLT  KNRDSYSLHW  ETQKMAYSFI
351  EHTFQVQYKK  KSDSWEDSKT  ENLDRAHSMD  LSQLEPDTSY  CARVRVKPIS
401  NYDGIWSKWS  EEYTWKTDWV  MPTLWIVLIL  VFLILTLLLI  LRFGCVSVYR
451  TYRKWKEKIP  NPSKSLLFQD  GGKGLWPPGS  MAAFATKNPA  LQGPQSRLLA
501  EQQGESYAHL  EDNNVSPLTI  EDPNIIRVPP  SGPDTTPAAS  SESTEQLPNV
551  QVEGPTPNRP  RKQLPSFDFN  GPYLGPPQSH  SLPDLPDQLG  SPQVGGSLKP
601  ALPGSLEYMC  LAPGGQVQLV  PLSQVMGQGQ  AMDVQCGSSL  ETSGSPSVEP
651  KENPPVELSM  EEQEARDNPV  TLPISSGGPE  GSMMASDYVT  PGDPVLTLPT
701  GPLSTSLGPS  LGLPSAQSPS  LCLKLPRVPS  GSPALGPPGF  EDYVELPPSV
751  SQAAKSPPGH  PAPPVASSPT  VIPGEPREEV  GPASPHPEGL  LVLQQVGDYC
801  FLPGLGPGSL  SPHSKPPSPS  LCSETEDLVQ  DLSVKKFPYQ  PMPQAPAIQF
851  FKSLKHQDYL  SLPPWDNSQS  GKVC
```

References

1 Ihle, J.N. (1991) In Peptide Growth Factors and their Receptors I, Sporn, M.B. and Roberts, A.B., eds, Springer-Verlag, New York, pp. 541–575.

2 Ihle, J.N. (1992) Chem. Immunol. 51, 65–106.

3 Miyatake, S. et al. (1985) Proc. Natl. Acad. Sci. USA 82, 316–320.

4 Otsuka, T. et al. (1988) J. Immunol. 140, 2288–2295.

5 Yang, Y-C. et al. (1986) Cell 47, 3–10.

6 Yokota, T. et al. (1984) Proc. Natl. Acad. Sci. USA 81, 1070–1074.

7 Fung, M.C. et al. (1984) Nature 307, 233–237.

8 Cosman, D. (1994) Cytokine 5, 95–106.

9 Hayashida, K. et al. (1990) Proc. Natl. Acad. Sci. USA 87, 9655–9659.

10 Gorman, D.M. et al. (1990) Proc. Natl. Acad. Sci. USA 87, 5459–5463.
11 Kitamura, T. et al. (1991) Proc. Natl. Acad. Sci. USA 88, 5082–5086.
12 Takaki, S. et al. (1991) EMBO J. 10, 2833–2838.
13 Park, L.S. et al. (1989) J. Biol. Chem. 264, 5420–5427.
14 Kitamura, T. et al. (1991) Cell 66, 1165–1174.
15 Hara, T. and Miyajima, A. (1992) EMBO J. 11, 1875–1884.
16 Isfort, R. et al. (1988) J. Biol. Chem. 263, 19203–19209.
17 Sorensen, P.H. et al. (1989) Blood 73, 406–418.
18 Murata, Y. et al. (1990) Biochem. Biophys. Res. Commun. 173, 1102–1108.
19 Sorensen, P. et al. (1989) J. Biol. Chem. 264, 19253–19258.
20 Itoh, N. et al. (1990) Science 247, 324–327.

Other names
B Cell stimulating factor 1 (BSF-1).

THE MOLECULE

Interleukin 4 is a pleiotropic cytokine derived from T cells and mast cells with multiple biological effects on B cells, T cells and many non-lymphoid cells including monocytes, endothelial cells and fibroblasts. It also induces secretion of IgG1 and IgE by mouse B cells and IgG4 and IgE by human B cells. The IL-4-dependent production of IgE and possibly IgG1 and IgG4 is due to IL-4-induced isotype switching [1-3]. IL-4 appears to share this property with IL-13.

Crossreactivity
Two regions of human IL-4 (amino acids 1–90 and 129–149) share approximately 50% sequence homology with the corresponding regions of mouse IL-4. In contrast, the region from amino acid positions 91–128 shares very little homology with the corresponding region of mouse IL-4. There is no cross-species reactivity between human and mouse IL-4.

Sources
Mast cells, T cells, some mouse B cell lymphomas, bone marrow stromal cells.

Bioassays
Human: Proliferation of PHA T cell blasts in the presence of blocking anti-IL-2 or anti-IL-2R antibody; proliferation of MO7 cell line; increased expression of CD23 or surface IgM on human tonsillar B cells.

Mouse: Proliferation of CTLL in the presence of anti-IL-2 or anti-IL-2R antibody. Increased expression of MHC class II on murine B cells.

Physicochemical properties of IL-4

Property	Human	Mouse
pI	10.5	6.5
Amino acids – precursor	153	140
– mature[a]	129	120
M_r (K) – predicted	15.0	13.6
– expressed	15–19	15–19
Potential N-linked glycosylation sites	2[b]	3
Disulphide bonds	3	3

[a] After removal of signal peptide.
[b] Asn38 is glycosylated.

3-D structure

The three-dimensional structure of IL-4 has been determined by NMR [4], and X-ray crystallography [5]. It has a compact globular structure with a predominantly hydrophobic core. A four α-helix bundle with the helices arranged in a left-handed antiparallel bundle with two overhand connections containing a two-stranded antiparallel β-sheet make up most of the molecule. The structure is similar to GM-CSF, M-CSF and IL-3.

Gene structure [6-7]

Scale

Exons 50 aa
[ ] Translated
[ ] Untranslated

Introns ⊢——⊣
1Kb

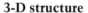

Chromosome

hIL-4   45 16   59   33   5q31

mIL-4   44 16   51   29   11

Amino acid sequence for human IL-4 [8]

Accession code: Swissprot P05112

```
-24  MGLTSQLLPP LFFLLACAGN FVHG
  1  HKCDITLQEI IKTLNSLTEQ KTLCTELTVT DIFAASKNTT EKETFCRAAT
 51  VLRQFYSHHE KDTRCLGATA QQFHRHKQLI RFLKRLDRNL WGLAGLNSCP
101  VKEANQSTLE NFLERLKTIM REKYSKCSS
```

Disulphide bonds between Cys3–127, 24–65 and 46–99. Asn38 is glycosylated.

Amino acid sequence for mouse IL-4 [9-10]

Accession code: Swissprot P07750

```
-20  MGLNPQLVVI LLFFLECTRS
  1  HIHGCDKNHL REIIGILNEV TGEGTPCTEM DVPNVLTATK NTTESELVCR
 51  ASKVLRIFYL KHGKTPCLKK NSSVLMELQR LFRAFRCLDS SISCTMNESK
101  STSLKDFLES LKSIMQMDYS
```

Disulphide bonds between Cys5–87, 27–67 and 49–94.

THE IL-4 RECEPTOR

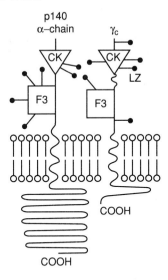

The IL-4 receptor is a complex consisting at least of two chains: a high affinity IL-4 binding (p140, α chain) (CD 124) chain and the IL-2R γ-chain also known as the common γ-chain (γc). The high affinity (K_d 10^{-10}M) IL-4 binding chain belongs to the cytokine receptor superfamily. It has a CKR domain and an FNIII domain containing the WSXWS motif in the extracellular region [11]. The cytoplasmic domain contains Ser/Pro-rich regions similar to those present in the IL-2R and GM-CSFR β-chains. A soluble form of the high affinity mouse IL-4 receptor is produced by alternative mRNA splicing [12]. The soluble form of the mouse IL-4R and a recombinant extracellular domain of the human IL-4R are both potent IL-4 antagonists [13]. The IL-2R γ-chain is a functional component of the IL-4R and augments IL-4 binding affinity [14,15]. A second low affinity (K_d 10^{-8}M) IL-4 receptor has also been identified and partially sequenced, but not yet cloned [16]. The high and low affinity receptors appear to be coupled to different signal transduction pathways [17].

Distribution

High affinity receptors for IL-4 are present in low numbers on pre B cells, resting B cells and resting T cells; and in high numbers after activation. They are also present on haematopoietic progenitor cells, mast cells, macrophages, myeloid cells, endothelial cells, epithelial cells, fibroblasts, muscle cells, neuroblasts, brain stroma and bone marrow stroma [18-21].

Physicochemical properties of the IL-4 receptor

Property		Human	Mouse
Amino acids	– precursor	825	810
	– mature[a]	800	785 (205)[b]
M_r (K)	– predicted	87	85.1 (23.9)[b]
	– expressed	140	138–145 (32–41)[b]
Potential N-linked glycosylation sites		6	5
Affinity K_d (M)		10^{-10}	10^{-10}

[a] After removal of predicted signal peptide.
[b] Secreted form of murine IL-4R in parenthesis.

Signal transduction

IL-4 binding to the high affinity receptor results in tyrosine phosphorylation of cellular proteins including 4PS which associates with the p85 subunit of PI 3-kinase after cytokine stimulation [22,23], and translocation of PKC [24]. Activation of a tyrosine phosphatase and dephosphorylation of an 80 000 molecular weight protein has also been reported [25]. Another signal transduction pathway for human IL-4 has been shown to involve breakdown of phosphatidylinositol bisphosphate (PIP₂) releasing IP₃ and intracellular calcium followed after a lag period of 10–15 min by a rise in intracellular cAMP [26]. This pathway may be coupled to a low affinity receptor [16,17].

Chromosomal location
The high affinity human IL-4 receptor is on chromosome 16p12.1–p11.2. The mouse IL-4 receptor is on chromosome 7.

Amino acid sequence for the human IL-4 receptor [27]
Accession code: Swissprot P24394

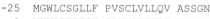

```
 -25  MGWLCSGLLF  PVSCLVLLQV  ASSGN
   1  MKVLQEPTCV  SDYMSISTCE  WKMNGPTNCS  TELRLLYQLV  FLLSEAHTCI
  51  PENNGGAGCV  CHLLMDDVVS  ADNYTLDLWA  GQQLLWKGSF  KPSEHVKPRA
 101  PGNLTVHTNV  SDTLLLTWSN  PYPPDNYLYN  HLTYAVNIWS  ENDPADFRIY
 151  NVTYLEPSLR  IAASTLKSGI  SYRARVRAWA  QCYNTTWSEW  SPSTKWHNSY
 201  REPFEQHLLL  GVSVSCIVIL  AVSLLCYVSI  TKIKKEWWDQ  IPNPARSRLV
 251  AIIIQDAQGS  QWEKRSRGQE  PAKCPHWKNC  LTKLLPCFLE  HNMKRDEDPH
 301  KAAKEMPFQG  SGKSAWCPVE  ISKTVLWPES  ISVVRCVELF  EAPVECEEEE
 351  EVEEEKGSFC  ASPESSRDDF  QEGREGIVAR  LTESLFLDLL  GEENGGFCQQ
 401  DMGESCLLPP  SGSTSAHMPW  DEFPSAGPKE  APPWGKEQPL  HLEPSPPASP
 451  TQSPDNLTCT  ETPLVIAGNP  AYRSFSNSLS  QSPCPRELGP  DPLLARHLEE
 501  VEPEMPCVPQ  LSEPTTVPQP  EPETWEQILR  RNVLQHGAAA  APVSAPTSGY
 551  QEFVHAVEQG  GTQASAVVGL  GPPGEAGYKA  FSSLLASSAV  SPEKCGFGAS
 601  SGEEGYKPFQ  DLIPGCPGDP  APVPVPLFTF  GLDREPPRSP  QSSHLPSSSP
 651  EHLGLEPGEK  VEDMPKPPLP  QEQATDPLVD  SLGSGIVYSA  LTCHLCGHLK
 701  QCHGQEDGGQ  TPVMASPCCG  CCCGDRSSPP  TTPLRAPDPS  PGGVPLEASL
 751  CPASLAPSGI  SEKSKSSSSF  HPAPGNAQSS  SQTPKIVNFV  SVGPTYMRVS
```

Amino acid sequence for the mouse IL-4 receptor [12]

Accession code: Swissprot P16382

```
-25   MGRLCTKFLT SVGCLILLLV TGSGS
  1   IKVLGEPTCF SDYIRTSTCE WFLDSAVDCS SQLCLHYRLM FFEFSENLTC
 51   IPRNSASTVC VCHMEMNRPV QSDRYQMELW AEHRQLWQGS FSPSGNVKPL
101   APDNLTLHTN VSDEWLLTWN NLYPSNNLLY KDLISMVNIS REDNPAEFIV
151   YNVTYKEPRL SFPINILMSG VYYTARVRVR SQILTGTWSE WSPSITWYNH
201   FQLPLIQRLP LGVTISCLCI PLFCLFCYFS ITKIKKIWWD QIPTPARSPL
251   VAIIIQDAQV PLWDKQTRSQ ESTKYPHWKT CLDKLLPCLL KHRVKKKTDF
301   PKAAPTKSLQ SPGKAGWCPM EVSRTVLWPE NVSVSVVRCM ELFEAPVQNV
351   EEEEDEIVKE DLSMSPENSG GCGFQESQAD IMARLTENLF SDLLEAENGG
401   LGQSALAESC SPLPSGSGQA SVSWACLPMG PSEEATCQVT EQPSHPGPLS
451   GSPAQSAPTL ACTQVPLVLA DNPAYRSFSD CCSPAPNPGE LAPEQQQADH
501   LEEEEPPSPA DPHSSGPPMQ PVESWEQILH MSVLQHGAAA GSTPAPAGGY
551   QEFVQAVKQG AAQDPGVPGV RPSGDPGYKA FSSLLSSNGI RGDTAAAGTD
601   DGHGGYKPFQ NPVPNQSPSS VPLFTFGLDT ELSPSPLNSD PPKSPPECLG
651   LELGLKGGDW VKAPPPADQV PKPFGDDLGF GIVYSSLTCH LCGHLKQHHS
701   QEEGGQSPIV ASPGCGCCYD DRSPSLGSLS GALESCPEGI PPEANLMSAP
751   KTPSNLSGEG KGPGHSPVPS QTTEVPVGAL GIAVS
```

Alternative mRNA splicing gives rise to three forms of the mouse IL-4 receptor. One is full length as shown, a second lacks the cytoplasmic domain (amino acids 233–285), and a third secreted form terminates with the sequence PSNENL which replaces HFQLPL at position 200–205 due to a 114 bp insertion at nucleotide number 598 [12].

References

[1] Ohara, J-I. (1989) In The Year in Immunology 1988: Immunoregulatory Cytokines and Cell Growth, Vol. 5, Cruse, J.M. and Lewis, R.E., eds, Karger, Basle, pp. 126–159.

[2] Callard, R.E. (1991) Br. J. Haematol. 78, 293–299.

[3] Paul, W.E. (1991) Blood 77, 1859–1870.

[4] Powers, R. et al. (1992) Science 256, 1673–1677.

[5] Walter, M.R. et al. (1992) J. Biol. Chem. 267, 20371–20376.

[6] Arai, N. et al. (1989) J. Immunol. 142, 274–282.

[7] Otsuka, T. et al. (1987) Nucl. Acids Res. 15, 333–344.

[8] Yokota, T. et al. (1986) Proc. Natl Acad. Sci. USA 83, 5894–5898.

[9] Noma, Y. et al. (1986) Nature 319, 640–646.

[10] Lee, F. et al. (1986) Proc. Natl Acad. Sci. USA. 83, 2061–2065.

[11] Beckmann, M.P. et al. (1992) Chem. Immunol. 51, 107–134.

[12] Mosley, B. et al. (1989) Cell 59, 335–348.

[13] Garrone, P. et al. (1991) Eur. J. Immunol. 21, 1365–1369.

[14] Russell, S.M. et al. (1993) Science 262, 1880–1883.

[15] Kondo, M. et al. (1993) Science 262, 1874–1877.

[16] Fanslow, W.C. et al. (1993) Blood 81, 2998–3005.

[17] Rigley, K.P. et al. (1991) Int. Immunol. 3, 197–203.

[18] Lowenthal, J.W. et al. (1988) J. Immunol. 140, 456–464.

[19] Ohara, J. and Paul, W.E. (1987) Nature 325, 537–540.

[20] Park, L.S. et al. (1987) Proc. Natl Acad. Sci. USA 84, 1669–1673.

21 Park, L.S. et al. (1987) J. Exp. Med. 166, 476–488.

22 Wang, L.-M. et al. (1992) EMBO J. 11, 4899–4908.

23 Wang, L.-M. et al. (1993) Proc. Natl Acad. Sci. USA 90, 4032–4036.

24 Harnett, M.M. et al. (1991) J. Immunol. 147, 3831–3836.

25 Mire-Sluis, A.R. and Thorpe, R. (1991) J. Biol. Chem. 266, 18113–18118.

26 Finney, M. et al. (1990) Eur. J. Immunol. 20, 151–156.

27 Idzerda, R.L. et al. (1990) J. Exp. Med. 171, 861–873.

IL-5

Other names

Eosinophil differentiation factor (EDF), eosinophil colony stimulating factor (E-CSF), B cell growth factor II (BCGFII), B cell differentiation factor for IgM (BCDFμ), IgA enhancing factor, T cell replacing factor (TRF).

THE MOLECULE

Interleukin 5 is a T cell-derived glycoprotein which stimulates eosinophil colony formation and is an eosinophil differentiation factor in humans and mice. It is also a growth and differentiation factor for mouse but not human B cells [1-3].

Crossreactivity

There is 71% homology between mouse and human IL-5 and significant crossreactivity in functional assays.

Sources

Mast cells, T cells and eosinophils.

Bioassays

Human: Eosinophil differentiation; proliferation of TF1 cell line.

Mouse: Eosinophil differentiation; proliferation of BCL1 or B13 B cell lines.

Physicochemical properties of IL-5

Property	Human	Mouse
pI	?	?
Amino acids – precursor	134	133
– mature[a]	115	113
M_r (K) – predicted	13.1	13.1
– expressed[b]	45	40–50
Potential N-linked glycosylation sites	2	3
Disulphide bonds[c]	2	2

[a] After removal of predicted signal peptide.
[b] Homodimer.
[c] Interchain.

3-D structure

IL-5 is an antiparallel disulphide-linked homodimer. The monomer is biologically inactive. The structure of the dimer has been determined at a resolution of 2.4 Å [4]. It has a novel two-domain structure with each domain showing significant structural homology to the cytokine fold in GM-CSF, M-CSF, IL-2, IL-4 and growth hormone. The IL-5 structure is made up of two left-handed bundles of four α-helices with two short β-sheets on opposite sides of the molecule. The C-terminal strand and helix of one chain of the dimer together with three helices and one strand at the N-terminal end of the other chain make up the bundle of four helices and a β-sheet. This dimeric structure of IL-5 is unique.

Gene structure [5-7]

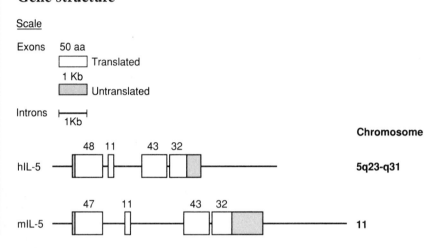

Scale

Exons
50 aa

[ ] Translated

1 Kb

[▨] Untranslated

Introns ⊢—⊣
1Kb

Chromosome

48 11   43 32

hIL-5

5q23-q31

47   11   43   32

mIL-5

11

Amino acid sequence for human IL-5 [5,8,9]

Accession code: Swissprot P05113

```
-19   MRMLLHLSLL ALGAAYVYA
  1   IPTEIPTSAL VKETLALLST HRTLLIANET LRIPVPVHKN HQLCTEEIFQ
 51   GIGTLESQTV QGGTVERLFK NLSLIKKYID GQKKKCGEER RRVNQFLDYL
101   QEFLGVMNTE WIIES
```

IL-5 is produced as an antiparallel homodimer formed by two interchain disulphide bonds between Cys44 and 86 of each chain.

Amino acid sequence for mouse IL-5 [10]

Accession code: Swissprot P04401

```
-20   MRRMLLHLSV LTLSCVWATA
  1   MEIPMSTVVK ETLTQLSAHR ALLTSNETMR LPVPTHKNHQ LCIGEIFQGL
 51   DILKNQTVRG GTVEMLFQNL SLIKKYIDRQ KEKCGEERRR TRQFLDYLQE
101   FLGVMSTEWA MEG
```

IL-5 is produced as an antiparallel homodimer formed by two interchain disulphide bonds between Cys42 and 84 of each chain.

THE IL-5 RECEPTOR

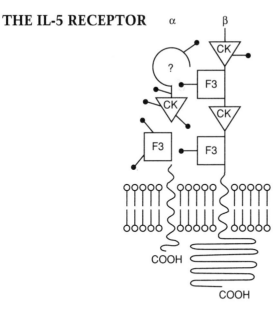

The IL-5 receptor consists of a low affinity (K_d 10^{-9}M) binding α-chain (CD 125) and a non-binding β-chain shared with the IL-3R and the GM-CSFR [11-14]. Both chains belong to the cytokine receptor superfamily. The extracellular region of the α-chain consists of an N-terminal region of about 100 amino acids with homology to a similar sequence in the α-chains of the IL-3 and GM-CSF receptors, followed by a CKR domain and an FNIII domain that contains the WSXWS motif. The human β-chain (KH97) and mouse β-chain (AIC2B) also belong to the CKR-SF. Both are described in the IL-3 entry. Soluble forms of the human and mouse IL-5R are produced by alternative mRNA splicing [13,15-17].

Distribution

In humans the IL-5 receptor is expressed on eosinophils and basophils. In mice it is expressed on eosinophils and B cells.

Physicochemical properties of the IL-5 receptor

Property	Human	Mouse
Amino acids – precursor	420	415
– mature[a]	400	398
M_r (K) – predicted	45.6	45.3
– expressed	60	60
Potential N-linked glycosylation sites	6	4
Affinity K_d (M)[b]	5×10^{-10}	5×10^{-9}

[a] After removal of predicted signal peptide.
[b] High affinity receptor formed by association of α-chain with human (KH97) and mouse (AIC2B) β-chains has K_d of 5×10^{-11} or 1.5×10^{-10}M respectively. The amino acid sequences and properties of the β-chains are given in the entry for IL-3.

Signal transduction
Mechanism unknown.

Chromosomal location
The IL-5R is on human chromosome 3p26 [18,19] and mouse chromosome 6 [16].

Amino acid sequence for human IL-5 receptor α-chain [17]

Accession code: GenEMBL X61176

```
-20  MIIVAHVLLI  LLGATEILQA
  1  DLLPDEKISL  LPPVNFTIKV  TGLAQVLLQW  KPNPDQEQRN  VNLEYQVKIN
 51  APKEDDYETR  ITESKCVTIL  HKGFSASVRT  ILQNDHSLLA  SSWASAELHA
101  PPGSPGTSVV  NLTCTTNTTE  DNYSRLRSYQ  VSLHCTWLVG  TDAPEDTQYF
151  LYYRYGSWTE  ECQEYSKDTL  GRNIACWFPR  TFILSKGRDW  LAVLVNGSSK
201  HSAIRPFDQL  FALHAIDQIN  PPLNVTAEIE  GTRLSIQWEK  PVSAFPIHCF
251  DYEVKIHNTR  NGYLQIEKLM  TNAFISIIDD  LSKYDVQVRA  AVSSMCREAG
301  LWSEWSQPIY  VGNDEHKPLR  EWFV̲I̲V̲I̲M̲A̲T̲  I̲C̲F̲I̲L̲L̲I̲L̲S̲L̲  I̲C̲K̲I̲C̲HLWIK
351  LFPPIPAPKS  NIKDLFVTTN  YEKAGSSETE  IEVICYIEKP  GVETLEDSVF
```

Two truncated soluble (extracellular) variants of the human IL-5 receptor have also been cloned [13-16]. Both differ from the membrane anchored isoform by a sequence switch at nucleotide position 1243. In humans, the major soluble isoform is encoded by a specific exon.

Amino acid sequence for mouse IL-5 receptor α-chain [15]

Accession code: Swissprot P21183

```
-17  MVPVLLILVG  ALATLQA
  1  DLLNHKKFLL  LPPVNFTIKA  TGLAQVLLHW  DPNPDQEQRH  VDLEYHVKIN
 51  APQEDEYDTR  KTESKCVTPL  HEGFAASVRT  ILKSSHTTLA  SSWVSAELKA
101  PPGSPGTSVT  NLTCTTHTVV  SSHTHLRPYQ  VSLRCTWLVG  KDAPEDTQYF
151  LYYRFGVLTE  KCQEYSRDAL  NRNTACWFPR  TFINSKGFEQ  LAVHINGSSK
201  RAAIKPFDQL  FSPLAIDQVN  PPRNVTVEIE  SNSLYIQWEK  PLSAFPDHCF
251  NYELKIYNTK  NGHIQKEKLI  ANKFISKIDD  VSTYSIQVRA  AVSSPCRMPG
301  RWGEWSQPIY  VGKERKSLVE  WH̲L̲I̲V̲L̲P̲T̲A̲A̲  C̲F̲V̲L̲L̲I̲F̲S̲L̲I̲  C̲R̲V̲C̲HLWTRL
351  FPPVPAPKSN  IKDLPVVTEY  EKPSNETKIE  VVHCVEEVGF  EVMGNSTF
```

Alternative soluble forms of the receptor with no transmembrane region due to deletions in nucleotides 986–1164 and 986–1079 have been identified. The amino acid sequences of these two forms from residue 312 are:

```
312  ETFE

312  GVIYGPGCFH  RFRPQRVTSK  ISLWLLNMRN  LRMKPKLKLY  IVWKRLDLKS
362  WEIPRFDGIL  PF
```

References

1 Sanderson, C.J. et al. (1988) Immunol. Rev. 102, 29–50.
2 McKenzie, A.N. and Sanderson, C.J. (1992) Chem. Immunol. 51, 135–152.
3 Takatsu, K. (1992) Curr. Opin. Immunol. 4, 299–306.
4 Milburn, M.V. et al. (1993) Nature 363, 172–176.
5 Campbell, H.D. et al. (1987) Proc. Natl. Acad. Sci. USA 84, 6629–6633.
6 Tanabe, T. et al. (1987) J. Biol. Chem. 262, 16580–16584.
7 Campbell, H.D. et al. (1988) Eur. J. Biochem. 174, 345–352.
8 Azuma, C. et al. (1986) Nucl. Acids Res. 14, 9149–9158.
9 Yokota, T. et al. (1987) Proc. Natl. Acad. Sci. USA 84, 7388–7392.
10 Kinashi, T. et al. (1986) Nature 324, 70–73.
11 Miyajima, A. (1992) Int. J. Cell Cloning 10, 126–134.
12 Kitamura, T. et al. (1991) Cell 66, 1165–1174.
13 Tavernier, J. et al. (1991) Cell 66, 1175–1184.
14 Mita, S. et al. (1991) Int. Immunol. 3, 665–672.
15 Takaki, S. et al. (1990) EMBO J. 9, 4367–4374.
16 Gough, N.M. and Raker, S. (1992) Genomics 12, 855–856.
17 Murata, Y. et al. (1992) J. Exp. Med. 175, 341–351.
18 Tuypens, T. et al. (1992) Eur. Cytokine Netw. 3, 451–459.
19 Isobe, M. et al. (1992) Genomics 14, 755–758.

Other names

Interferon-β2 (IFNβ2), 26-kDa protein, B cell stimulatory factor 2 (BSF-2), hybridoma/plasmacytoma growth factor (HPGF or IL-HP1), hepatocyte stimulating factor (HSF), monocyte granulocyte inducer type 2 (MGI-2), cytotoxic T cell differentiation factor and thrombopoietin.

THE MOLECULE

Interleukin 6 is a multifunctional cytokine secreted by both lymphoid and non-lymphoid cells which regulates B and T cell function, haematopoiesis and acute phase reactions [1-3].

Crossreactivity

There is 42% homology between mouse and human IL-6. Human IL-6 is functional on mouse cells but mouse IL-6 has no activity on human cells.

Sources

IL-6 is made by lymphoid cells (T cells, B cells), and many non-lymphoid cells including macrophages, bone marrow stromal cells, fibroblasts, keratinocytes, mesangium cells, astrocytes and endothelial cells.

Bioassays

Proliferation by IL-6-dependent B9 cell line. Increased Ig secretion by CESS or other EBV-transformed human lymphoblastoid B cell lines.

Physicochemical properties of IL-6

Property	Human	Mouse
Amino acids – precursor	212	211
– mature[a]	183[b]	187
M_r (K) – predicted	20.8	21.7
– expressed	26	22–29
Potential N-linked glycosylation sites	2	0[c]
Disulphide bonds[d]	2	2[d]

[a] After removal of predicted signal peptide.

[b] N-Terminal amino acids of human IL-6 derived from a T cell line, an osteosarcoma cell line and a liposarcoma cell line are Pro, Ala and Val respectively, indicating heterogeneity in the signal peptide cleavage site.

[c] There are several potential O-linked glycosylation sites.

[d] Potential disulphide bonds between Cys43–49, 72–82 in man and 46–52, 75–85 in mouse. These four Cys residues are conserved between human and mouse IL-6, G-CSF, LIF and CNTF.

3-D structure

Not known.

Gene structure [4,5]

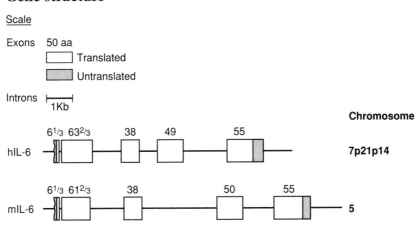

Scale

Exons   50 aa

[   ] Translated

[▨] Untranslated

Introds ├───┤
1Kb

Chromosome

hIL-6   6¹/₃ 63²/₃   38   49   55

7p21p14

mIL-6   6¹/₃ 61²/₃   38   50   55   **5**

Note that one base coding for amino acid 7 is in exon one and the other two bases of this codon are in exon two for both human and mouse IL-6.

Amino acid sequence for human IL-6 [6,7]

Accession code: Swissprot P05231

```
 -29   MNSFSTSAFG PVAFSLGLLL VLPAAFPAP
   1   VPPGEDSKDV AAPHRQPLTS SERIDKQIRY ILDGISALRK ETCNKSNMCE
  51   SSKEALAENN LNLPKMAEKD GCFQSGFNEE TCLVKIITGL LEFEVYLEYL
 101   QNRFESSEEQ ARAVQMSTKV LIQFLQKKAK NLDAITTPDP TTNASLLTKL
 151   QAQNQWLQDM TTHLILRSFK EFLQSSLRAL RQM
```

The N-terminal amino acid of IL-6 from different sources has been reported as Ala, Pro and Val, indicating some heterogeneity in the signal peptide cleavage site.

Amino acid sequence for mouse IL-6 [8]

Accession code: Swissprot P08505

```
 -24   MKFLSARDFH PVAFLGLMLV TTTA
   1   FPTSQVRRGD FTEDTTPNRP VYTTSQVGGL ITHVLWEIVE MRKELCNGNS
  51   DCMNNDDALA ENNLKLPEIQ RNDGCYQTGY NQEICLLKIS SGLLEYHSYL
 101   EYMKNNLKDN KKDKARVLQR DTETLIHIFN QEVKDLHKIV LPTPISNALL
 151   TDKLESQKEW LRTKTIQFIL KSLEEFLKVT LRSTRQT
```

THE IL-6 RECEPTOR

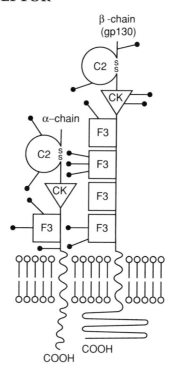

High affinity (K_d 10^{-11}M) IL-6 receptors are formed by the non-covalent association of two subunits [3,9]. The IL-6R α-chain (CD126) binds IL-6 with low affinity (K_d 10^{-9}M) but does not signal. The extracellular region consists of an IgSF C2 set domain at the N-terminus followed by a CKR-SF domain and an FNIII domain which includes the WSXWS motif. The β-chain (gp130) (CD130) does not itself bind IL-6, but associates with the α-chain/IL-6 complex and is responsible for signal transduction [9]. The extracellular domain of gp130 consists of an IgSF C2 set domain at the N-terminus followed by a CKR-SF domain and four FNIII domains, only the first of which contains the WSXWS motif. gp130 is also an oncostatin M receptor and an affinity converter (β-chain) for the LIF and CNTF receptors [3,10]. A mouse variant of the IL-6 receptor has been cloned in which the intracellular domain has been replaced by part of a long terminal repeat (LTR) sequence from the intracisternal A particle (IAP) gene [11]. Cells transfected with this variant bind IL-6 and respond in proliferation assays.

Distribution

The IL-6 receptor is expressed on activated but not resting B cells, plasma cells, T cells, monocytes and many other non-lymphoid cells including epithelial cells, fibroblasts, hepatocytes and neural cells.

Physicochemical properties of the IL-6 receptor

Property	IL-6R α-chain		gp130	
	Human	Mouse	Human	Mouse
Amino acids – precursor	468	460	918	917
– mature[a]	449	441	896	895
M_r – predicted	49.9	48.6	101	100
– expressed	80	80	130	130
Potential N-linked glycosylation sites	5	3	10	9
Affinity K_d (M)[b]	10^{-9}	2.5×10^{-9}	none	none

[a] After removal of predicted signal peptide.
[b] The high affinity (K_d 10^{-11}M) receptor is formed by association of the IL-6R α-chain with gp130.

Signal transduction

The signal transducing molecule in the IL-6 receptor is the gp130 chain [3]. IL6 binds to the IL-6R (α-chain) and the IL-6/IL-6R complex then binds two gp130 molecules to form a gp130 disulphide linked homodimer [12]. Dimerization results in tyrosine phosphorylation of gp130. IL-6 has also been shown to induce phosphorylation of the CD40 B cell surface antigen [13]. A motif of about 60 amino acids proximal to the transmembrane domain in the cytoplasmic domain of gp130 is required for signal transduction. Two short segments within this motif are highly conserved among many cytokine receptor signal transducers and may be important for association with a tyrosine kinase.

Chromosomal location

The IL-6R α-chain is on human chromosome 1. In humans, gp130 has two distinct chromosomal loci on chromosomes 5 and 17. The presence of two distinct gp130 gene sequences is restricted to primates and is not found in other vertebrates [14].

Amino acid sequence for human IL-6 receptor α-chain [15]

Accession code: Swissprot P08887

```
 -19   MLAVGCALLA ALLAAPGAA
   1   LAPRRCPAQE VARGVLTSLP GDSVTLTCPG VEPEDNATVH WVLRKPAAGS
  51   HPSRWAGMGR RLLLRSVQLH DSGNYSCYRA GRPAGTVHLL VDVPPEEPQL
 101   SCFRKSPLSN VVCEWGPRST PSLTTKAVLL VRKFQNSPAE DFQEPCQYSQ
 151   ESQKFSCQLA VPEGDSSFYI VSMCVASSVG SKFSKTQTFQ GCGILQPDPP
 201   ANITVTAVAR NPRWLSVTWQ DPHSWNSSFY RLRFELRYRA ERSKTFTTWM
 251   VKDLQHHCVI HDAWSGLRHV VQLRAQEEFG QGEWSEWSPE AMGTPWTESR
 301   SPPAENEVST PMQALTTNKD DDNILFRDSA NATSLPVQDS SSVPLPTFLV
 351   AGGSLAFGTL LCIAIVLRFK KTWKLRALKE GKTSMHPPYS LGQLVPERPR
 401   PTPVLVPLIS PPVSPSSLGS DNTSSHNRPD ARDPRSPYDI SNTDYFFPR
```

Amino acids 24–81 form an Ig-like domain with potential disulphide bonds between Cys28 and Cys77.

Amino acid sequence for human IL-6 receptor β-chain (gp130) [16]

Accession code: Genbank M57230

```
 -22  MLTLQTWVVQ  ALFIFLTTES  TG
   1  ELLDPCGYIS  PESPVVQLHS  NFTAVCVLKE  KCMDYFHVNA  NYIVWKTNHF
  51  TIPKEQYTII  NRTASSVTFT  DIASLNIQLT  CNILTFGQLE  QNVYGITIIS
 101  GLPPEKPKNL  SCIVNEGKKM  RCEWDGGRET  HLETNFTLKS  EWATHKFADC
 151  KAKRDTPTSC  TVDYSTVYFV  NIEVWVEAEN  ALGKVTSDHI  NFDPVYKVKP
 201  NPPHNLSVIN  SEELSSILKL  TWTNPSIKSV  IILKYNIQYR  TKDASTWSQI
 251  PPEDTASTRS  SFTVQDLKPF  TEYVFRIRCM  KEDGKGYWSD  WSEEASGITY
 301  EDRPSKAPSF  WYKIDPSHTQ  GYRTVQLVWK  TLPPFEANGK  ILDYEVTLTR
 351  WKSHLQNYTV  NATKLTVNLT  NDRYLATLTV  RNLVGKSDAA  VLTIPACDFQ
 401  ATHPVMDLKA  FPKDNMLWVE  WTTPRESVKK  YILEWCVLSD  KAPCITDWQQ
 451  EDGTVHRTYL  RGNLAESKCY  LITVTPVYAD  GPGSPESIKA  YLKQAPPSKG
 501  PTVRTKKVGK  NEAVLEWDQL  PVDVQNGFIR  NYTIFYRTII  GNETAVNVDS
 551  SHTEYTLSSL  TSDTLYMVRM  AAYTDEGGKD  GPEFTFTTPK  FAQGEIEAIV
 601  VPVCLAFLLT  TLLGVLFCFN  KRDLIKKHIW  PNVPDPSKSH  IAQWSPHTPP
 651  RHNFNSKDQM  YSDGNFTDVS  VVEIEANDKK  PFPEDLKSLD  LFKKEKINTE
 701  GHSSGIGGSS  CMSSSRPSIS  SSDENESSQN  TSSTVQYSTV  VHSGYRHQVP
 751  SVQVFSRSES  TQPLLDSEER  PEDLQLVDHV  DGGDGILPRQ  QYFKQNCSQH
 801  ESSPDISHFE  RSKQVSSVNE  EDFVRLKQQI  SDHISQSCGS  GQMKMFQEVS
 851  AADAFGPGTE  GQVERFETVG  MEAATDEGMP  KSYLPQTVRQ  GGYMPQ
```

Amino acid sequence for mouse IL-6 receptor α-chain [11]

Accession code: Swissprot P22272

```
 -19  MLTVGCTLLV  ALLAAPAVA
   1  LVLGSCRALE  VANGTVTSLP  GATVTLICPG  KEAAGNVTIH  WVYSGSQNRE
  51  WTTTGNTLVL  RDVQLSDTGD  YLCSLNDHLV  GTVPLLVDVP  PEEPKLSCFR
 101  KNPLVNAICE  WRPSSTPSPT  TKAVLFAKKI  NTTNGKSDFQ  VPCQYSQQLK
 151  SFSCQVEILE  GDKVYHIVSL  CVANSVGSKS  SHNEAFHSLK  MVQPDPPANL
 201  VVSAIPGRPR  WLKVSWQHPE  TWDPSYYLLQ  FQLRYRPVWS  KEFTVLLLPV
 251  AQYQCVIHDA  LRGVKHVVQV  RGKEELDLGQ  WSEWSPEVTG  TPWIAEPRTT
 301  PAGILWNPTQ  VSVEDSANHE  DQYESSTEAT  SVLAPVQESS  SMSLPTFLVA
 351  GGSLAFGLLL  CVFIILRLKQ  KWKSEAEKES  KTTSPPPPPY  SLGPLKPTFL
 401  LVPLLTPHSS  GSDNTVNHSC  LGVRDAQSPY  DNSNRDYLFP  R
```

Amino acids 24–77 form an Ig-like domain with potential disulphide bonds between Cys28 and Cys73. Conflicting sequence A->R at position 355.

Amino acid sequence for mouse IL-6 receptor β-chain (gp130) [17]

Accession code: Genbank M83336

```
 -22  MSAPRIWLAQ  ALLFFLTTES  IG
   1  QLLEPCGYIY  PEFPVVQRGS  NFTAICVLKE  ACLQHYYVNA  SYIVWKTNHA
  51  AVPREQVTVI  NRTTSSVTFT  DVVLPSVQLT  CNILSFGQIE  QNVYGVTMLS
 101  GFPPDKPTNL  TCIVNEGKNM  LCQWDPGRET  YLETNYTLKS  EWATEKFPDC
 151  QSKHGTSCMV  SYMPTYYVNI  EVWVEAENAL  GKVSSESINF  DPVDKVKPTP
 201  PYNLSVTNSE  ELSSILKLSW  VSSGLGGLLD  LKSDIQYRTK  DASTWIQVPL
 251  EDTMSPRTSF  TVQDLKPFTE  YVFRIRSIKD  SGKGYWSDWS  EEASGTTYED
 301  RPSRPPSFWY  KTNPSHGQEY  RSVRLIWKAL  PLSEANGKIL  DYEVILTQSK
 351  SVSQTYTVTG  TELTVNLTND  RYVASLAARN  KVGKSAAAVL  TIPSPHVTAA
 401  YSVVNLKAFP  KDNLLWVEWT  PPPKPVSKYI  LEWCVLSENA  PCVEDWQQED
 451  ATVNRTHLRG  RLLESKCYQI  TVTPVFATGP  GGSESLKAYL  KQAAPARGPT
 501  VRTKKVGKNE  AVLAWDQIPV  DDQNGFIRNY  SISYRTSVGK  EMVVHVDSSH
 551  TEYTLSSLSS  DTLYMVRMAA  YTDEGGKDGP  EFTFTTPKFA  QGEIEAIVVP
 601  VCLAFLLTTL  LGVLFCFNKR  DLIKKHIWPN  VPDPSKSHIA  QWSPHTPPRH
 651  NFNSKDQMYS  DGNFTDVSVV  EIEANNKKPC  PDDLKSVDLF  KKEKVSTEGH
 701  SSGIGGSSCM  SSSRPSISSN  EENESAQSTA  STVEYSTVVH  SGYRHQVPSV
 751  QVFSRSESTQ  PLLDSEERPE  DLQLVDSVDG  GDEILPRQPY  FKQNCSQPEA
 801  CPEISHFERS  NQVLSGNEED  FVRLKQQQVS  DHISQPYGSE  QRRLFQEGST
 851  ADALGTGADG  QMERFESVGM  ETTIDEEIPK  SYLPQTVRQG  GYMPQ
```

References

1 Hirano, T. (1991) In The Cytokine Handbook, Thomson, A. W., ed., Academic Press, London, pp. 169–190.
2 Kishimoto, T. (1989) Blood 74, 1–10.
3 Kishimoto, T. et al. (1992) Science 258, 593–597.
4 Yasukawa, K. et al. (1987) EMBO J. 6, 2939–2945.
5 Tanabe, O. et al. (1988) J. Immunol. 141, 3875–3881.
6 Hirano, T. et al. (1986) Nature 324, 73–76.
7 May, L.T. et al. (1986) Proc. Natl. Acad. Sci. USA 83, 8957–8961.
8 van Snick, J. et al. (1988) Eur. J. Immunol. 18, 193–197.
9 Taga, T. et al. (1989) Cell 58, 573–581.
10 Gearing, D.P. et al. (1992) Science 255, 1434–1437.
11 Sugita, T. et al. (1990) J. Exp. Med. 171, 2001–2009.
12 Murakami, M. et al. (1993) Science 260, 1808–1810.
13 Clark, E.A. and Shu, G. (1990) J. Immunol. 145, 1400–1406.
14 Kidd, V.J. et al. (1992) Somat. Cell Mol. Genet. 18, 477–483.
15 Yamasaki, K. et al. (1988) Science 241, 825–828.
16 Hibi, M. et al. (1990) Cell 63, 1149–1157.
17 Saito, M. et al. (1992) J. Immunol. 148, 4066–4071.

IL-7

Other names
Lymphopoietin 1 (LP-1), pre-B cell growth factor.

THE MOLECULE

Interleukin 7 is a stromal cell-derived growth factor for progenitor B cells and T cells. The main population in the thymus responsive to IL-7 is CD4−CD8−. IL-7 also stimulates proliferation and differentiation of mature T cells [1,2].

Crossreactivity
There is 60% homology between human and mouse IL-7 and significant cross-species reactivity.

Sources
Bone marrow, thymic stromal cells and spleen cells.

Bioassays
Proliferation of B cell precursors, 2bx murine pre-B cell line, or mitogen-stimulated T cells.

Physicochemical properties of IL-7

Property	Human	Mouse
pI	9	?
Amino acids – precursor	177	154
– mature[a]	152	129
M_r (K) – predicted	17.4	14.9
– expressed	20–28	25
Potential N-linked glycosylation sites	3	2
Disulphide bonds[b]	3	3

[a] After removal of predicted signal peptide.
[b] All six Cys residues probably form disulphide bonds.

3-D structure
Not known.

Gene structure [3]

Scale

Exons 50 aa
☐ Translated
1 Kb
▨ Untranslated

Introrns ⊢⊣
1Kb

~15kb   **Chromosome**

hIL-7   3¹/₃   45²/₃ 27   44   18 39   **8q12-q13**

mIL-7   3¹/₃ 44²/₃   27 44   35   **?**

The human IL-7 gene spans at least 33 kb. Intron 2 has not been fully sequenced and the 5′ initiation site has not been identified. The 18 amino acids coded for by exon 5 are not found in mouse IL-7.

The mouse IL-7 gene spans 56 kb or more. The 3′ end has not been cloned, and the position and size of exon 5 have not been established. Sizes of introns 1, 2 and 4 are not known.

Amino acid sequence for human IL-7 [4]

Accession code: Swissprot P13232

```
-25   MFHVSFRYIF GLPPLILVLL PVASS
  1   DCDIEGKDGK QYESVLMVSI DQLLDSMKEI GSNCLNNEFN FFKRHICDAN
 51   KEGMFLFRAA RKLRQFLKMN STGDFDLHLL KVSEGTTILL NCTGQVKGRK
101   PAALGEAQPT KSLEENKSLK EQKKLNDLCF LKRLLQEIKT CWNKILMGTK
151   EH
```

The 18 amino acids from positions 96-113 are absent in murine IL-7 and are coded for by an extra exon in the human IL-7 gene.

Amino acid sequence for mouse IL-7 [5]

Accession code: Swissprot P10168

```
-25   MFHVSFRYIF GIPPLILVLL PVTSS
  1   ECHIKDKEGK AYESVLMISI DELDKMTGTD SNCPNNEPNF FRKHVCDDTK
 51   EAAFLNRAAR KLKQFLKMNI SEEFNVHLLT VSQGTQTLVN CTSKEEKNVK
101   EQKKNDACFL KRLLREIKTC WNKILKGSI
```

THE IL-7 RECEPTOR

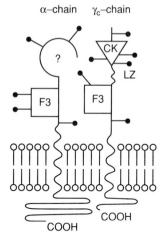

The IL-7 receptor is a complex consisting at least of an IL-7 binding chain (CD127) and the IL-2R γ-chain (γc-chain). The extracellular domain of the IL-7R binding chain consists of an N-terminal region of about 100 amino acids with no clear sequence homology to other proteins, followed by an FNIII domain containing the WSXWS motif. Overall homology with the CKR-SF is poor, however, and it is unclear whether it should be included as a member of the CKR superfamily [6]. A soluble form of the IL-7R is produced by alternative splicing of the IL-7R gene [7]. The IL-2R γ-chain is a functional component of the IL-7R and augments IL-7 binding [8]. This may explain the two classes of IL-7 binding sites which have been described on human and murine cells with high ($K_d \sim 10^{-10}$M) and low ($K_d \sim 10^{-8}$M) affinity [9]. Similar high and low affinity binding sites have also been described on cells transfected with IL-7R cDNA [7]. A low affinity IL-7 receptor has also been identified but not yet cloned [10].

Distribution

Thymocytes, T and B cell progenitors, mature T cells, monocytes, and some lymphoid and myeloid cell lines.

Physicochemical properties of the IL-7 receptor

Property		Human	Mouse
Amino acids	– precursor	459	459
	– mature[a]	439	439
M_r (K)	– predicted	49.5	49.6
	– expressed	68	68
Potential N-linked glycosylation sites		5	3
Affinity K_d (M)	– high	2×10^{-10}	2×10^{-10}
	– low	10^{-8}	10^{-8}

[a] After removal of predicted signal peptide.

Signal transduction

IL-7 stimulates tyrosine phosphorylation of cellular proteins and tyrosine kinase-dependent activation of PI-specific phospholipase C with hydrolysis of PIP_2 and release of IP_3 [11]. IL-7R activates PI-3' kinase [12] and has been shown to associate with and activate p59fyn [13].

Chromosomal location

The IL-7R gene is on human chromosome 5p13 [14], and mouse chromosome 15.

Amino acid sequence for human IL-7 receptor [7]

Accession code: Swissprot P16871

```
-20    MTILGTTFGM VFSLLQVVSG
  1    ESGYAQNGDL EDAELDDYSF SCYSQLEVNG SQHSLTCAFE DPDVNTTNLE
 51    FEICGALVEV KCLNFRKLQE IYFIETKKFL LIGKSNICVK VGEKSLTCKK
101    IDLTTIVKPE APFDLSVIYR EGANDFVVTF NTSHLQKKYV KVLMHDVAYR
151    QEKDENKWTH VNLSSTKLTL LQRKLQPAAM YEIKVRSIPD HYFKGFWSEW
201    SPSYYFRTPE INNSSGEMDP ILLTISILSF FSVALLVILA CVLWKKRIKP
251    IVWPSLPDHK KTLEHLCKKP RKNLNVSFNP ESFLDCQIHR VDDIQARDEV
301    EGFLQDTFPQ QLEESEKQRL GGDVQSPNCP SEDVVVTPES FGRDSSLTCL
351    AGNVSACDAP ILSSSRSLDC RESGKNGPHV YQDLLLSLGT TNSTLPPPFS
401    LQSGILTLNP VAQGQPILTS LGSNQEEAYV TMSSFYQNQ
```

Fibronectin type III domain 108–204. Thr residue at position 262 is a PKC phosphorylation site. A soluble form of the human IL-7 receptor resulting from a 93 bp deletion terminates with the sequence

```
216    GLSLSYGPVS PIIRRLWNIF VRNQEKI
```

Amino acid sequence for mouse IL-7 receptor [7]

Accession code: Swissprot P16872

```
-20    MMALGRAFAI VFCLIQAVSG
  1    ESGNAQDGDL EDADADDHSF WCHSQLEVDG SQHLLTCAFN DSDINTANLE
 51    FQICGALLRV KCLTLNKLQD IYFIKTSEFL LIGSSNICVK LGQKNLTCKN
101    MAINTIVKAE APSDLKVVYR KEANDFLVTF NAPHLKKKYL KKVKHDVAYR
151    PARGESNWTH VSLFHTRTTI PQRKLRPKAM YEIKVRSIPH NDYFKGFWSE
201    WSPSSTFETP EPKNQGGWDP VLPSVTILSL FSVFLLVILA HVLWKKRIKP
251    VVWPSLPDHK KTLEQLCKKP KTSLNVSFIP EIFLDCQIHE VKGVEARDEV
301    EIFLPNDLPA QPEELETQGH RAAVHSANRS PETSVSPPET VRRESPLRCL
351    ARNLSTCNAP PLLSSRSPDY RDGDRNRPPV YQDLLPNSGN TNVPVPVPQP
401    LPFQSGILIP FSQRQPISTS SVLNQEEAYV TMSSFYQNK
```

Fibronectin type III domain 108–205. Thr residue at position 262 is a PKC phosphorylation site.

References

1 Goodwin, R.G. and Namen, A. E. (1991) In The Cytokine Handbook, Thomson, A.W. ed., Academic Press, London, pp. 191–200.
2 Henney, C.S. (1989) Immunol. Today 10, 170–173.
3 Lupton, S.D. et al. (1990) J. Immunol. 144, 3592–3601.
4 Goodwin, R.G. et al. (1989) Proc. Natl. Acad. Sci. USA 86, 302–306.
5 Namen, A.E. et al. (1988) Nature 333, 571–573.
6 Barclay, A.N. et al. (1993) The Leucocyte Antigen FactsBook, Academic Press, London.
7 Goodwin, R.G. et al. (1990) Cell 60, 941–951.
8 Noguchi, M. et al. (1993) Science 262, 1877–1880.
9 Park, L.S. et al. (1990) J. Exp. Med. 171, 1073–1089.
10 Armitage, R.J. et al. (1992) Blood 79, 1738–1745.
11 Uckun, F.M. et al. (1991) Proc. Natl Acad. Sci. USA 88, 3589–3593.
12 Dadi, H.K. et al. (1993) Biochem. Biophys. Res. Commun. 192, 459–464.
13 Venkitaraman, A.R. and Cowling, R.J. (1992) Proc. Natl Acad. Sci. USA 89, 12083–12087.
14 Lynch, M. et al. (1992) Hum. Genet. 89, 566–568.

Other names

Neutrophil attractant/activating protein (NAP-1), monocyte derived neutrophil activating peptide (MONAP), monocyte derived neutrophil chemotactic factor (MDNCF), neutrophil activating factor (NAF), leucocyte adhesion inhibitor (LAI), Granulocyte chemotactic protein (GCP).

THE MOLECULE

IL-8 is an inflammatory cytokine, produced by many cell types, which mainly functions as a neutrophil chemoattractant, and activating factor [1–3]. It also attracts basophils and a subpopulation of lymphocytes. IL-8 is a potent angiogenic factor [4].

Crossreactivity

There is no obvious murine homologue of human IL-8, although murine MIP-2 can compete with IL-8 for binding to its receptors on neutrophils [3]. IL-8 exhibits limited reactivity on neutrophils from other species [5].

Sources

IL-8 is secreted by multiple cell types including, monocytes, lymphocytes, granulocytes, fibroblasts, endothelial cells, bronchial epithelial cells, keratinocytes, hepatocytes, mesangial cells and chondrocytes.

Bioassays

IL-8 can be measured in neutrophil chemotaxis and activation assays [6,7].

Physicochemical properties

Property	Human
pI	8.6
Amino acids – precursor	99
– mature[ab]	77–72
M_r (K) – predicted	11.1
– expressed	6–8
Potential N-linked glycosylation sites	0
Disulphide bonds[c]	2

[a] IL-8 appears to exist as a dimer in solution.
[b] Several distinct N-termini are found in the natural protein [8].
[c] Disulphide bonds link residues 7–33 and 9–49.

3-D structure

X-ray crystallography and NMR studies have given compatible structures for IL-8 [9,10] The monomer unit consists of a triple-stranded antiparallel β-sheet in a Greek key, with a long C-terminal helix. The monomers are joined by hydrogen bonds from residues 25–29, 27–27 and 29–25 respectively.

Gene structure [11]

Scale

Exons   50 aa

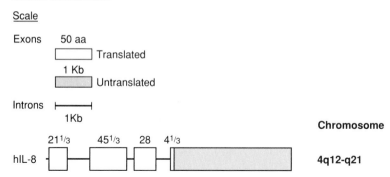

Introns ├────────┤
           1Kb

Chromosome

21¹/₃ 45¹/₃ 28 4¹/₃

hIL-8

4q12-q21

Amino acid sequence for human IL-8 [2]

Accession code: Swissprot P10145

```
27   MTSKLAVALL AAFLISAALC EGAVLPR
 1   SAKELRCQCI KTYSKPFHPK FIKELRVIES GPHCANTEII VKLSDGRELC
51   LDPKENWVQR VVEKFLKRAE NS
```

Conflicting sequence E->L at position 28.

THE IL-8 RECEPTOR

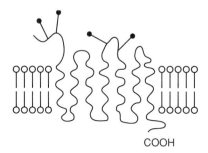

COOH

There have been two sequences for IL-8 receptors published, one high affinity (CDw128) and another of lower affinity [12,13]. Both are seven transmembrane spanning, G-protein-linked receptors of the rhodopsin superfamily. The high affinity receptor has a predicted M_r of 40 000, and glycosylation at five potential N-linked sites would bring the weight up to that measured on neutrophils of 58 000–67 000. Its affinity for IL-8 has been measured as 3.6×10^{-9}M. The high affinity receptor is 77% identical to the low affinity receptor. The low affinity receptor has an unglycosylated molecular weight of 32 000. Its affinity for IL-8 has not been determined but in transfected cells its EC_{50} of 20nM was 20-fold lower than that for IL-8 on neutrophils. The high affinity receptor only binds IL-8, whereas the low affinity receptor binds GRO/MGSA and NAP-2 [14].

Distribution

Neutrophils, basophils, lymphocytes have functional receptors. Saturable binding sites on monocytes, eosinophils, endothelial cells and erythrocytes have been demonstrated.

Physicochemical properties of the IL-8 receptors

Properties	High affinity Human	Low affinity Human
Amino acids – precursor	350	355
– mature	?	?
M_r (K) – predicted	40	32
– expressed	58–67	?
Potential N-linked glycosylation sites	4	3
Affinity K_d (M) 3.6×10^{-9}	20×10^{-9} (EC$_{50}$)	

Signal transduction

Stimulation of neutrophils by IL-8 causes an immediate increase in intracellular Ca^{2+} which is pertussis toxin-sensitive. Inhibitors of PKC block neutrophil activation by IL-8.

Chromosomal location

The genes for both receptors are located on chromosome 2q35 [15].

Amino acid sequence for human high affinity IL-8 receptor [12,13]

Accession code: Genbank M68932

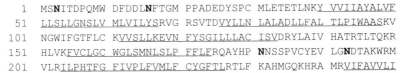

```
  1   MSNITDPQMW  DFDDLNFTGM  PPADEDYSPC  MLETETLNKY  VVIIAYALVF
 51   LLSLLGNSLV  MLVILYSRVG  RSVTDVYLLN  LALADLLFAL  TLPIWAASKV
101   NGWIFGTFLC  KVVSLLKEVN  FYSGILLLAC  ISVDRYLAIV  HATRTLTQKR
151   HLVKFVCLGC  WGLSMNLSLP  FFLFRQAYHP  NNSSPVCYEV  LGNDTAKWRM
201   VLRILPHTFG  FIVPLFVMLF  CYGFTLRTLF  KAHMGQKHRA  MRVIFAVVLI
251   FLLCWLPYNL  VLLADTLMRT  QVIQETCERR  NNIGRALDAT  EILGFLHSCL
301   NPIIYAFIGQ  NFRHGFLKIL  AMHGLVSKEF  LARHRVTSYT  SSSVNVSSNL
```

Amino acid sequence for human low affinity IL-8 receptor [12,13]

Accession code: Genbank M73969

```
  1 MESDSFEDFW KGEDLSNYSY SSTLPPFLLD AAPCEPESLE INKYFVVILY
 51 ALVFLLSLLG NSLVMLVILY SRVGRSVTDV YLLNLALADL LFALTLPIWA
101 ASAVNGWIFG TFLCKVVSLI KEVNFYSGIL LLACISVDRY LAIVHATRTL
151 TQKRYLVKFI CLSIWGLSLL LALPVLLFRR TVYSSNVSPA CYEDMGNNTA
201 NWRMLLRILP QSFGFIVPLL IMLFCYGFTL RTLFKAHMGQ KHRAMRVIFA
251 VVLIFLLCWL PYNLVLLADT LMRTQVIQET CERRNHIDRA LDATEILGIL
301 HSCLNPLIYA FIGQKFRHGL LKILAIHGLI SKDSLPKDSR PSFVGSSSGH
351 TSTTL
```

References

1 Matsushima, K. and Oppenheim J.J. (1989) Cytokine 1, 2–13.
2 Matsushima, K. et al. (1988) J. Exp. Med. 167, 1883–1893.
3 Oppenheim, J.J. et al. (1991) Annu. Rev. Immunol. 9, 617–648.
4 Koch, A.E. et al. (1993) Science 258, 1798–1801.
5 Rot, A. (1991) Cytokine 3, 21–27.
6 Van Damme, J. and Conings, R. (1991) In Cytokines: A Practical Approach, Balkwill, F.R., ed., IRL Press, Oxford, pp. 187–196.
7 Westwick, J. (1991) In Cytokines: A Practical Approach, Balkwill, F.A. ed., IRL Press, Oxford, pp. 197–204.
8 Van Damme, J. et al. (1989) J. Exp. Med. 167, 1364–1376.
9 Clore, G.M. and Gronenborn A.M. (1991) J. Mol. Biol. 217, 611–620.
10 Baldwin, E.T. et al. (1991) Proc. Natl Acad. Sci. USA 88, 502–506.
11 Mukaida, N. et al.(1989) J. Immunol. 143, 1366–1371.
12 Holmes, W.E. et al. (1991) Science 253, 1278–1280.
13 Murphy, P.M. and Tiffany, H.L. (1991) Science 253, 1280–1283.
14 LaRosa, G.J. et al. (1992) J. Biol. Chem. 267, 25402–25406.
15 Morris, S.W. et al. (1992) Genomics 14, 685–691.

IL-9

Other names

Human IL-9 has been known as P40. Mouse IL-9 has been known as P40, mast cell growth-enhancing activity and T cell growth factor III.

THE MOLECULE

Interleukin 9 is a cytokine which enhances the proliferation of T lymphocytes, mast cell lines, megakaryoblastic leukaemia cell lines and erythroid precursors [1-7].

Cross reactivity

There is about 55 % homology between human and mouse IL-9 [8]. Mouse IL-9 functions on human cells, human IL-9 is inactive on mouse cells [9].

Sources

IL-9 is produced by IL-2 activated TH2 lymphocytes and Hodgkin's lymphoma cells [10].

Bioassays

Mouse and human IL-9 can be assayed using the proliferation of PHA- plus IL-4-stimulated human lymphoblast lines [4]

Physicochemical properties of IL-9

Property	Human	Mouse
pI	?	6.2–7.3
Amino acids – precursor	144	144
– mature	126	126
M_r (K) – predicted	14.1	14.0
– expressed	32–39	30–40
Potential N-linked glycosylation sites	4	4
Disulphide bonds	5	5

3-D structure

No information.

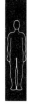

Gene structure [8,11]

Scale

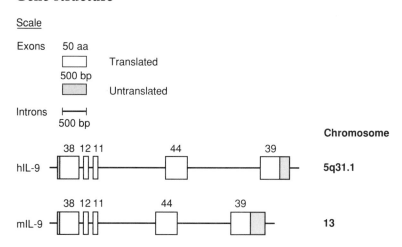

Amino acid sequence for human IL-9 [1,8]

Accession code: Swissprot P15248

```
-24   MLLAMVLTSA LLLCSVAGQG CPTL
  1   AGILDINFLI NKMQEDPASK CHCSANVTSC LCLGIPSDNC TRPCFSERLS
 51   QMTNTTMQTR YPLIFSRVKK SVEVLKNNKC PYFSCEQPCN QTTAGNALTF
101   LKSLLEIFQK EKMRGMRGKI
```

Amino acid sequence for mouse IL-9 [3]

Accesion code: Swissprot P15247

```
-24   MLVTYILASV LLFSSVLGQR CSTT
  1   WGIRDTNYLI ENLKDDPPSK CSCSGNVTSC LCLSVPTDDC TTPCYREGLL
 51   QLTNATQKSR LLPVFHRVKR IVEVLKNITC PSFSCEKPCN QTMAGNTLSF
101   LKSLLGTFQK TEMQRQKSRP
```

THE IL-9 RECEPTOR

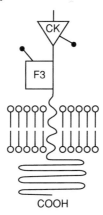

A single receptor type is detected on mouse T cell lines with a K_d of 6.7×10^{-11}M, and a M_r of 64 000, which is reduced to 54 000 after N-glycosidase F treatment [12]. The recombinant mouse receptor has a K_d of 1.9×10^{-10}M [13]. Both membrane-bound and soluble forms of the receptor exist [13]. The IL-2R γ-chain may associate with the IL-9R.

Distribution

IL-9 receptors are found on T helper clones, macrophages, some T cell tumours and mast cell lines.

Physicochemical properties of the IL-9 receptor

Properties		Human	Mouse
Amino acids	– precursor	522	468
	– mature	482	431
M_r (K)	– predicted	57	52
	– expressed	?	64
Potential N-linked glycosylation sites		2	2
Affinity K_d (M)		?	1.9×10^{-10}

Signal transduction

IL-9 causes tyrosine phosphorylation of four major proteins in MO7e cells, but not MAP kinase or Raf-1 [14].

Chromosomal location
Not yet determined.

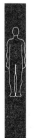

Amino acid sequence for human IL-9 receptor [13]

Accession code: Swissprot Q01113

```
-40   MGLGRCIWEG  WTLESEALRR  DMGTWLLACI  CICTCVCLGV
  1   SVTGEGQGPR  SRTFTCLTNN  ILRIDCHWSA  PELGQGSSPW  LLFTSNQAPG
 51   GTHKCILRGS  ECTVVLPPEA  VLVPSDNFTI  TFHHCMSGRE  QVSLVDPEYL
101   PRRHVKLDPP  SDLQSNISSG  HCILTWSISP  ALEPMTTLLS  YELAFKKQEE
151   AWEQAQHRDH  IVGVTWLILE  AFELDPGFIH  EARLRVQMAT  LEDDVVEEER
201   YTGQWSEWSQ  PVCFQAPQRQ  GPLIPPWGWP  GNTLVAVSIF  LLLTGPTYLL
251   FKLSPRVKRI  FYQNVPSPAM  FFQPLYSVHN  GNFQTWMGAH  RAGVLLSQDC
301   AGTPQGALEP  CVQEATALLT  CGPARPWKSV  ALEEEQEGPG  TRLPGNLSSE
351   DVLPAGCTEW  RVQTLAYLPQ  EDWAPTSLTR  PAPPDSEGSR  SSSSSSSSSN
401   NNNYCALGCY  GGWHLSALPG  NTQSSGPIPA  LACGLSCDHQ  GLETQQGVAW
451   VLAGHCQRPG  LHEDLQGMLL  PSVLSKARSW  TF
```

Amino acid sequence for mouse IL-9 receptor [13]

Accession code: Swissprot Q01114

```
-37   MALGRCIAEG  WTLERVAVKQ  VSWFLIYSWV  CSGVCRG
  1   VSVPEQGGGG  QKAGAFTCLS  NSIYRIDCHW  SAPELGQESR  AWLLFTSNQV
 51   TEIKHKCTFW  DSMCTLVLPK  EEVFLPFDNF  TITLHRCIMG  QEQVSLVDSQ
101   YLPRRHIKLD  PPSDLQSNVS  SGRCVLTWGI  NLALEPLITS  LSYELAFKRQ
151   EEAWEARHKD  RIVGVTWLIL  EAVELNPGSI  YEARLRVQMT  LESYEDKTEG
201   EYYKSHWSEW  SQPVSFPSPQ  RRQGLLVPRW  QWSASILVVV  PIFLLLTGFV
251   HLLFKLSPRL  KRIFYQNIPS  PEAFFHPLYS  VYHGDFQSWT  GARRAGPQAR
301   QNGVSTSSAG  SESSIWEAVA  TLTYSPACPV  QFACLKWEAT  APGFPGLPGS
351   EHVLPAGCLE  LEGQPSAYLP  QEDWAPLGSA  RPPPPDSDSG  SSDYCMLDCC
401   EECHLSAFPG  HTESPELTLA  QPVALPVSSR  A
```

References

1 Renauld, J.-C. et al. (1990) Cytokine 2, 9–12.
2 Uyttenhove, C. et al. (1988) Proc. Natl Acad. Sci. USA. 85, 6934–6938.
3 Van Snick, J. et al. (1989) J. Exp. Med. 169, 363–368.
4 Yang, Y. et al. (1989) Blood 74, 1880–1884.
5 Yang, Y.C. (1992) Leuk. Lymphoma 8, 441–447.
6 Moeller, J. (1990) J. Immunol. 144, 4231–4234.
7 Williams, D.E. et al. (1990) Blood 76, 906–914.
8 Renauld, J.-C. et al. (1990) J. Immunol. 144, 4235–4241.
9 Birner, A. et al. (1992) Exp. Hematol. 20, 541--545.
10 Gruss, H.J. et al. (1992) Cancer Res 52, 1026–1031.
11 Kelleher, K. et al. (1991) Blood 77, 1436–1441.
12 Druez, C. et al. (1990) J. Immunol. 145, 2494–2499.
13 Renauld, J.C. et al. (1992) Proc. Natl Acad. Sci. USA 89, 5690–5694.
14 Miyazawa, K. et al. (1992) Blood 80, 1685–1692.

IL-10

Other names
Cytokine synthesis inhibitory factor (CSIF).

THE MOLECULE

Interleukin 10 is an acid-labile cytokine secreted by TH0 and TH2 subsets of CD4+ T lymphocytes that blocks activation of cytokine synthesis by TH1 T cells, activated monocytes and NK cells [1-3]. IL-10 also stimulates and/or enhances proliferation of B cells, thymocytes and mast cells [1,2,4], and it cooperates with TGFβ to stimulate IgA production by human B cells [5]. There is a high degree of homology (70%) between IL-10 and an open reading frame (BCRF1), in the EBV genome. The protein encoded by BCRF1 exhibits some of the activities of IL-10 and has been designated vIL-10.

Crossreactivity
There is 72% homology between human and mouse mature IL-10. Human IL-10 is active on mouse cells, but murine IL-10 is not active on human cells.

Sources
TH0 and TH2 subsets of CD4+ murine T cells, activated CD4+ and CD8+ human T cells, and murine Ly-1+ B cells, monocytes, macrophages, keratinocytes.

Bioassays
Inhibition of IFNγ synthesis by mitogen/antigen-activated TH1 clones or activated PBMC. Proliferation of MC/9 mouse mast cell line.

Physicochemical properties of IL-10

Property	Human	Mouse
pI	8	8.1
Amino acids – precursor	178	178
– mature[a]	160	160
M_r (K) – predicted	18.6	18.8
– expressed	35–40	17–21
Potential N-linked glycosylation sites	1	2
Disulphide bonds[b]	2	2

[a] After removal of predicted signal peptide.
[b] Possible disulphide bonds.

3-D structure
Not known.

Gene structure [6]

Scale

Exons 50 aa

    □ Translated

    ▨ Untranslated

Introns ⊢—⊣
    500bp

Chromosome

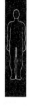

mIL-10 — 55 20 51 22 30   1

Human Il-10 is on syntenic region of chromosome 1

Amino acid sequence for human IL-10 [7]

Accession code: Swissprot P22301

```
-18   MHSSALLCCL VLLTGVRA
  1   SPGQGTQSEN SCTHFPGNLP NMLRDLRDAF SRVKTFFQMK DQLDNLLLKE
 51   SLLEDFKGYL GCQALSEMIQ FYLEEVMPQA ENQDPDIKAH VNSLGENLKT
101   LRLRLRRCHR FLPCENKSKA VEQVKNAFNK LQEKGIYKAM SEFDIFINYI
151   EAYMTMKIRN
```

Amino acid sequence for mouse IL-10 [8]

Accession code: Swissprot P18893

```
-18   MPGSALLCCL LLLTGMRI
  1   SRGQYSREDN NCTHFPVGQS HMLLELRTAF SQVKTFFQTK DQLDNILLTD
 51   SLMQDFKGYL GCQALSEMIQ FYLVEVMPQA EKHGPEIKEH LNSLGEKLKT
101   LRMRLRRCHR FLKCENKSKA VEQVKSDFNK LEDQGVYKAM NEFDIFINCI
151   EAYMMIKMKS
```

THE IL-10 RECEPTOR

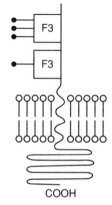

COOH

The IL-10 receptor belongs to the class II CKR family which also includes the IFNγ receptor, IFNα/β receptor and tissue factor [9-11]. The extracellular region of 220 amino acids consists of two homologous FNIII domains. The first of these has two conserved tryptophans and a pair of conserved cysteines whereas the second has a unique disulphide loop formed from the second pair of conserved cysteines, but no WSXWS motif characteristic of class I cytokine receptors [12].

Distribution

IL-10R mRNA is expressed in B cells, thymocytes, the mast cell line MC/9 and the macrophage cell line IG.18LA. Human IL-10R mRNA is restricted mostly to haematopoietic cells and cell lines.

Physicochemical properties of the IL-10 receptor

Property		Human	Mouse
Amino acids	– precursor	578	575
	– mature[a]	557	559
M_r (K)	– predicted	61	63
	– expressed	90–110	110
Potential N-linked glycosylation sites		6	4
Affinity K_d (M)		2×10^{-10}	7×10^{-11}

[a] After removal of predicted signal peptide.

Signal transduction

Not known, but likely to involve JAK family of kinases.

Chromosomal location

hIL-10R is on chromosome 11.

Amino acid sequence for human IL-10 receptor [13]

Accession code: Genbank U00672

```
 -21  MLPCLVVLLA ALLSLRLGSD A
   1  HGTELPSPPS VWFEAEFFHH ILHWTPIPNQ SESTCYEVAL LRYGIESWNS
  51  ISNCSQTLSY DLTAVTLDLY HSNGYRARVR AVDGSRHSNW TVTNTRFSVD
 101  EVTLTVGSVN LEIHNGFILG KIQLPRPKMA PANDTYESIF SHFREYEIAI
 151  RKVPGNFTFT HKKVKHENFS LLTSGEVGEF CVQVKPSVAS RSNKGMWSKE
 201  ECISLTRQYF TVTNVIIFFA FVLLLSGALA YCLALQLYVR RRKKLPSVLL
 251  FKKPSPFIFI SQRPSPETQD TIHPLDEEAF LKVSPELKNL DLHGSTDSGF
 301  GSTKPSLQTE EPQFLLPDPH PQADRTLGNG EPPVLGDSCS SGSSNSTDSG
 351  ICLQEPSLSP STGPTWEQQV GSNSRGQDDS GIDLVQNSEG RAGDTQGGSA
 401  LGHHSPPEPE VPGEEDPAAV AFQGYLRQTR CAEEKATKTG CLEEESPLTD
 451  GLGPKFGRCL VDEAGLHPPA LAKGYLKQDP LEMTLASSGA PTGQWNQPTE
 501  EWSLLALSSC SDLGISDWSF AHDLAPLGCV AAPGGLLGSF NSDLVTLPLI
 551  SSLQSSE
```

Amino acid sequence for mouse IL-10 receptor [14]

Accession code: GenEMBL L12120

```
 -16 MLSRLLPFLV TISSLS
   1 LEFIAYGTEL PSPSYVWFEA RFFQHILHWK PIPNQSESTY YEVALKQYGN
  51 STWNDIHICR KAQALSCDLT TFTLDLYHRS YGYRARVRAV DNSQYSNWTT
 101 TETRFTVDEV ILTVDSVTLK AMDGIIYGTI HPPRPTITPA GDEYEQVFKD
 151 LRVYKISIRK FSELKNATKR VKQETFTLTV PIGVRKFCVK VLPRLESRIN
 201 KAEWSEEQCL LITTEQYFTV TNLSILVISM LLFCGILVCL VLQWYIRHPG
 251 KLPTVLVFKK PHDFFPANPL CPETPDAIHI VDLEVFPKVS LELRDSVLHG
 301 STDSGFGSGK PSLQTEESQF LLPGSHPQIQ GTLGKEESPG LQATCGDNTD
 351 SGICLQEPGL HSSMGPAWKQ QLGYTHQDQD DSDVNLVQNS PGQPKYTQDA
 401 SALGHVCLLE PKAPEEKDQV MVTFQGYQKQ TRWKAEAAGP AECLDEEIPL
 451 TDAFDPELGV HLQDDLAWPP PALAAGYLKQ ESQGMASAPP GTPSRQWNQL
 501 TEEWSLLGVV SCEDLSIESW RFAHKLDPLD CGAAPGGLLD SLGSNLVTLP
 551 LISSLQVEE
```

The Cys pairs 59,67 and 188,209; Trp residues 29 and 53; and Tyr residue 154 are conserved in the cytokine receptor class II super family.

References

1 Moore, K.W. et al. (1993) Annu. Rev. Immunol. 11, 165–190.
2 Malefyt, R.D.W. et al. (1992) Curr. Opin. Immunol. 4, 314–320.
3 Howard, M. and O'Garra, A. (1992) Immunol. Today 13, 198–200.
4 Go, N.F. et al. (1990) J. Exp. Med. 172, 1625–1631.
5 Defrance, T. et al. (1992) J. Exp. Med. 175, 671–682.
6 Kim, J.M. et al. (1992) J. Immunol. 148, 3618–3623.
7 Vieira, P. et al. (1991) Proc. Natl Acad. Sci. USA 88, 1172–1176.
8 Moore, K.W. et al. (1990) Science 248, 1230–1234.
9 Bazan, J.F. (1990) Proc. Natl Acad. Sci. USA 87, 6934–6938.
10 Aguet, M. (1991) Br. J. Haematol. 79, 6–8.
11 Lutfalla, G. et al. (1992) J. Biol. Chem. 267, 2802–2809.
12 Bazan, J.F. (1990) Cell 61, 753–754.
13 Liu, Y. et al. (1994) J. Immunol. 152, 1821–1829.
14 Ho, A.S.Y. et al. (1993) Proc. Natl Acad. Sci. USA 90, 11267–11271.

IL-11

Other names
Adipogenesis inhibitory factor [1].

THE MOLECULE

Interleukin 11 is a growth factor for plasmacytomas, haematopoietic multipotential and commited megakaryocytic and macrophage progenitor cells, and inhibits adipogenesis in mouse pre-adipocytes [1-5]. IL-11 is distantly related to IL-6, LIF and OSM [6].

Crossreactivity
Human IL-11 is active on mouse cells.

Sources
IL-1-stimulated fibroblasts, bone marrow stromal cell lines.

Bioassays
IL-11 can be assayed by its proliferative effects on some murine IL-6-dependent plasmacytoma lines such as T1165 [7].

Physicochemical properties of IL-11

Property	Human
Amino acids – precursor	199
– mature	179
M_r (K) – predicted	20
– expressed	23
Potential N-linked glycosylation sites	0
Disulphide bonds	0

3-D structure
No information.

Gene structure
Located on chromosome 19q13.3-13.4 [6,8].

Amino acid sequence for Human IL-11 [2]

Accesion code: Swissprot P20809

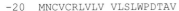

```
-20   MNCVCRLVLV VLSLWPDTAV
  1   APGPPPGPPR VSPDPRAELD STVLLTRSLL ADTRQLAAQL RDKFPADGDH
 51   NLDSLPTLAM SAGALGALQL PGVLTRLRAD LLSYLRHVQW LRRAGGSSLK
101   TLEPELGTLQ ARLDRLLRRL QLLMSRLALP QPPPDPPAPP LAPPSSAWGG
151   IRAAHAILGG LHLTLDWAVR GLLLLKTRL
```

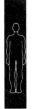

THE IL-11 RECEPTOR

A single class of specific receptor has been shown on mouse cells, with a K_d of 3.5×10^{-10}M and an apparent M_r of 151 000 [9]. Ligand interaction causes the tyrosine phosphorylation of four proteins at 152 000, 94 000, 47 000 and 44 000. The IL-6 signal transducer gp130 may be involved in IL-11R function [8].

References

1 Kawashima, I. et al. (1991) FEBS Lett. 283, 199–202.
2 Paul, S.R. et al. (1990) Proc. Natl Acad. Sci. USA 87, 7512–7516.
3 Musashi, M. et al. (1991) Proc. Natl Acad. Sci. USA 88, 765–769.
4 Quesniaux, V.F. et al. (1993) Int. Rev. Exp. Pathol. 34, 205–214.
5 Musashi, M. et al. (1991) Blood 78, 1448–1451.
6 Bruce, A.G. et al. (1992) Prog. Growth Factor Res. 4, 157–170.
7 Gearing, A.J.H. et al. (1994) In The Cytokine Handbook, 2nd edn, Ed Thomson A.W., ed., Academic Press, London (in press).
8 Yang, Y.C. and Lin, T. (1992) Biofactors 4, 15–21.
9 Yin, T. et al. (1992) J. Biol. Chem. 267, 8347–8351.

IL-12

Other names

Human IL-12 has been known as natural killer cell stimulatory factor (NKSF) and cytotoxic lymphocyte maturation factor (CLMF) [1].

THE MOLECULE

Interleukin 12 is a heterodimeric cytokine made up of two chains (p35 and p40) important in defence against intracellular pathogens [2]. It induces IFNγ production by T cells and NK cells, enhances NK and ADCC activity, and co-stimulates peripheral blood lymphocyte proliferation [1,3–7]. IL-12 also stimulates proliferation and induces the differentiation of the TH1 subset of T lymphocytes [8,9].

Crossreactivity

There is 70% homology between human and mouse p40, and 60% homology between the p35 chains of IL-12 [10]. Human IL-12 is inactive on mouse cells, mouse IL-12 is active on human cells [10].

Sources

B Lymphoblastoid cells, monocyte/macrophages, B cells [11].

Bioassays

Proliferation of PHA-activated lymphoblasts in the presence of monoclonal antibodies to IL-2, or stimulation of IFNγ production by spleen cells [7].

Physicochemical properties of IL-12

Property	p35[a]		p40[a,b]	
	Human	Mouse	Human	Mouse
pI	6.5	?	5.4	?
Amino acids – precursor	253	215	328	335
– mature	196	193	306	313
M_r (K) – predicted	27.5	24.3	34.7	38.3
– expressed	30–33	?	35–44	?
Potential N-linked glycosylation sites	3	1	4	5
Disulphide bonds[c]	3	3	5	6

[a] Neither chain alone has biological activity

[b] The p40 chain shares extensive sequence homology with the extracellular immunoglobulin and hematopoietin domains of the IL-6 receptor [12].

[c] Possible disulphide bonds.

3-D structure

No information.

Gene structure

No information.

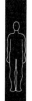

Amino acid sequence for human IL-12 p35 chain [3,6]

Accession code: Genbank M65271, M38443

```
-56  MWPPGSASQP PPSPAAATGL HPAARPVSLQ CRLSMCPARS LLLVATLVLL
 -6  DHLSLA
  1  RNLPVATPDP GMFPCLHHSQ NLLRAVSNML QKARQTLEFY PCTSEEIDHE
 51  DITKDKTSTV EACLPLELTK NESCLNSRET SFITNGSCLA SRKTSFMMAL
101  CLSSIYEDLK MYQVEFKTMN AKLLMDPKRQ IFLDQNMLAV IDELMQALNF
151  NSETVPQKSS LEEPDFYKTK IKLCILLHAF RIRAVTIDRV TSYLNAS
```

Amino acid sequence for human IL-12 p40 chain [3,6]

Accession code: Genbank M65272, M38443, M38444

```
-22  MCHQQLVISW FSLVFLASPL VA
  1  IWELKKDVYV VELDWYPDAP GEMVVLTCDT PEEDGITWTL DQSSEVLGSG
 51  KTLTIQVKEF GDAGQYTCHK GGEVLSHSLL LLHKKEDGIW STDILKDQKE
101  PKNKTFLRCE AKNYSGRFTC WWLTTISTDL TFSVKSSRGS SDPQGVTCGA
151  ATLSAERVRG DNKEYEYSVE CQEDSACPAA EESLPIEVMV DAVHKLKYEN
201  YTSSFFIRDI IKPDPPKNLQ LKPLKNSRQV EVSWEYPDTW STPHSYFSLT
251  FCVQVQGKSK REKKDRVFTD KTSATVICRK NASISVRAQD RYYSSSWSEW
301  ASVPCS
```

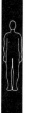

Amino acid sequence for mouse IL-12 p35 chain [10]

Accession code: Genbank M86672

```
-22  MCQSRYLLFL ATLALLNHLS LA
  1  RVIPVSGPAR CLSQSRNLLK TTDDMVKTAR EKLKHYSCTA EDIDHEDITR
 51  DQTSTLKTCL PLELHKNESC LATRETSSTT RGSCLPPQKT SLMMTLCLGS
101  IYEDLKMYQT EFQAINAALQ NHNHQQIILD KGMLVAIDEL MQSLNHNGET
151  LRQKPPVGEA DPYRVKMKLC ILLHAFSTRV VTINRVMGYL SSA
```

Amino acid sequence for mouse IL-12 p40 chain [10]

Accession code: Genbank M86771

```
-22  MCPQKLTISW FAIVLLVSPL MA
  1  MWELEKDVYV VEVDWTPDAP GETVNLTCDT PEEDDITWTS DQRHGVIGSG
 51  KTLTITVKEF LDAGQYTCHK GGETLSHSHL LLHKKENGIW STEILKNFKN
101  KTFLKCEAPN YSGRFTCSWL VQRNMDLKFN IKSSSSPPDS RAVTCGMASL
151  SAEKVTLDQR DYEKYSVSCQ EDVTCPTAEE TLPIELALEA RQQNKYENYS
201  TSFFIRDIIK PDPPKNLQMK PLKNSQVEVS WEYPDSWSTP HSYFSLKFFV
251  RIQRKKEKMK ETEEGCNQKG AFLVEKTSTE VQCKGGNVCV QAQDRYYNSS
301  CSKWACVPCR VRS
```

THE IL-12 RECEPTOR

The receptor for IL-12 is an M_r 180 000 glycoprotein with a K_d of $5–10 \times 10^{-11}$M found on T cells and NK cells [13]. One component of the IL-12 receptor complex has recently been cloned and shown to be related to gp130, GCSFR and LIFR [14]. The cloned receptor has an affinity of $2–5 \times 10^{-9}$M. Genbank accession code W03187.

References

1 Gately, M.K. et. al. (1991) J. Immunol. 147, 874–882.

2 Locksley, R.M. (1993) Proc. Natl Acad. Sci. USA 90, 5879–5880.

3 Wolf, S.F. et al. (1991) J. Immunol. 146, 3074–3081.

4 Lieberman, M.D. et al. (1991) J. Surg. Res. 50, 410–415.

5 Chan, S.H. et al. (1991) J. Exp. Med. 173, 869–879.

6 Gubler, U. et al. (1991) Proc. Natl Acad. Sci. USA 88, 4143–4147.

7 Stern, A. et al. (1990) Proc. Natl Acad. Sci. USA 87, 6808–6812.

8 Hsieh, C.-S. et al. (1993) Science 260, 547–549.

9 Manetti, R. et al. (1993) J. Exp. Med. 177, 1199–1204.

10 Schoenhaut, D.S. et al. (1992) J. Immunol. 148, 3433.

11 D'Andrea, A. et al. (1992) J. Exp. Med. 176, 1387–1398.

12 Gearing, D.P. and Cosman, D. (1991) Cell 66, 9–10.

13 Truitt, T et al. (1991) J. Cell. Biochem. Suppl. 15F, 120.

14 Chua, A.O. et al. (1994) J. Immunol. 153, 128–136.

IL-13

Other names
Mouse IL-13 is also known as P600.

THE MOLECULE

Interleukin 13 is secreted by activated T cells and inhibits the production of inflammatory cytokines (IL-1β, IL-6, TNFα, IL-8) by LPS-stimulated monocytes [1]. Human and mouse IL-13 induce CD23 expression on human B cells, promote B cell proliferation in combination with anti-Ig or CD40 antibodies, and stimulate secretion of IgM, IgE and IgG4 [2-4]. IL-13 has also been shown to prolong survival of human monocytes and increase surface expression of MHC class II and CD23 [3]. Human and mouse IL-13 have no known activity on mouse B cells.

Crossreactivity
There is 58% amino acid sequence identity between human and mouse IL-13 and significant cross-species reactivity.

Sources
Activated T cells.

Bioassays
Proliferation of human B cells co-stimulated with anti-IgM or CD40 antibody.

Physicochemical properties of IL-13

Property	Human	Mouse
Amino acids – precursor	132	131
– mature[a]	112	113
M_r (K) – predicted	12.3	12.4
– expressed[b]	9/17	?
Potential N-linked glycosylation sites	4	3
Disulphide bonds	2	?

[a] After removal of signal peptide. Human IL-13 expressed in COS and Chinese hamster cells has N-terminal Gly. Mouse signal peptide is computer predicted.

[b] The 17 000 molecular weight form is glycosylated. Unglycosylated IL-13 has a predicted M_r of 12 000 (confirmed by electrospray mass spectrometry), but it migrates as a 9 000 protein on SDS–PAGE.

3-D structure
Not known.

Gene structure [5]

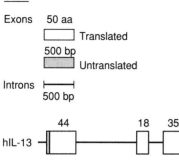

Scale

Exons 50 aa
☐ Translated
500 bp
▨ Untranslated

Introrns |———|
500 bp

Chromosome

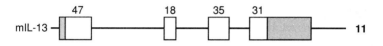

hIL-13 44 18 35 35 **5q31**

↑
*

mIL-13 47 18 35 31 **11**

Alternative splicing (marked *) gives rise to a second mRNA species in human T cells containing an additional codon for Gln at the 5' end of exon 4 [3].

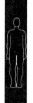

Amino acid sequence for human IL-13 [1,3]

Accession code: GenEMBL X69079, L06801

```
-34   MHPLLNPLLL ALGL
-20   MALLLTTVIA LTCLGGFASP
  1   GPVPPSTALR ELIEELVNIT QNQKAPLCNG SMVWSINLTA GMYCAALESL
 51   INVSGCSAIE KTQRMLSGFC PHKVSAGQFS SLHVRDTKIE VAQFVKDLLL
101   HLKKLFREGR FN
```

There are two possible ATG initiation codons giving rise to Met –34 and Met –20. The second is the most likely initiation site. The protein secreted by transfected COS and Chinese hamster cells has Gly at the N-terminus [1]. Two mRNAs encoding one and two Gln residues at position 78 are expressed by activated T cells [3]. Disulphide bonds between Cys 28–56 and 44–70.

Amino acid sequence for mouse IL-13 (p600) [3,6]

Accession code: GenEMBL M23504

```
-18   MALWVTAVLA LACLGGLA
  1   APGPVPRSVS LPLTLKELIE ELSNITQDQT PLCNGSMVWS VDLAAGGFCV
 51   ALDSLTNISN CNAIYRTQRI LHGLCNRKAP TTVSSLPDTK IEVAHFITKL
101   LSYTKQLFRH GPF
```

Computer-predicted signal peptide –1 to –18. Signal peptide in Swissprot database is given as –1 to –21 by similarity with human IL-13. Possible disulphide bonds between Cys33–61 and 49–75 by similarity with human IL-13.

THE IL-13 RECEPTOR

The receptor for IL-13 has not yet been cloned. IL-13 may share some receptor components with IL-4 [7].

Distribution

Not known.

Signal transduction

Not known.

Chromosomal location
Not known.

References
1 Minty, A. et al. (1993) Nature 362, 248–250.
2 Punnonen, J. et al. (1993) Proc. Natl Acad. Sci. USA 90, 3730–3734.
3 McKenzie, A.N.J. et al. (1993) Proc. Natl Acad. Sci. USA 90, 3735–3739.
4 Cocks, B.G. et al. (1993) Int. Immunol. 5, 657–663.
5 McKenzie, A.N.J. et al. (1993) J. Immunol. 150, 5436–5444.
6 Brown, K.D. et al. (1989) J. Immunol. 142, 679–687.
7 Zurawski, S.M. et al. (1993) EMBO J. 12, 2663–2670.

IL-14

Other names
Human IL-14 has been known as high molecular weight B cell growth factor (HMW-BCGF) [1].

THE MOLECULE

Interleukin 14 is a cytokine which enhances the proliferation of activated B cells, and inhibits immunoglobulin synthesis [1-4]. IL-14 is unrelated to any other cytokines, but shares homology with complement factor Bb [2,3].

Crossreactivity
There are no reports of murine IL-14.

Sources
IL-14 is produced by T cells and some B cell tumours [2].

Bioassays
Human IL-14 can be assayed by proliferation of *Staphylococcus aureus* activated B cells [4].

Physicochemical properties of IL-14

Property	Human
pI	6.7–7.8
Amino acids – precursor	498
– mature	483
M_r (K) – predicted	53
– expressed	60
Potential N-linked glycosylation sites	3
Disulphide bonds[a]	?

[a] IL-14 has 34 Cys residues some of which may form disulphide bonds.

3-D structure
No information.

Gene structure
No information.

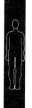

Amino acid sequence for human IL-14 [2]

Accession code: Genbank L15344

```
 -15  MIRLLRSIIG LVLAL
   1  PKGRGSDAKG LLTSTSSHAK TFSRSLVSRQ EIPSSERPAR LCLGTPFLRS
  51  REVKVSLPEQ LGGPELDLSK PCSSRQMQFN DLGVLLVLSS EGQGGVIEPQ
 101  SQTEKCSSHF CQLTVMAATD DSPSQDSSAH RQATDFICTH PHPQCKLHCT
 151  LTGINAFARP CKMPYVRKTD PQKCQNCKCQ MPARSEHAWL QQWAAQHGSL
 201  LWARLAGLPL PSQHDPTPGS LGPGGGGLLR PVWPDASVLG CSWVARRFCD
 251  PGGAGCLMPQ CPSGLLSGPL SVREPWPPAL RSCTLLFRSL RSVCSARHSF
 301  SSRWIFTCRP SSSLSRTVFS SAISSRALLL LSHRDRYMVV SFSSFLIFLV
 351  IFSISCLNVV NTSLLLESVF WNSSNFSVYR ASCCFRWVSC CFISSHILWD
 401  STASFRRKSF SRWCRSSASF SISWACWSLA STSCCCRSLC LKTLSICSSR
 451  SSYCSISFLS LSASSMFSWR SLELRSLCCS ICS
```

THE IL-14 RECEPTOR

A single receptor type with an affinity of 20×10^{-9}M is detected on B cells and B cell leukaemias [5,6]. IL-14 causes upregulation of its receptor on B cells. IL-14 receptors also bind complement fragment Bb [3].

Signal transduction

IL-14 causes increases in intracellular cAMP, DAG and calcium [3].

References
1 Kehrl, J. et al. (1984) Immunol. Rev. 78, 75-96.
2 Ambrus, J.L. Jr et al. (1993) Proc. Natl Acad. Sci. USA 90, 6330–6334.
3 Ambrus, J.L. Jr et al. (1991) J. Biol. Chem. 266, 3702–3708.
4 Ambrus, J.L. Jr et al. (1990) J. Immunol. 145, 3949–3955.
5 Uckun, F. et al. (1989) J. Clin. Invest. 84, 1595–1608.
6 Ambrus, J.L. Jr et al. (1988) J. Immunol. 141, 861–869.

IL-15

Other names
None.

THE MOLECULE

Interleukin 15 was isolated and cloned from the simian kidney epithelial cell line CV1/EBNA [1]. It shares many of the biological properties of IL-2 including stimulation of CTLL proliferation, and *in vitro* generation of alloantigen-specific cytotoxic T cells and non-antigen specific lymphokine activated killer (LAK) cells.

Crossreactivity
Human IL-15 is active on mouse CTLL cells.

Sources
IL-15 mRNA is found in a wide variety of human cell types including peripheral blood mononuclear cells (PBMC), placenta, skeletal muscle, kidney, lung, liver, heart, and the IMTLH bone marrow stromal cell line. It is produced most abundantly by epithelial cells and monocytes.

Bioassays
Proliferation of activated T cells.

Physicochemical properties of IL-15

Property	Simian
Amino acids – precursor	162
– mature	114
M_r (K) – predicted	12.9
– expressed	14–15
Potential N-linked glycosylation sites	2
Disulphide bonds[a]	2

[a] Disulphide bonds predicted by three-dimensional modelling

3-D structure
Computer modelling of IL-15 indicates a four α-helical bundle structure similar to IL-2.

Gene structure

Not yet determined.

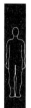

Amino acid sequence for human IL-15 [1]

Accession code: U03099

```
-48 MRISKPHLRS ISIQCYLCLL LKSHFLTEAG IHVFILGCFS AGLPKTEA
  1 NWVNVISDLK KIEDLIQSMH IDATLYTESD VHPSCKVTAM KCFLLELQVI
 50 SHESGDTDIH DTVENLIILA NNILSSNGNI TESGCKECEE LEEKNIKEFL
101 QSFVHIVQMF INTS
```

THE IL-15 RECEPTOR

IL-2 receptor β and γ chains are both components of the IL15R but the α chain (Tac) is not. [2]

Distribution

Not known.

Signal transduction

Not known.

Chromosomal location

Not known.

References
1 Grabstein, K. et al. (1994) Science 264, 965–968.
2 Giri, J.G. et al. (1994) EMBO J. 13, 2822–2830.

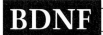 The Neurotrophin Family

Other names
None.

THE MOLECULE

Brain derived neurotrophic factor is important in the development and maintenance of the vertebrate nervous system. It promotes the survival of neuronal populations located either in the central nervous system or directly connected to it, and helps to maintain neurons and their differentiated phenotype in the adult. It is similar to NGF and NT-3 but with its own neuronal specificities [1,2].

Crossreactivity
The amino acid sequences of mature BDNF from mouse, human and pig are identical, with complete cross-species reactivity.

Sources
High levels of BDNF mRNA are found in pyramidal and granule cells of the hippocampus, and specific regions of the cortex, and cerebellum of the CNS. Low levels are detectable in the spinal cord [3]. Also in heart, lung and skeletal muscle in adult.

Bioassays
Survival and outgrowth of neurites from embryo chicken dorsal root ganglia. Survival and differentiation of trkB transfected cell lines.

Physicochemical properties of BDNF

Property	Human	Mouse
pI	9.99	9.99
Amino acids – precursor	247	249
– mature[a]	119	119
M_r (K) – predicted	13.5	13.5
– expressed[b]	27	27
Potential N-linked glycosylation sites[c]	0	0
Disulphide bonds[d]	3	3

[a] After removal of propeptide.
[b] Non-covalently linked dimer.
[c] One N-linked glycosylation site in the propeptide.
[d] Conserved between NGF, BDNF, NT-3 and NT-4.

3-D structure
The molecule has 70% β-sheet and is expressed as a tightly associated homodimer [4]. Crystal structure is not yet known, but is likely to be similar to NGF.

Gene structure [5]

Scale

Exons   50 aa
☐ Translated
1 Kb
▦ Untranslated

Introns ├──┤
1 Kb

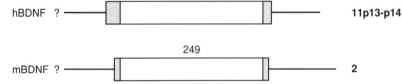

Chromosome

247

hBDNF ?

11p13-p14

249

mBDNF ?

2

There is some evidence for more than one mRNA species arising from alternative splicing and other ATG initiation sites on additonal upstream exons (similar to NGF).

Amino acid sequence for human BDNF [5,6]

Accession Code: Swissprot P23560

```
-18   MTILFLTMVI SYFGCMKA
  1   APMKEANIRG QGGLAYPGVR THGTLESVNG PKAGSRGLTS LADTFEHVIE
 51   ELLDEDQKVR PNEENNKDAD LYTSRVMLSS QVPLEPPLLF LLEEYKNYLD
101   AANMSMRVRR HSDPARRGEL SVCDSISEWV TAADKKTAVD MSGGTVTVLE
151   KVPVSKGQLK QYFYETKCNP MGYTKEGCRG IDKRHWNSQC RTTQSYVRAL
201   TMDSKKRIGW RFIRIDTSCV CTLTIKRGR
```

Variant sequence V->M at position 48. Mature BDNF is formed by removal of a predicted signal peptide and propeptide (in italics, 1–110). Other precursor forms with extended N-terminal sequences similar to NGF may also exist. Disulphide bonds between Cys123–190, 168–219 and 178–221 by similarity.

Amino acid sequence for mouse BDNF [3]

Accession Code: Swissprot P21237

```
-18   MTILFLTMVI SYFGCMKA
  1   APMKEVNVHG QGNLAYPGVR THGTLESVNG PRAGSRGLTT TSLADTFEHV
 51   IEELLDEDQK VRPNEENHKD ADLYTSRVML SSQVPLEPPL LFLLEEYKNY
101   LDAANMSMRV RRHSDPARRG ELSVCDSISE WVTAADKKTA VDMSGGTVTV
151   LEKVPVSKGQ LKQYFYETKC NPMGYTKEGC RGIDKRHWNS QCRTTQSYVR
201   ALTMDSKKRI GWRFIRIDTS CVCTLTIKRG R
```

Mature BDNF is formed by removal of a predicted signal peptide and propeptide (in italics, 1–112). Other precursor forms with extended N-terminal sequences similar to NGF may also exist. Disulphide bonds between Cys125–192, 170–221 and 180–223 by similarity.

THE BDNF RECEPTORS

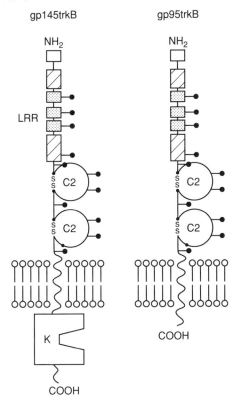

BDNF binds to low affinity and high affinity cell surface receptors. The low affinity receptor is LNGFR, which also binds the other members of the NGF neurotrophin family, NGF, NT-3 and NT-4 [7-9] (see NGF entry). Cells expressing LNGFR do not respond to BDNF. Rather, BDNF mediates its neurotrophic properties through gp145trkB (trkB) [10-12]. Although there are no conclusive BDNF binding studies to trkB receptors, most BDNF responsive cells express gp145trkB but not LNGFR transcripts [13]. The trkB receptor is a member of the trk family of tyrosine kinases described in the entry for NGF receptors. Two classes of trkB receptors have been identified. These are gp145trkB and a truncated isoform gp95trkB which lacks the cytoplasmic kinase domain [14-15]. Additional trkB receptors may also exist [15-16]. Both gp145trkB and gp95trkB have identical extracellular and transmembrane domains, but gp95trkB has a short 23 amino acid cytoplasmic domain including 11 C-terminal residues which are different to those on the gp145trkB receptor [15,16]. gp145trkB is also a functional receptor for NT-4 and NT-3 but not NGF [17-18].

Distribution

TrkB mRNA has been shown by *in situ* hybridization studies to be expressed widely throughout the central and peripheral nervous system including non-neuronal cells such as glia and Schwann cells [13]. It has also been shown to be present by Northern blotting in brain, lung, muscle and ovaries [14].

Physicochemical properties of the BDNF receptor (trkB)

	Mouse gp 145[trkB]	Mouse gp95[trkB]
Amino acids – precursor	821	476
– mature[a]	790	445
M_r (K) – predicted	88.6	52
– expressed	145	95
Potential N-linked glycosylation sites	11	11
Affinity K_d (M)[b,c]	10^{-9}	ND
Kinase activity	yes	no

[a] After removal of predicted signal peptide.

[b] TrkB binds NT-3 with similar affinity [11]. This low affinity binding was measured for trkB expressed in NIH 3T3 pJM8 cells which are unresponsive to BDNF and NT-3. It is possible that high affinity binding would be observed in responsive cells similar to NGF binding to trkA.

[c] High affinity receptor may be formed by a combination of trkB and LNGFR.

Signal transduction by gp145[trkB]

gp145[trkB] has intrinsic protein tyrosine kinase activity. Both BDNF and NT-3 stimulate receptor autophosphorylation [11], and phosphorylation of PLC-γ1 resulting in PIP$_2$ hydrolysis with release of IP$_3$ and DAG [19]. LNGFR is not required for signal transduction [17,20].

Chromosomal location

LNGFR is on chromosome 17q21–q22. The location of *trkB* has not been established.

Amino acid sequence for the mouse BDNF receptor (trkB) [14]

(Human trkB has not yet been cloned)
Accession Number: Swissprot P15209

```
-31   MSPWLKWHGP AMARLWGLCL LVLGFWRASL A
  1   CPTSCKCSSA RIWCTEPSPG IVAFPRLEPN SVDPENITEI LIANQKRLEI
 51   INEDDVEAYV GLRNLTIVDS GLKFVAYKAF LKNSNLRHIN FTRNKLTSLS
101   RRHFRHLDLS DLILTGNPFT CSCDIMWLKT LQETKSSPDT QDLYCLNESS
151   KNMPLANLQI PNCGLPSARL AAPNLTVEEG KSVTLSCSVG GDPLPTLYWD
```

```
201    VGNLVSKHMN ETSHTQGSLR ITNISSDDSG KQISCVAENL VGEDQDSVNL
251    TVHFAPTITF LESPTSDHHW CIPFTVRGNP KPALQWFYNG AILNESKYIC
301    TKIHVTNHTE YHGCLQLDNP THMNNGDYTL MAKNEYGKDE RQISAHFMGR
351    PGVDYETNPN YPEVLYEDWT TPTDIGDTTN KSNEIPSTDV ADQSNREHLS
401    VYAVVVIASV VGFCLLVMLL LLKLARHSKF GMKGPASVIS NDDDSASPLH
451    HISNGSNTPS SSEGGPDAVI IGMTKIPVIE NPQYFGITNS QLKPDTFVQH
501    IKRHNIVLKR ELGEGAFGKV FLAECYNLCP EQDKILVAVK TLKDASDNAR
551    KDFHREAELL TNLQHEHIVK FYGVCVEGDP LIMVFEYMKH GDLNKFLRAH
601    GPDAVLMAEG NPPTELTQSQ MLHIAQQIAA GMVYLASQHF VHRDLATRNC
651    LVGENLLVKI GDFGMSRDVY STDYYRVGGH TMLPIRWMPP ESIMYRKFTT
701    ESDVWSLGVV LWEIFTYGKQ PWYQLSNNEV IECITQGRVL QRPRTCPQEV
751    YELMLGCWQR EPHTRKNIKS IHTLLQNLAK ASPVYLDILG
```

Variable splicing at position 435 (PASVISNDDDS->FVLFHKIPLDG) gives rise to a gp95^{trkB} variant missing the cytoplasmic kinase domain [15]. Tyr 674 is site of autophosphorylation.

The sequences for human and rat LNGFR are given in the NGF entry.

References

1 Yancopoulos, G.D. et al. (1990) Cold Spring Harbor Symp. Quant. Biol. LV, 371–379.
2 Ebendal, T. (1992) J. Neurosci. Res. 32, 461–470.
3 Hofer, M. et al. (1990) EMBO J. 9, 2459–2464.
4 Radziejewski, C. et al. (1992) Biochemistry 31, 4431–4436.
5 Maisonpierre, P.C. et al. (1991) Genomics 10, 558–568.
6 Jones, K.R. and Reichardt, L.F. (1990) Proc. Natl. Acad. Sci. USA 87, 8060–8064.
7 Rodriguez-Tebar, A. et al. (1992) EMBO J. 11, 917–922.
8 Chao, M.V. (1991) Curr. Topics Microbiol. Immunol. 165, 39–53.
9 Meakin, S.O. and Shooter, E.M. (1992) Trends Neurosci. 15, 323–331.
10 Squinto, S.P. et al. (1991) Cell 65, 885–893.
11 Soppet, D. et al. (1991) Cell 65, 895–903.
12 Klein, R. et al. (1991) Cell 66, 395–403.
13 Klein, R. et al. (1990) Development 109, 845–850.
14 Klein, R. et al. (1989) EMBO J. 8, 3701–3709.
15 Klein, R. et al. (1990) Cell 61, 647–656.
16 Middlemas, D.S. et al. (1991) Mol. Cell Biol. 11, 143–153.
17 Glass, D.J. et al. (1991) Cell 66, 405–413.
18 Klein, R. et al. (1992) Neuron 8, 947–956.
19 Widmer, H.R. et al. (1992) J. Neurochem. 59, 2113–2124.
20 Barker, P.A. and Murphy, R.A. (1992) Mol. Cell. Biochem. 110, 1–15.

CNTF

Other names
None.

THE MOLECULE

Ciliary neurotrophic factor promotes the survival and/or differentiation of neuronal cells. CNTF has no homology with the other neurotrophic growth factors, NGF, BDNF and NT-3. The absence of a signal peptide and N-linked glycosylation sites is consistent with CNTF being a cytosolic protein.

Crossreactivity
There is 84% homology between human and rat CNTF, and both human and rat CNTF are active on neurons from chicken dorsal root ganglia.

Sources
CNTF has been purified from embryonic chick eye, and rat and rabbit sciatic nerve.

Bioassays
Activity of CNTF from human and rat can be determined by its ability to maintain neurons from embryonic chickens.

Physicochemical properties of CNTF

Property	Human	Mouse
pI	6.0	6.0
Amino acids – precursor	200	200
– mature[a]	200	200
M_r (K) – predicted	22.9	22.9
– expressed	22	22.5
Potential N-linked glycosylation sites	0	0
Disulphide bonds	0	0

[a] CNTF has no signal peptide.

3-D structure
The 3-D structure of CNTF is not known, but it has significant homologies with IL-6, LIF, oncostatin M and G-CSF. It is thought that these molecules share a four helix bundle structure [1].

Gene structure [2]

Scale

Exons   50 aa

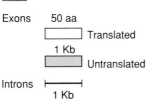

Introns

Chromosome

hCNTF

11

Amino acid sequence for human CNTF [3]

Accession code: Swissprot P26441

```
  1  MAFTEHSPLT PHRRDLCSRS IWLARKIRSD LTALTESYVK HQGLNKNINL
 51  DSADGMPVAS TDQWSELTEA ERLQENLQAY RTFHVLLARL LEDQQVHFTP
101  TEGDFHQAIH TLLLQVAAFA YQIEELMILL EYKIPRNEAD GMPINVGDGG
151  LFEKKLWGLK VLQELSQWTV RSIHDLRFIS SHQTGIPARG SHYIANNKKM
```

Amino acid sequence for rat CNTF [4]

Accession code: Swissprot P20294

```
  1  MAFAEQTPLT LHRRDLCSRS IWLARKIRSD LTALMESYVK HQGLNKNINL
 51  DSVDGVPVAS TDRWSEMTEA ERLQENLQAY RTFQGMLTKL LEDQRVHFTP
101  TEGDFHQAIH TLMLQVSAFA YQLEELMVLL EQKIPENEAD GMPATVGDGG
151  LFEKKLWGLK VLQELSQWTV RSIHDLRVIS SHQMGISALE SHYGAKDKQM
```

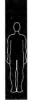

THE CNTF RECEPTOR

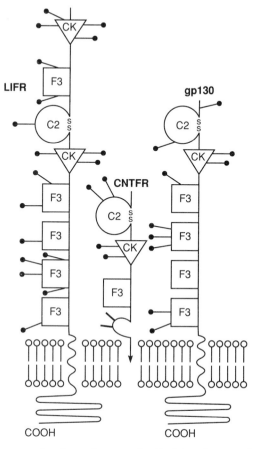

The CNTF receptor has homology to the IL-6R and is unrelated to receptors for NGF, BDNF and NT-3 [5]. Unlike all other cytokine receptors, the CNTF receptor is anchored to cell membranes by a glycosyl-phosphatidylinositol (GPI) linkage [6]. Associated chains are the LIFR, and gp130 (see IL-6) which is shared with receptors for IL-6, LIF and oncostatin M [7-11]. Complexes of CNTF and soluble CNTF receptor can act through gp130/LIFR to activate cells which do not express CNTF receptor [12].

Distribution

The CNTF receptor is expressed mostly within the nervous system and skeletal muscle. Expressed at lower levels in sciatic nerve, adrenal gland, skin, liver, kidney and testes.

Physicochemical properties of the CNTF receptor

Properties		Human	Rat
Amino acids	– precursor	372	372
	– mature[a]	352	352
M_r (K)	– predicted	38.9	40
	– expressed	72	?
Potential N-linked glycosylation sites		4	5
Affinity K_d (M)		?	?

[a] After removal of predicted signal peptide. Actual cleavage site is not known.

Signal transduction

The signal transduction components of the CNTFR (gp130 and LIFR) are tyrosine phosphorylated in response to CNTF binding [9,10]. Signalling probably requires hetero-dimerization of gp130 and LIFR [9]. May also involve activation of PKC [13].

Chromosomal location
Not known.

Amino acid sequence for human CNTF receptor [6]

Accession code: Genbank M73238

```
-20   MAAPVPWACC AVLAAAAAVV
  1   YAQRHSPQEA PHVQYERLGS DVTLPCGTAN WDAAVTWRVN GTDLAPDLLN
 51   GSQLVLHGLE LGHSGLYACF HRDSWHLRHQ VLLHVGLPPR EPVLSCRSNT
101   YPKGFYCSWH LPTPTYIPNT FNVTVLHGSK IMVCEKDPAL KNRCHIRYMH
151   LFSTIKYKVS ISVSNALGHN ATAITFDEFT IVKPDPPENV VARPVPSNPR
201   RLEVTWQTPS TWPDPESFPL KFFLRYRPLI LDQWQHVELS DGTAHTITDA
251   YAGKEYIIQV AAKDNEIGTW SDWSVAAHAT PWTEEPRHLT TEAQAAETTT
301   STTSSLAPPP TTKICDPGEL GSGGGPSAPF LVSVPITLAL AAAAATASSL
351   LI
```

The exact cleavage site for the signal peptide has not been established. The C-terminal hydrophobic sequence (in italics, 327–352) is typical of GPI linked proteins and may be removed although the exact cleavage site is not known.

Amino acid sequence for rat CNTF receptor [14]

Accession code: GenEMBL S54212
(Mouse CNTF receptor sequence has not been reported.)

```
-20   MAASVPWACC AVLAAAAAAV
  1   YTQKHSPQEA PHVQYERLGT DVTLPCGTAS WDAAVTWRVN GTDLAPDLLN
 51   GSQLILRSLE LGHSGLYACF HRDSWHLRHQ VLLHVGLPPR EPVLSCRSNT
101   YPKGFYCSWH LSAPTYIPNT FNVTVLHGSK MMVCEKDPAL KNRCHIRYMH
151   LFSTIKYKVS ISVSNALGHN TTAITFDEFT IVKPDPPENV VARPVPSNPR
201   RLEVTWQTPS TWPDPESFPL KFFLRYRPLI LDQWQHVELS NGTAHTITDA
251   YAGKEYIIQV AAKDNEIGTW SDWSVAAHAT PWTEEPRHLT TEAQAPETTT
301   STTSSLAPPP TTKICDPGEL SSGGGP*SIPF LTSVPVTLVL AAAAATANNL*
351   *LI*
```

The exact cleavage site for the signal peptide has not been established. The C-terminal hydrophobic sequence (in italics, 327–352) is typical of GPI-linked proteins and may be removed although the exact cleavage site is not known.

References

1 Bazan, J.F. (1991) Neuron 7, 197–208.
2 Lam, A. et al. (1991) Gene 102, 271–276.
3 Negro, A. et al. (1991) Eur. J. Biochem. 201, 289–294.
4 Stockli, K.A. et al. (1989) Nature 342, 920–923.
5 Davis, S. and Yancopoulos, G.D. (1993) Curr. Opin. Cell. Biol. 5, 281–285.
6 Davis, S. et al. (1991) Science 253, 59–63.
7 Kishimoto, T. et al. (1992) Science 258, 593–597.
8 Ip, N.Y. et al. (1992) Cell 69, 1121–1132.
9 Davis, S. et al. (1993) Science 260, 1805–1808.
10 Stahl, N. et al. (1993) J. Biol. Chem. 268, 7628–7631.
11 Baumann, H. et al. (1993) J. Biol. Chem. 268, 8414–8417.
12 Davis, S. et al. (1993) Science 259, 1736–1739.
13 Kalberg, C. et al. (1993) J. Neurochem. 60, 145–152.
14 Ip, N.Y. et al. (1993) Neuron 10, 89–102.

Other names

Human EGF has been known as β-urogastrone [1].

THE MOLECULE

Epidermal growth factor is a 53 amino acid cytokine which is proteolytically cleaved from a large integral membrane protein precursor [2]. EGF acts to stimulate growth of epithelial cells, accelerates tooth eruption and eyelid opening in mice, inhibits gastric acid secretion and is involved in wound healing [3].

Crossreactivity

There is about 70% homology between mature 53 amino acid human and mouse EGF [4-6]. Neither factor acts across species. EGF is closely structurally related to TGFα and to vaccinia growth factor, both of which bind to the EGF receptor [7,8,9].

Sources

EGF is made by ectodermal cells, monocytes, kidney and duodenal glands.

Bioassays

Proliferation of the A431 carcinoma line

Physicochemical properties of EGF

Property	Human	Mouse
pI	4.6	4.6
Amino acids – precursor[a]	1207	1217
– mature	53	53
M_r (K) – predicted	6	6
– expressed	6	6
Potential N-linked glycosylation sites[b]	0	0
Disulphide bonds[c]	3	3

[a] The full length protein is composed of eight extracellular EGF-like domains, only one of which has EGF activity.

[b] Processed mature molecule.

[c] In active EGF, disulphide bonds link residues 6–20, 14–31 and 33–42 in human and mouse EGF (numbering for processed active molecule only beginning at amino acid Asn949 of precursor for human and Asn977 for mouse).

3-D structure

Structure determined by NMR shows a major antiparallel β-sheet from residues 19–23 and 28–32, and a minor antiparallel β-sheet from residues 37–38 and 44–45. Residues 41 and 47 are involved in receptor binding (numbering for processed active molecule only beginning at amino acid Asn949 for human and Asn977 for mouse precursor).

Gene structure

The gene for human EGF is on chromosome 4q25

Amino acid sequence for human EGF [5]

Accession code: Swissprot P01133

```
-22    MLLTLIILLP VVSKFSFVSL SA
  1    PQHWSCPEGT LAGNGNSTCV GPAPFLIFSH GNSIFRIDTE GTNYEQLVVD
 51    AGVSVIMDFH YNEKRIYWVD LERQLLQRVF LNGSRQERVC NIEKNVSGMA
101    INWINEEVIW SNQQEGIITV TDMKGNNSHI LLSALKYPAN VAVDPVERFI
151    FWSSEVAGSL YRADLDGVGV KALLETSEKI TAVSLDVLDK RLFWIQYNRE
201    GSNSLICSCD YDGGSVHISK HPTQHNLFAM SLFGDRIFYS TWKMKTIWIA
251    NKHTGKDMVR INLHSSFVPL GELKVVHPLA QPKAEDDTWE PEQKLCKLRK
301    GNCSSTVCGQ DLQSHLCMCA EGYALSRDRK YCEDVNECAF WNHGCTLGCK
351    NTPGSYYCTC PVGFVLLPDG KRCHQLVSCP RNVSECSHDC VLTSEGPLCF
401    CPEGSVLERD GKTCSGCSSP DNGGCSQLCV PLSPVSWECD CFPGYDLQLD
451    EKSCAASGPQ PFLLFANSQD IRHMHFDGTD YGTLLSQQMG MVYALDHDPV
501    ENKIYFAHTA LKWIERANMD GSQRERLIEE GVDVPEGLAV DWIGRRFYWT
551    DRGKSLIGRS DLNGKRSKII TKENISQPRG IAVHPMAKRL FWTDTGINPR
601    IESSSLQGLG RLVIASSDLI WPSGITIDFL TDKLYWCDAK QSVIEMANLD
651    GSKRRRLTQN DVGHPFAVAV FEDYVWFSDW AMPSVIRVNK RTGKDRVRLQ
701    GSMLKPSSLV VVHPLAKPGA DPCLYQNGGC EHICKKRLGT AWCSCREGFM
751    KASDGKTCLA LDGHQLLAGG EVDLKNQVTP LDILSKTRVS EDNITESQHM
801    LVAEIMVSDQ DDCAPVGCSM YARCISEGED ATCQCLKGFA GDGKLCSDID
851    ECEMGVPVCP PASSKCINTE GGYVCRCSEG YQGDGIHCLD IDECQLGVHS
901    CGENASCTNT EGGYTCMCAG RLSEPGLICP DSTPPPHLRE DDHHYSVRNS
951    DSECPLSHDG YCLHDGVCMY IEALDKYACN CVVGYIGERC QYRDLKWWEL
1001   RHAGHGQQQK VIVVAVCVVV LVMLLLLSLW GAHYYRTQKL LSKNPKNPYE
1051   ESSRDVRSRR PADTEDGMSS CPQPWFVVIK EHQDLKNGGQ PVAGEDGQAA
1101   DGSMQPTSWR QEPQLCGMGT EQGCWIPVSS DKGSCPQVME RSFHMPSYGT
1151   QTLEGGVEKP HSLLSANPLW QQRALDPPHQ MELTQ
```

Propeptide is in italics. Soluble mature EGF amino acids Asn949-Arg1001.

Amino acid sequence for mouse EGF [6]

Accession code: Swissprot P01132

```
  1    MPWGRRPTWL LLAFLLVFLK ISILSVTAWQ TGNCQPGPLE RSERSGTCAG
 51    PAPFLVFSQG KSISRIDPDG TNHQQLVVDA GISADMDIHY KKERLYWVDV
101    ERQVLLRVFL NGTGLEKVCN VERKVSGLAI DWIDDEVLWV DQQNGVITVT
151    DMTGKNSRVL LSSLKHPSNI AVDPIERLMF WSSEVTGSLH RAHLKGVDVK
201    TLLETGGISV LTLDVLDKRL FWVQDSGEGS HAYIHSCDYE GGSVRLIRHQ
251    ARHSLSSMAF FGDRIFYSVL KSKAIWIANK HTGKDTVRIN LHPSFVTPGK
301    LMVVHPRAQP RTEDAAKDPD PELLKQRGRP CRFGLCERDP KSHSSACAEG
351    YTLSRDRKYC EDVNECATQN HGCTLGCENT PGSYHCTCPT GFVLLPDGKQ
401    CHELVSCPGN VSKCSHGCVL TSDGPRCICP AGSVLGRDGK TCTGCSSPDN
451    GGCSQICLPL RPGSWECDCF PGYDLQSDRK SCAASGPQPL LLFANSQDIR
501    HMHFDGTDYK VLLSRQMGMV FALDYDPVES KIYFAQTALK WIERANMDGS
```

```
 551  QRERLITEGV  DTLEGLALDW  IGRRIYWTDS  GKSVVGGSDL  SGKHHRIIIQ
 601  ERISRPRGIA  VHPRARRLFW  TDVGMSPRIE  SASLQGSDRV  LIASSNLLEP
 651  SGITIDYLTD  TLYWCDTKRS  VIEMANLDGS  KRRRLIQNDV  GHPFSLAVFE
 701  DHLWVSDWAI  PSVIRVNKRT  GQNRVRLQGS  MLKPSSLVVV  HPLAKPGADP
 751  CLYRNGGCEH  ICQESLGTAR  CLCREGFVKA  WDGKMCLPQD  YPILSGENAD
 801  LSKEVTSLSN  STQAEVPDDD  GTESSTLVAE  IMVSGMNYED  DCGPGGCGSH
 851  ARCVSDGETA  ECQCLKGFAR  DGNLCSDIDE  CVLARSDCPS  TSSRCINTEG
 901  GYVCRCSEGY  EGDGISCFDI  DECQRGAHNC  AENAACTNTE  GGYNCTCAGR
 951  PSSPGRSCPD  STAPSLLGED  GHHLDRNSYP  GCPSSYDGYC  LNGGVCMHIE
1001  SLDSYTCNCV  IGYSGDRCQT  RDLRWWELRH  AGYGQKHDIM  VVAVCMVALV
1051  LLLLLGMWGT  YYYRTRKQLS  NPPKNPCDEP  SGSVSSSGPD  SSSGAAVASC
1101  PQPWFVVLEK  HQDPKNGSLP  ADGTNGAVVD  AGLSPSLQLG  SVHLTSWRQK
1151  PHIDGMGTGQ  SCWIPPSSDR  GPQEIEGNSH  LPSYRPVGPE  KLHSLQSANG
1201  SCHERAPDLP  RQTEPVK
```

Propeptide in italics, signal sequence is not known. Soluble mature EGF amino acids Asn977-Arg1029.

THE EGF RECEPTOR

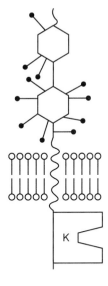

The EGF receptor (also known as c-erbB) is a class I receptor tyrosine kinase [10,11]. The receptor is also shared with TGFα, and with vaccinia virus growth factor. A viral oncogene v-*erbB* encodes a truncated EGF receptor lacking most of the extracellular domains. The EGF receptor is involved in bacterial and viral invasion of cells [12,13].

Distribution

Most cells.

Physicochemical properties of the EGF receptor

Properties	Human	Rat[a]
Amino acids – precursor	1210	644[a]
– mature	1186	620[a]
M_r (K) – predicted	132	soluble form
– expressed	170	only described
Potential N-linked glycosylation sites	11	11[a]
Affinity K_d (M)	$3\text{–}10 \times 10^{-9}$	10^{-10}

[a] Only the soluble form of rat EGFR has been described.

Signal transduction

Binding of EGF to its receptor triggers oligomerization and an increase in receptor affinity. The tyrosine kinase domain then autophosphorylates the receptor [11]. Subsequent events include Tyr phosphorylation of other proteins, including the neu p185 receptor, breakdown of inositol lipids, increase in calcium concentration and activation of Ser/Thr protein kinases. Ser/Thr phosphorylation of the receptor, which can occur by transmodulation from the PDGF receptor, downregulates its affinity. Only the soluble form of the rat receptor has been cloned to date, this has no signal transduction capability [14].

Chromosomal location
The human receptor gene is found on chromosome 7.

Amino acid sequence for human EGF receptor [10]

Accession code: Swissprot P00533

```
 -24   MRPSGTAGAA  LLALLAALCP  ASRA
   1   LEEKKVCQGT  SNKLTQLGTF  EDHFLSLQRM  FNNCEVVLGN  LEITYVQRNY
  51   DLSFLKTIQE  VAGYVLIALN  TVERIPLENL  QIIRGNMYYE  NSYALAVLSN
 101   YDANKTGLKE  LPMRNLQEIL  HGAVRFSNNP  ALCNVESIQW  RDIVSSDFLS
 151   NMSMDFQNHL  GSCQKCDPSC  PNGSCWGAGE  ENCQKLTKII  CAQQCSGRCR
 201   GKSPSDCCHN  QCAAGCTGPR  ESDCLVCRKF  RDEATCKDTC  PPLMLYNPTT
 251   YQMDVNPEGK  YSFGATCVKK  CPRNYVVTDH  GSCVRACGAD  SYEMEEDGVR
 301   KCKKCEGPCR  KVCNGIGIGE  FKDSLSINAT  NIKHFKNCTS  ISGDLHILPV
 351   AFRGDSFTHT  PPLDPQELDI  LKTVKEITGF  LLIQAWPENR  TDLHAFENLE
 401   IIRGRTKQHG  QFSLAVVSLN  ITSLGLRSLK  EISDGDVIIS  GNKNLCYANT
 451   INWKKLFGTS  GQKTKIISNR  GENSCKATGQ  VCHALCSPEG  CWGPEPRDCV
 501   SCRNVSRGRE  CVDKCKLLEG  EPREFVENSE  CIQCHPECLP  QAMNITCTGR
 551   GPDNCIQCAH  YIDGPHCVKT  CPAGVMGENN  TLVWKYADAG  HVCHLCHPNC
 601   TYGCTGPGLE  GCPTNGPKIP  SIATGMVGAL  LLLLVVALGI  GLFMRRRHIV
 651   RKRTLRRLLQ  ERELVEPLTP  SGEAPNQALL  RILKETEFKK  IKVLGSGAFG
 701   TVYKGLWIPE  GEKVKIPVAI  KELREATSPK  ANKEILDEAY  VMASVDNPHV
 751   CRLLGICLTS  TVQLITQLMP  FGCLLDYVRE  HKDNIGSQYL  LNWCVQIAKG
```

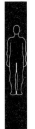

```
 801   MNYLEDRRLV  HRDLAARNVL  VKTPQHVKIT  DFGLAKLLGA  EEKEYHAEGG
 851   KVPIKWMALE  SILHRIYTHQ  SDVWSYGVTV  WELMTFGSKP  YDGIPASEIS
 901   SILEKGERLP  QPPICTIDVY  MIMVKCWMID  ADSRPKFREL  IIEFSKMARD
 951   PQRYLVIQGD  ERMHLPSPTD  SNFYRALMDE  EDMDDVVDAD  EYLIPQQGFF
1001   SSPSTSRTPL  LSSLSATSNN  STVACIDRNG  LQSCPIKEDS  FLQRYSSDPT
1051   GALTEDSIDD  TFLPVPEYIN  QSVPKRPAGS  VQNPVYHNQP  LNPAPSRDPH
1101   YQDPHSTAVG  NPEYLNTVQP  TCVNSTFDSP  AHWAQKGSHQ  ISLDNPDYQQ
1151   DFFPKEAKPN  GIFKGSTAEN  AEYLRVAPQS  SEFIGA
```

Tyr1068, Tyr1148, Tyr1173, Tyr1086 and Thr654 are phosphorylated.

Amino acid sequence for rat EGF receptor (soluble form only) [14]

Accession code: GenEMBL M37394

```
 -24   MRPSGTARTK  LLLLLAALCA  AGGA
   1   LEEKKVCQGT  SNRLTQLGTF  EDHFLSLQRM  FNNCEVVLGN  LEITYVQRNY
  51   DLSFLKTIQE  VAGYVLIALN  TVERIPLENL  QIIRGNALYE  NTYALAVLSN
 101   YGTNKTGLRE  LPMRNLQEIL  IGAVRFSNNP  ILCNMETIQW  RDIVQDVFLS
 151   NMSMDVQRHL  TGCPKCDPSC  PNGSCWGRGE  ENCQKLTKII  CAQQCSRRCR
 201   GRSPSDCCHN  QCAAGCTGPR  ESDCLVCHRF  RDEATCKDTC  PPLMLYNPTT
 251   YQMDVNPEGK  YSFGATCVKK  CPRNYVVTDH  GSCVRACGPD  YYEVEEDGVS
 301   KCKKCDGPCR  KVCNGIGIGE  FKDTLSINAT  NIKHFKYCTA  ISGDLHILPV
 351   AFKGDSFTRT  PPLDPRELEI  LKTVKEITGF  LLIQAWPENW  TDLHAFENLE
 401   IIRGRTKQHG  QFSLAVVGLN  ITSLGLRSLK  EISDGDVIIS  GNRNLCIANT
 451   INWKKLFGTP  NQKTKIMNNR  AEKDCKATNH  VCNPLCSSEG  CWGPEPTDCV
 501   SCQNVSRGRE  CVDKCNILEG  EPREFVENSE  CIQCHPECLP  QTMNITCTGR
 551   GPDNCIKCAH  YVDGPHCVKT  CPSGIMGENN  TLVWKFADAN  NVCHLCHANC
 601   TYGCAGPGLK  GCQQPEGSNY
```

Sequence is for soluble form only.

References
1 Gregory, H. (1975) Nature 257, 325–327.
2 Carpenter, G. and Cohen, S. (1990) J. Biol. Chem. 265, 7709–7712.
3 Burgess, A.W. (1989) In Br. Med. Bull. 45, Growth Factors, Waterfield, M.D., ed., Churchill Livingstone, Edinburgh, pp. 401–424.
4 Bell, G.I. et al. (1986) Nucl. Acids Res. 14, 8427–8446.
5 Gray, A., Dull, T.J. and Ullrich, A. (1983) Nature 303, 722–725.
6 Scott, J. et al. (1983) Science 221, 236–240.
7 Montelione, G.T. et al. (1986) Proc. Natl Acad. Sci. USA 83, 8594–8598.
8 Stroobant, P. et al. (1985) Cell: 42, 383–393.
9 Lee, C.L. et al. (1985) Nature 313, 489–491.
10 Ullrich, A. et al. (1984) Nature 309, 418–425.
11 Ullrich, A. and Schlessinger J (1990) Cell 61, 203–212.
12 Galan, J.E. et al. (1992) Nature 357, 588–589.
13 Eppstein, D.A. et al. (1985) Nature 318, 663–665.
14 Petch, L.A. et al. (1990) Mol. Cell. Biol. 10, 2973–2982.

Epo

Other names
No other names.

THE MOLECULE

Erythropoietin is an unusual cytokine in that it is not produced by haematopoietic cells, only by kidney or liver. It acts as a true hormone, stimulating erythroid precursors to generate red blood cells. It also stimulates platelet generation [1-4].

Crossreactivity
There is about 80% homology between human and mouse Epo [4]. Human Epo is active on murine cells and vice versa.

Sources
Kidney or liver in response to hypoxia or anaemia [5].

Bioassays
Bone marrow erythroid colony formation in methylcellulose, or stimulation of proliferation of TF-1 cell line [6,7].

Physicochemical properties of Epo

Property	Human	Mouse
pI	4–5	4–5
Amino acids – precursor	193	192
– mature[a]	166	165
M_r (K) – predicted	21	21
– expressed	36	34
Potential N-linked glycosylation sites[b]	3	3
Disulphide bonds[c]	2	2

[a] Mature human Epo has C-terminal arginine removed post-translationally.
[b] Human Epo also has 1 O-linked site (Ser126).
[c] disulphide bonds link Cys7–161 and 29–33.

3-D structure
No information.

Gene structure for Human and Mouse Epo [8]

Scale

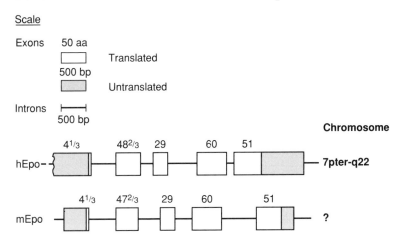

Exons   50 aa

☐   Translated

500 bp

▨   Untranslated

Introns   ├──┤
500 bp

Chromosome

| 4¹/₃ | 48²/₃ | 29 | 60 | 51 |

hEpo─   7pter-q22

| 4¹/₃ | 47²/₃ | 29 | 60 | 51 |

mEpo   ?

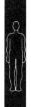

Amino acid sequence for human Epo [3,9]

Accession code: Swissprot P01588

```
-27   MGVHECPAWL  WLLLSLLSLP  LGLPVLG
  1   APPRLICDSR  VLERYLLEAK  EAENITTGCA  EHCSLNENIT  VPDTKVNFYA
 51   WKRMEVGQQA  VEVWQGLALL  SEAVLRGQAL  LVNSSQPWEP  LQLHVDKAVS
101   GLRSLTTLLR  ALGAQKEAIS  PPDAASAAPL  RTITADTFRK  LFRVYSNFLR
151   GKLKLYTGEA  CRTGDR
```

Amino acid sequence for mouse Epo [4]

Accession code: Swissprot P07321

```
-26   MGVPERPTLL  LLLSLLLIPL  GLPVLC
  1   APPRLICDSR  VLERYILEAK  EAENVTMGCA  EGPRLSENIT  VPDTKVNFYA
 51   WKRMEVEEQA  IEVWQGLSLL  SEAILQAQAL  LANSSQPPET  LQLHIDKAIS
101   GLRSLTSLLR  VLGAQKELMS  PPDTTPPAPL  RTLTVDTFCK  LFRVYANFLR
151   GKLKLYTGEV  CRRGDR
```

115

THE EPO RECEPTOR

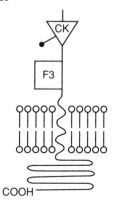

A single class of receptor for Epo, which is a member of the haematopoietin receptor family, has been identified on mouse and human cells [10-12]. The recombinant receptor alone forms high and low affinity structures on COS cells, probably by self-association.

Physicochemical properties of the Epo receptor

Properties	Human	Mouse
Amino acids – precursor	508	507
– mature	484	483
M_r (K) – predicted	55	55
– expressed	85–100	85–100
Potential N-linked glycosylation sites	1	1
Affinity K_d (M)	$0.1–1.1\times10^{-9}$	$0.3–2\times10^{-10}$

Signal transduction

The Epo receptor couples directly to the JAK2 kinase to cause tyrosine phosphorylation [13].

Chromosomal location
The gene for the human Epo receptor is on chromosome 19p [14].

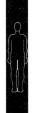

Amino acid sequences for the human Epo receptor [10]

Accession code: Swissprot P19235

```
-24  MDHLGASLWP QVGSLCLLLA GAAW
  1  APPPNLPDPK FESKAALLAA RGPEELLCFT ERLEDLVCFW EEAASAGVGP
 51  GNYSFSYQLE DEPWKLCRLH QAPTARGAVR FWCSLPTADT SSFVPLELRV
101  TAASGAPRYH RVIHINEVVL LDAPVGLVAR LADESGHVVL RWLPPPETPM
151  TSHIRYEVDV SAGNGAGSVQ RVEILEGRTE CVLSNLRGRT RYTFAVRARM
201  AEPSFGGFWS AWSEPVSLLT PSDLDPLILT LSLILVVILV LLTVLALLSH
251  RRALKQKIWP GIPSPESEFE GLFTTHKGNF QLWLYQNDGC LWWSPCTPFT
301  EDPPASLEVL SERCWGTMQA VEPGTDDEGP LLEPVGSEHA QDTYLVLDKW
351  LLPRNPPSED LPGPGGSVDI VAMDEGSEAS SCSSALASKP SPEGASAASF
401  EYTILDPSSQ LLRPWTLCPE LPPTPPHLKY LYLVVSDSGI STDYSSGDSQ
```

Residues 112–128 are also predicted to be a transmembrane spanning sequence. Disulphide bonds between Cys28–38 and 67–83.

Amino acid sequences for the mouse Epo receptor [11]

Accession code: Swissprot P14753

```
-24  MDKLRVPLWP RVGPLCLLLA GAAW
  1  APSPSLPDPK FESKAALLAS RGSEELLCFT QRLEDLVCFW EEAASSGMDF
 51  NYSFSYQLEG ESRKSCSLHQ APTVRGSVRF WCSLPTADTS SFVPLELQVT
101  EASGSPRYHR IIHINEVVLL DAPAGLLARR AEEGSHVVLR WLPPPGAPMT
151  THIRYEVDVS AGNRAGGTQR VEVLEGRTEC VLSNLRGGTR YTFAVRARMA
201  EPSFSGFWSA WSEPASLLTA SDLDPLILTL SLILVLISLL LTVLALLSHR
251  RTLQQKIWPG IPSPESEFEG LFTTHKGNFQ LWLLQRDGCL WWSPGSSFPE
301  DPPAHLEVLS EPRWAVTQAG DPGADDEGPL LEPVGSEHAQ DTYLVLDKWL
351  LPRTPCSENL SGPGGSVDPV TMDEASETSS CPSDLASKPR PEGTSPSSFE
401  YTILDPSSQL LCPRALPPEL PPTPPHLKYL YLVVSDSGIS TDYSSGGSQG
451  VHGDSSDGPY SHPYENSLVP DSEPLHPGYV ACS
```

Residues 111–127 are also predicted to be a transmembrane spanning sequence. Disulphide bonds between Cys28–38 and 66–82.

References
1 Krantz, S.B. (1991) Blood 77, 419–434.
2 Spivak, J.L. (1989) Nephron 52, 289–294.
3 Jacobs, K. et al (1985) Nature 313, 806–810.
4 Shoemaker, C.B. and Mitsock, L.D. (1986) Mol. Cell. Biol. 6, 849–858.
5 Schuster, S.J. et al (1987) Blood 70, 316–318.
6 Krumwieh, D. et al. (1988) In Cytokines: Laboratory and Clinical Evaluation., Vol. 69, Developments in Biological Standardisation, Gearing, A.J.H. and Hennessen, W. eds, Karger, Basle, pp. 15–22.
7 Gearing, A.J.H. et al (1994) In The Cytokine Handbook, Thomson, A.W., ed., Academic press, London (in press).
8 Law, M.L. et al (1986) Proc. Natl. Acad. Sci. USA 83, 6920–6924.
9 Lin, F.-K. et al (1985) Proc. Natl. Acad. Sci. USA 82, 7580–7584.
10 Jones, S.S. et al (1990) Blood 76, 31–35.

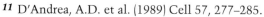

11 D'Andrea, A.D. et al. (1989) Cell 57, 277–285.

12 Kuramochi, S. et al. (1990) J. Mol. Biol. 216, 567–575.

13 Witthuhn, B.A. et al (1993) Cell 74, 227–236.

14 Winkelmann, J.C. et al (1990) Blood 76, 24–30.

FGF

Other names

aFGF: Heparin binding growth factor (HBGF-1), endothelial cell growth factor (ECGF), embryonic kidney-derived angiogenesis factor I, astroglial growth factor I, retina-derived growth factor, eye derived growth factor II, prostatropin.

bFGF: Leukaemia growth factor, macrophage growth factor, embryonic kidney-derived angiogenesis factor 2, prostatic growth factor, astroglial growth factor 2, endothelial growth factor, tumour angiogenesis factor, hepatoma growth factor, chondrosarcoma growth factor, cartilage-derived growth factor, eye-derived growth factor I, heparin binding growth factors class II, myogenic growth factor, human placenta purified factor, uterine-derived growth factor, embryonic carcinoma-derived growth factor, human pituitary growth factor, pituitary-derived chondrocyte growth factor, adipocyte growth factor, prostatic osteoblastic factor, mammary tumour-derived growth factor.

THE MOLECULES

Basic FGF (bFGF) and acidic FGF (aFGF) are modulators of cell proliferation, motility, differentiation and angiogenesis [1]. Both factors have a high affinity for heparin and are found associated with the extracellular matrix [1-3]. Several cellular proto-oncogenes with sequence homology (40-50%) to aFGF and bFGF have been identified in humans [4,5] and mice [6] (see FGF family below). Some of these such as INT-2, are expressed primarily during embryogenesis and are under tight temporal control suggesting that they play an important role in early development. Only aFGF and bFGF are described in detail below.

Crossreactivity

There is 95% homology between human and mouse aFGF and bFGF, and complete cross-species reactivity.

Sources

aFGF: Detected in large amounts only in the brain; lesser amounts in retina, bone matrix, osteoblasts, astrocytes, kidney, endothelial cells and foetal vascular smooth muscle cells.

bFGF: Brain, retina, pituitary, kidney, placenta, testis, corpus luteum, adrenal glands, monocytes, prostate, bone, liver, cartilage, endothelial cells, epithelial cells.

Bioassays

Proliferation of vascular endothelial cells.

THE FGF FAMILY

Name	Amino acids (human)[a]	Secreted form	Major tissue localization[b]	Human chromosome	Known receptors	Swissprot accession codes Human	Mouse
aFGF (FGF-1)	155	Not secreted	Adult tissue	5q31.3–q33.2	FGFR-1,2,3,4	P05230 P07502	P10935
bFGF (FGF-2)	155	Not secreted	Adult and embryonic tissue	4q25–q27	FGFR-1,2	P09038	P15655
INT-2 (FGF-3)	239	ND	Embryonic tissue	11q13		P11487	P05524
K-FGF/HST (FGF-4)	206	176	Embryonic tissue	11q13.3	FGFR-1,2	P08620	P11403
FGF-5	267	ND	Neonatal brain	4q21		P12034	P15656
FGF-6	208	ND	Embryonic	12p13	FGFR-2 (variant)	P10767	P21658
KGF (FGF-7)	194	163	Dermis, kidney gastrointestinal tract	Unassigned		P21781	Unassigned

[a] Primary translation product.
[b] References 4, 5.

Physicochemical properties of acidic and basic FGF

Property	aFGF Human	Mouse	bFGF Human	Mouse
pI	5.4	5.4	9.6	9.6
Amino acids – precursor	155	155	155 196[a] 201[a] 210[a]	154
– mature[b]	155 140	155 140	155 146[c]	154 145
M_r (K) – predicted[d]	17.5	17.4	17.3	17.2
– expressed	16	16–18	16.5[e] 18 22.5[a] 23.1[a] 24.2[a]	16.5[e]
Potential N-linked glycosylation sites	1	1	0	0
Disulphide bonds	0	0	0	0

[a] Long forms arising by translation from upstream CUG initiation sites (see sequence).

[b] The predominant form of aFGF is 155 amino acids in length and the predominant form of bFGF is 155 (human), 154 (mouse) amino acids. There is no typical signal peptide. Removal of N-terminal propeptide (15 amino acids in aFGF and 9 amino acids in bFGF) gives rise to truncated forms which are still active. Another truncated form coded for by exon 1 with an additional four C-terminal amino acids has been described and shown to be an antagonist to the full length form [7] (see sequence).

[c] Smaller truncated forms which retain biological activity have been isolated from different tissues, but it is not known whether these are due to in vivo processing or artefacts of extraction and purification.

[d] Primary translation product

[e] For 146 and 145 amino acid product.

3-D structure

X-Ray crystallography to a resolution of 1.8 Å has shown that bFGF is composed entirely of a β-sheet structure with a threefold repeat of a four stranded antiparallel β-meander which forms a barrel-like structure with three loops. The topology of bFGF is very similar to IL-1. The receptor and heparin binding sites are adjacent but separate determinants on the β-barrel [8,9].

Gene structure [10–13]

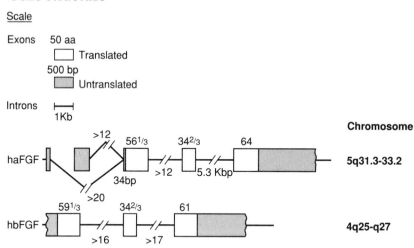

Scale

Exons   50 aa

□ Translated

500 bp

▨ Untranslated

Introns ⊢⊣
    1Kb

Chromosome

haFGF   5q31.3-33.2

hbFGF   4q25-q27

Different sized aFGF mRNA species containing alternative 5′ untranslated sequences coded for by additional upstream exons have been described and shown to be expressed in a tissue-specific manner [14].

The gene structures for mouse FGFs have not been described.

Note: A new amino acid numbering system for the FGFs has been proposed in which the amino acid immediately following the initiation Met is designated as amino acid number 1. For consistency with the rest of this book we have not followed this proposal but designated the initiation Met itself as number 1.

Amino acid sequence for human aFGF (FGF-1) [10–13]

Accession code: Swissprot P05230, P07502

```
  1  MAEGEITTFT ALTEKFNLPP GNYKKPKLLY CSNGGHFLRI LPDGTVDGTR
 51  DRSDQHIQLQ LSAESVGEVY IKSTETGQYL AMDTDGLLYG SQTPNEECLF
101  LERLEENHYN TYISKKHAEK NWFVGLKKNG SCKRGPRTHY GQKAILFLPL
151  PVSSD
```

aFGF has no signal sequence. Truncated forms of 140 and 134 amino acids in length arise by cleavage between amino acids Lys15/Phe16 and Gly21/Asn22. An FGF antagonist has been identified consisting of the first 56 amino acids coded for by exon 1 and an additional four amino acids (TDTK) forming the C-terminus [7]. Cys residues at positions 31 and 98 are conserved in all members of the FGF family but do not form disulphide bonds.

Amino acid sequence for human bFGF (FGF-2) [15,16]

Accession code: Swissprot P09038

```
-55   LGDRGRGRAL PGGRLGGRGR GRAPQRVGGR GRGRGTAAPR AAPAARGSRP
 -5   GPAGT
  1   MAAGSITTLP ALPEDGGSGA FPPGHFKDPK RLYCKNGGFF LRIHPDGRVD
 51   GVREKSDPHI KLQLQAEERG VVSIKGVCAN RYLAMKEDGR LLASKCVTDE
101   CFFFERLESN NYNTYRSRKY TSWYVALKRT GQYKLGSKTG PGQKAILFLP
151   MSAKS
```

bFGF has no signal sequence. High molecular weight forms (M_r 24 200, 23 100, 22 500) arise by initiation of translation at CUG triplets coding for Leu residues (bold) at positions –55, –46, and –41 [17,18]. Truncated form arises by cleavage between amino acids Lys9/Pro10. It is not clear whether these are formed *in vivo* or are artefacts of purification. Cys residues at positions 34 and 101 are conserved in all members of the FGF family, but do not form disulphide bonds.

Amino acid sequence for mouse aFGF (FGF-1) [6,19]

Accession code: Swissprot P10935

```
  1   MAEGEITTFA ALTERFNLPL GNYKKPKLLY CSNGGHFLRI LPDGTVDGTR
 51   DRSDQHIQLQ LSAESAGEVY IKGTETGQYL AMDTEGLLYG SQTPNEECLF
101   LERLEENHYN TYTSKKHAEK NWFVGLKKNG SCKRGPRTHY GQKAILFLPL
151   PVSSD
```

aFGF has no signal sequence. Truncated form arises by cleavage between amino acids Arg15/Phe16. Cys residues at positions 31 and 98 are conserved in all members of the FGF family, but do not form disulphide bonds.

Amino acid sequence for mouse bFGF (FGF-2) [6]

Accession code: Swissprot P15655

```
  1   MAASGITSLP ALPEDGGAAF PPGHFKDPKR LYCKNGGFFL RIHPDGRVDG
 51   VREKSDPHVK LQLQAEERGV VSIKGVCANR YLAMKEDGRL LASKCVTEEC
101   FFFERLESNN YNTYRSRKYS SWYVALKRTG QYKLGSKTGP GQKAILFLPM
151   SAKS
```

bFGF has no signal sequence. Truncated form arises by cleavage between amino acids Lys9/Pro10. Cys 33 and 100 are conserved in all members of the FGF family, but do not form disulphide bonds.

THE FGF RECEPTORS

FGFR-1

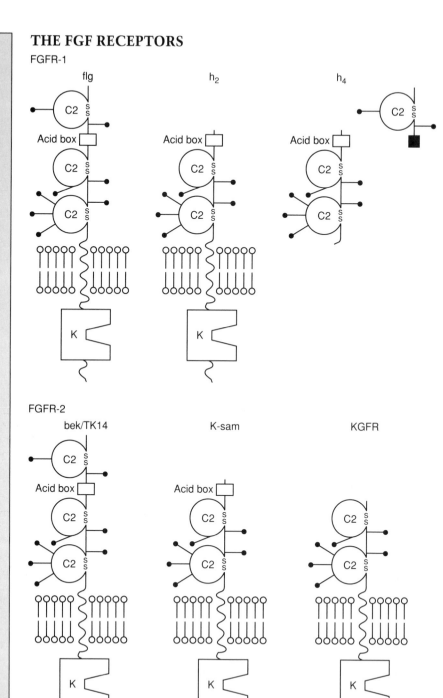

FGFR-2

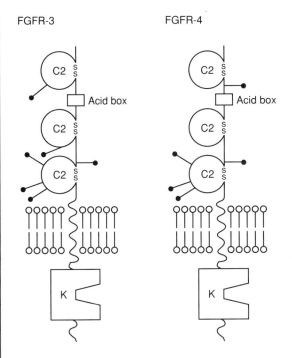

FGFR-3   FGFR-4

FGF binds to both low affinity and high affinity receptors [20]. Low affinity receptors are heparan sulphate proteoglycans. Binding of FGF to heparin and other glycosaminoglycans (GAGs) protects FGF from degradation and can hold FGF in the extracellular matrix as a reservoir. FGF also binds to cell surface heparan sulphate proteoglycans, but it is not clear whether these can signal. FGF binds simultaneously to low affinity heparan sulphate proteoglycan and to the high affinity receptor [21].

High affinity FGF receptors are members of a complex family of receptors characterized by between 1 and 3 extracellular Ig-SF domains determined by alternative mRNA splicing, and an intracellular tyrosine kinase split by a short inserted sequence of 14 amino acids [20]. Between the first and second Ig-SF domains there is a unique motif that has not been seen in other growth factor receptors consisting of eight consecutive acidic residues called the "acid box". There are at least four distinct receptors: FGFR-1 (flg), FGFR-2 (bek), FGFR-3 and FGFR-4 coded for by separate genes. For FGFR-1 and FGFR-2, at least, alternative splicing gives rise to multiple forms, including soluble receptors [22]. The different names given to these receptors and their splice variants are shown in the table below and in the receptor diagram. The receptors have distinct patterns of expression on different tissues. On binding aFGF or bFGF the receptors form dimers. Dimerization is required for signal transduction involving auto- or inter-chain phosphorylation [23]. FGF receptors have been shown to be receptors for Herpes Simplex virus type 1 [24].

Physicochemical properties of the FGF receptors

Properties	FGFR-1 (flg)		FGFR-2 (bek)		FGFR-3		FGFR-4	
	Human	Mouse	Human	Mouse	Human	Mouse	Human	Mouse
amino acids – precursor[a]	822	822	821	820	806	801	802	808
– mature	801	802	800	800	784	781	778	790
M_r (K) – predicted[b]	89.4	89.7	89.7	89.8	85.8	85.8	85.5	87.8
– expressed[b]	160	145	135	150	135	?	140	?
				125	125			
					97			
Potential N-linked glycosylation sites	8	8	8	9	6	6	5	5
Affinity (K_d)	Usually between 2×10^{-9} M and 5×10^{-10} M							

[a] There are multiple forms of FGFR-1 and FGFR-2 which arise from alternative mRNA splicing (see sequence).
[b] M_r given are for full length forms. Variants of human FGFR-3 are due to glycosylation.

Names given to the different FGF receptors [20]

FGFR-1	FGFR-2	FGFR-3	FGFR-4
flg	bek	Cek2	FGFR-4
bFGFR	Cek3	FGFR-3	
Cek1	K-sam		
N-bFGFR	TK14		
h2, h3	TK25		
h4, h5	KGFR		
FGFR-1	FGFR-2		

There is a very high degree of homology between human and mouse FGF receptors: 98% for FGFR-1 with only three amino acid differences in the intracellular domain.

Distribution [25,26]

FGFR-1 (flg) mRNA is highly expressed in human foetal brain, skin, growth plates of developing bones and calvarial bones with lesser amounts in other tissues. FGFR-2 (bek) mRNA is expressed in brain, choroid plexus, liver, lung, intestine, kidney, skin, growth plates of developing bone, and calvarial bone. FGFR-3 mRNA is expressed in brain, lung, intestine, kidney, skin, growth plates of developing bones and calvarial bone. FGFR-4 mRNA is expressed in human foetal adrenals, lung, kidney, liver, pancreas, intestine, striated muscle and spleen.

Signal transduction

The FGF receptors belong to the split tyrosine kinase receptor family which includes PDGFR and c-kit. Ligand binding induces dimerization and inter-chain and/or autophosphorylation [27]. The receptor binds to and activates PLC-γ through Tyr766 (FGFR-1) and stimulates the PI second messenger pathway. Receptors are internalized, and degradation is slow and partial.

Chromosomal location

	Human	Mouse
FGFR-1	8p12	8
FGFR-2	10q25.3–q26	7
FGFR-3	4p16.3	
FGFR-4	5q33–qter	

Amino acid sequence for human FGFR-1 (flg) [28–31]

Accession code: Swissprot P11362, P17049

```
-21  MWSWKCLLFW AVLVTATLCT A
  1  RPSPTLPEQA QPWGAPEVEVE SFLVHPGDLL QLRCRLRDDV QSINWLRDGV
 51  QLAESNRTRI TGEEVEVQDS VPADSGLYAC VTSSPSGSDT TYFSVNVSDA
101  LPSSEDDDDD DDSSSEEKET DNTKPNRMPV APYWTSPEKM EKKLHAVPAA
151  KTVKFKCPSS GTPNPTLRWL KNGKEFKPDH RIGGYKVRYA TWSIIMDSVV
201  PSDKGNYTCI VENEYGSINH TYQLDVVERS PHRPILQAGL PANKTVALGS
251  NVEFMCKVYS DPQPHIQWLK HIEVNGSKIG PDNLPYVQIL KTAGVNTTDK
301  EMEVLHLRNV SFEDAGEYTC LAGNSIGLSH HSAWLTVLEA LEERPAVMTS
351  PLYLEIIIYC TGAFLISCMV GSVIVYKMKS GTKKSDFHSQ MAVHKLAKSI
401  PLRRQVTVSA DSSASMNSGV LLVRPSRLSS SGTPMLAGVS EYELPEDPRW
451  ELPRDRLVLG KPLGEGCFGQ VVLAEAIGLD KDKPNRVTKV AVKMLKSDAT
501  EKDLSDLISE MEMMKMIGKH KNIINLLGAC TQDGPLYVIV EYASKGNLRE
551  YLQARRPPGL EYCYNPSHNP EEQLSSKDLV SCAYQVARGM EYLASKKCIH
601  RDLAARNVLV TEDNVMKIAD FGLARDIHHI DYYKKTTNGR LPVKWMAPEA
651  LFDRIYTHQS DVWSFGVLLW EIFTLGGSPY PGVPVEELFK LLKEGHRMDK
701  PSNCTNELYM MMRDCWHAVP SQRPTFKQLV EDLDRIVALT SNQEYLDLSM
751  PLDQYSPSFP DTRSSTCSSG EDSVFSHEPL PEEPCLPRHP AQLANGGLKR
801  R
```

There are several alternative forms of the FGFR-1 receptor derived by alternative splicing [20] (see receptor diagram). Two full length forms vary only by the presence or absence of two amino acids (Arg and Met) at positions 127–128. Short forms are missing amino acids 31–119 comprising the first Ig domain. These also vary by the presence or absence of the Arg–Met dipeptide at positions 127–128. Soluble forms have been described in which the C-terminal 510 amino acids have been replaced by the unique 79 amino acid C-terminal sequence:

```
VIMAPVFVGQ STGKETTVSG AQVPVGRLSC PRMGSFLTLQ AHTLHLSRDL
ATSPRTSNRG HKVEVSWEQR AAGMGGAGL
```

Another soluble form has a complete Ig domain 1 followed by 32 unique amino acids and a stop codon. Conflicting amino acid sequence ALFDRI->IYLTGS at positions 650–655 and G->R at position 796. Phosphorylated tyrosines at positions 632, 745. Tyr745 is required for PLC-γl association and activation.

Amino acid sequence for human FGFR-2 (bek) [29]

Accession code: Swissprot P21802

```
-21  MVSWGRFICL VVVTMATLSL A
  1  RPSFSLVEDT TLEPEEPPTK YQISQPEVYV AAPGESLEVR CLLKDAAVIS
 51  WTKDGVHLGP NNRTVLIGEY LQIKGATPRD SGLYACTASR TVDSETWYFM
101  VNVTDAISSG DDEDDTDGAE DFVSENSNNK RAPYWTNTEK MEKRLHAVPA
151  ANTVKFRCPA GGNPMPTMRW LKNGKEFKQE HRIGGYKVRN QHWSLIMESV
201  VPSDKGNYTC VVENEYGSIN HTYHLDVVER SPHRPILQAG LPANASTVVG
251  GDVEFVCKVY SDAQPHIQWI KHVEKNGSKY GPDGLPYLKV LKAAGVNTTD
301  KEIEVLYIRN VTFEDAGEYT CLAGNSIGIS FHSAWLTVLP APGREKEITA
```

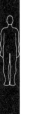

```
351   SPDYLEIAIY CIGVFLIACM VVTVILCRMK NTTKKPDFSS QPAVHKLTKR
401   IPLRRQVTVS AESSSSMNSN TPLVRITTRL SSTADTPMLA GVSEYELPED
451   PKWEFPRDKL TLGKPLGEGC FGQVVMAEAV GIDKDKPKEA VTVAVKMLKD
501   DATEKDLSDL VSEMEMMKMI GKHKNIINLL GACTQDGPLY VIVEYASKGN
551   LREYLRARRP PGMEYSYDIN RVPEEQMTFK DLVSCTYQLA RGMEYLASQK
601   CIHRDLAARN VLVTENNVMK IADFGLARDI NNIDYYKKTT NGRLPVKWMA
651   PEALFDRVYT HQSDVWSFGV LMWEIFTLGG SPYPGIPVEE LFKLLKEGHR
701   MDKPANCTNE LYMMMRDCWH AVPSQRPTFK QLVEDLDRIL TLTTNEEYLD
751   LSQPLEQYSP SYPDTRSSCS SGDDSVFSPD PMPYEPCLPQ YPHINGSVKT
```

There are several alternative forms of the FGFR-2 receptor derived by alternative splicing using different exons [32] (see receptor diagram). One of the alternative forms is a receptor for KGF and aFGF (FGFR-2 does not bind KGF) and is expressed only on epithelial cells. It is identical to FGFR-2 except for two missing amino acids (Ala–Ala) at positions 293–294 followed immediately by a divergent 38 amino acid sequence (HSGINSSNAE VLALFNVTEA DAGEYICKVS NYIGQANQ) from position 295–332 corresponding to the second half of the third Ig domain, an insert of three amino acids (Lys–Gln–Gln) between residues 340 and 341, and a G->R substitution at position 592. The second variant (K-SAM) [33] has a deletion of 87 amino acids from positions 18–104 which includes the first Ig domain, and a deletion of two amino acids (Val–Thr) at positions 407–408. As with the KGF receptor, it has two missing amino acids (Ala–Ala) at positions 293–294, followed by the divergent 38 amino acid sequence from positions 295–332, and the Lys–Gln–Gln insert between residues 340 and 341. It also has a truncated C-terminus ending with a divergent 12 amino acid sequence (PPNPSLMSIF RK) from position 740. Tyr 635 is autophosphorylated.

Amino acid sequence for human FGFR-3 [34,35]

Accession code: Swissprot P22607

```
-22   MGAPACALAL CVAVAIVAGA SS
  1   ESLGTEQRVV GRAAEVPGPE PGQQEQLVFG SGDAVELSCP PPGGGPMGPT
 51   VWVKDGTGLV PSERVLVGPQ RLQVLNASHE DSGAYSCRQR LTQRVLCHFS
101   VRVTDAPSSG DDEDGEDEAE DTGVDTGAPY WTRPERMDKK LLAVPAANTV
151   RFRCPAAGNP TPSISWLKNG REFRGEHRIG GIKLRHQQWS LVMESVVPSD
201   RGNYTCVVEN KFGSIRQTYT LDVLERSPHR PILQAGLPAN QTAVLGSDVE
251   FHCKVYSDAQ PHIQWLKHVE VNGSKVGPDG TPYVTVLKTA GANTTDKELE
301   VLSLHNVTFE DAGEYTCLAG NSIGFSHHSA WLVVLPAEEE LVEADEAGSV
351   YAGILSYGVG FFLFILVVAA VTLCRLRSPP KKGLGSPTVH KISRFPLKRQ
401   VSLESNASMS SNTPLVRIAR LSSGEGPTLA NVSELELPAD PKWELSRARL
451   TLGKPLGEGC FGQVVMAEAI GIDKDRAAKP VTVAVKMLKD DATDKDLSDL
501   VSEMEMMKMI GKHKNIINLL GACTQGGPLY VLVEYAAKGN LREFLRARRP
551   PGLDYSFDTC KPPEEQLTFK DLVSCAYQVA RGMEYLASQK CIHRDLAARN
601   VLVTEDNVMK IADFGLARDV HNLDYYKKTT NGRLPVKWMA PEALFDRVYT
651   HQSDVWSFGV LLWEIFTLGG SPYPGIPVEE LFKLLKEGHR MDKPANCTHD
701   LYMIMRECWH AAPSQRPTFK QLVEDLDRVL TVTSTDEYLD LSAPFEQYSP
751   GGQDTPSSSS SGDDSVFAHD LLPPAPPSSG GSRT
```

Tyr625 is site of autophosphorylation by similarity.

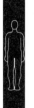

Amino acid sequence for human FGFR-4 [25,35]

Accession code: Swissprot P22455

```
 -24  MRLLLALLGV  LLSVPGPPVL  SLEA
   1  SEEVELEPCL  APSLEQQEQE  LTVALGQPVR  LCCGRAERGG  HWYKEGSRLA
  51  PAGRVRGWRG  RLEIASFLPE  DAGRYLCLAR  GSMIVLQNLT  LITGDSLTSS
 101  NDDEDPKSHR  DPSNRHSYPQ  QAPYWTHPQR  MEKKLHAVPA  GNTVKFRCPA
 151  AGNPTPTIRW  LKDGQAFHGE  NRIGGIRLRH  QHWSLVMESV  VPSDRGTYTC
 201  LVENAVGSIR  YNYLLDVLER  SPHRPILQAG  LPANTTAVVG  SDVELLCKVY
 251  SDAQPHIQWL  KHIVINGSSF  GAVGFPYVQV  LKTADINSSE  VEVLYLRNVS
 301  AEDAGEYTCL  AGNSIGLSYQ  SAWLTVLPEE  DPTWTAAAPE  ARYTDIILYA
 351  SGSLALAVLL  LLAGLYRGQA  LHGRHPRPPA  TVQKLSRFPL  ARQFSLESGS
 401  SGKSSSSLVR  GVRLSSSGPA  LLAGLVSLDL  PLDPLWEFPR  DRLVLGKPLG
 451  EGCFGQVVRA  EAFGMDPARP  DQASTVAVKM  LKDNASDKDL  ADLVSEMEVM
 501  KLIGRHKNII  NLLGVCTQEG  PLYVIVECAA  KGNLREFLRA  RRPPGPDLSP
 551  DGPRSSEGPL  SFPVLVSCAY  QVARGMQYLE  SRKCIHRDLA  ARNVLVTEDN
 601  VMKIADFGLA  RGVHHIDYYK  KTSNGRLPVK  WMAPEALFDR  VYTHQSDVWS
 651  FGILLWEIFT  LGGSPYPGIP  VEELFSLLRE  GHRMDRPPHC  PPELYGLMRE
 701  CWHAAPSQRP  TFKQLVEALD  KVLLAVSEEY  LDLRLTFGPY  SPSGGDASST
 751  CSSSDSVFSH  DPLPLGSSSF  PFGSGVQT
```

Tyr618 is potential site of autophosphorylation by similarity.

Amino acid sequence for mouse FGFR-1 (flg) [36–38]

Accession code: Swissprot P16092

```
 -20  MWGWKCLLFW  AVLVTATLCT
   1  ARPAPTLPEQ  AQPWGVPVEV  ESLLVHPGDL  LQLRCRLRDD  VQSINWLRDG
  51  VQLVESNRTR  ITGEEVEVRD  SIPADSGLYA  CVTSSPSGSD  TTYFSVNVSD
 101  ALPSSEDDDD  DDDSSSEEKE  TDNTKPNRRP  VAPYWTSPEK  MEKKLHAVPA
 151  AKTVKFKCPS  SGTPNPTLRW  LKNGKEFKPD  HRIGGYKVRY  ATWSIIMDSV
 201  VPSDKGNYTC  IVENEYGSIN  HTYQLDVVER  SPHRPILQAG  LPANKTVALG
 251  SNVEFMCKVY  SDPQPHIQWL  KHIEVNGSKI  GPDNLPYVQI  LKTAGVNTTD
 301  KEMEVLHLRN  VSFEDAGEYT  CLAGNSIGLS  HHSAWLTVLE  ALEERPAVMT
 351  SPLYLEIIIY  CTGAFLISCM  LGSVIIYKMK  SGTKKSDFHS  QMAVHKLAKS
 401  IPLRRQVTVS  ADSSASMNSG  VLLVRPSRLS  SSGTPMLAGV  SEYELPEDPR
 451  WELPRDRLVL  GKPLGEGCFG  QVVLAEAIGL  DKDKPNRVTK  VAVKMLKSDA
 501  TEKDLSDLIS  EMEMMKMIGK  HKNIINLLGA  CTQDGPLYVI  VEYASKGNLR
 551  EYLQARRPPG  LEYCYNPSHN  PEEQLSSKDL  VSCAYQVARG  MEYLASKKCI
 601  HRDLAARNVL  VTEDNVMKIA  DFGLARDIHH  IDYYKKTTNG  RLPVKWMAPE
 651  ALFDRIYTHQ  SDVWSFGVLL  WEIFTLGGSP  YPGVPVEELF  KLLKEGHRMD
 701  KPSNCTNELY  MMMRDCWHAV  PSQRPTFKQL  VEDLDRIVAL  TSNQEYLDLS
 751  IPLDQYSPSF  PDTRSSTCSS  GEDSVFSHEP  LPEEPCLPRH  PTQLANSGLK
 801  RR
```

Splice variants using three alternative exons for the third Ig domain give
rise to different receptor forms (a) with a divergent sequence (SGINSSDAEV
LTLFNVTEAQ SGEYVCKVSN YIGEANQSAW LTV) from position 296–338 and (b)
with a divergent sequence (VLLTSFLG) followed by a stop codon, which have

different tissue expression and binding affinities for bFGF [39]. The second of these (b) codes for a secreted receptor that lacks transmembrane and cytoplasmic sequences including part of the third Ig domain. In another splice variant, 89 amino acids (11–99), including the first Ig domain, are missing [38]. Tyr 633 is a potential site of autophosphorylation by similarity.

Conflicting amino acid sequences T->S at position 209, ILQ->HPS at positions 236–238, G->A at position 250, G->A at position 420, I->M at position 524, VL->LV at positions 609–610, R->H at position 736, and E->D at position 745. In addition, the dipeptide Arg–Arg at positions 128 and 129 is missing in one sequence [37]. This may be a splice variant similar to that described for human FGFR-1.

Amino acid sequence for mouse FGFR-2 (bek) [40]

Accession code: GenEMBL X55441 and Swissprot P21803 for splice variant missing amino acids 19–132.

```
 -21   MVSWGRFICL VLVTMATLSL A
   1   RPSFSLVEDT TLEPEEPPTK YQISQPEAYV VVPRGSLELQ CMLKDAAVIS
  51   WTKDGVHLGP NNRTVLIGRY LQIKGATPRD SGLYACTAAR TVDSETWYFM
 101   VNVTDAISSG DDEDDTDSSE RVSENRSNQR APYWTNTEKM EKRLHAVPAA
 151   NTVKFRCPAG GNPTPTMRWL KNGKEFKQEH RIGGYKVRNQ HRSLIMESVV
 201   PSDKGNITCL VENEYGSINH TYHLDVVERS PHRPILQAGL PANASTVVGG
 251   DVRFVCKVYS DAQPHIQWIK HVEKNGSKYG PDGLPYLKVL KAAGVNTTDK
 301   EIEVLYIRNV TFEDAGEYTC LAGNSIGISF HSAWLTVLPA PVREKEITAS
 351   PDYLEIAIYC IGVFLIACMV VTVIFCRMKT TTKKPDFSSQ PAVHKLTKRI
 401   PLRRQVTVSA ESSSSMNSNT PLVRITTRLS STADTPMLAG VSEYELPEDP
 451   KWEFPRDKLT LGKPLGEGCF GQVVMAEAVG IDKDKPKEAV TVAVKMLKDD
 501   ATEKDLSDLV SEMEMMKMIG KHKNIINLLG ACTQDGPLYV IVEYASKGNL
 551   REYLRARRPP GMEYSYDINR VPEEQMTFKD LVSCTYQLAR GMEYLASQKC
 601   IHRDLAARNV LVTENNVMKI ADFGLARDIN NIDYYKKTTN GRLPVKWMAP
 651   EALFDRVYTH QSDVWSFGVL MWEIFTLGGS PYPGIPVEEL FKLLKEGHRM
 701   DKPTNCTNEL YMMMRDCWHA VPSQRPTFKQ LVEDLDRILT LTTNEEYLDL
 751   TQPLEQYSPS YPDTSSSCSS GDDSVFSPDP MPYEPCLPQY PHINGSVKT
```

There is a variant similar to human K-SAM (see human FGFR-2 above) [32] which is missing 114 amino acids including the first Ig domain at positions 19–132, and has an I->Y substitution at position 207, an R->E substitution at position 253, two missing amino acids (Ala–Ala) at positions 292–293 followed by a divergent 38 amino acid sequence (HSGINSSNAE VLALFNVTEM DAGEYICKVS NYIGQANQ) from positions 294–331, and a Lys–Gln–Gln insert between amino acids 339 and 340. Tyr634 is a potential site of autophosphorylation by similarity.

Amino acid sequence for mouse FGFR-3 [41]

Accession code: GenEMBL M81342

```
 -20  MVVPACVLVF  CVAVVAGATS
   1  EPPGPEQRVV  RRAAEVPGPE  PSQQEQVAFG  SGDTVELSCH  PPGGAPTGPT
  51  VWAKDGTGLV  ASHRILVGPQ  RLQVLNASHE  DAGVYSCQHR  LTRRVLCHFS
 101  VRVTDAPSSG  DDEDGEDVAE  DTGAPYWTRP  ERMDKKLLAV  PAANTVRFRC
 151  PAAGNPTPSI  SWLKNGKEFR  GEHRIGGIKL  RHQQWSLVME  SVVPSDRGNY
 201  TCVVENKFGS  IRQTYTLDVL  ERSPHRPILQ  AGLPANQTAI  LGSDVEFHCK
 251  VYSDAQPHIQ  WLKHVEVNGS  KVGPDGTPYV  TVLKTAGANT  TDKELEVLSL
 301  HNVTFEDAGE  YTCLAGNSIG  FSHHSAWLVV  LPAEEELMET  DEAGSVYAGV
 351  LSYGVVFFLF  ILVVAAVILC  RLRSPPKKGL  GSPTVHKVSR  FPLKRQVSLE
 401  SNSSMNSNTP  LVRIARLSSG  EGPVLANVSE  LELPADPKWE  LSRTRLTLGK
 451  PLGEGCFGQV  VMAEAIGIDK  DRTAKPVTVA  VKMLKDDATD  KDLSDLVSEM
 501  EMMKMIGKHK  NIINLLGACT  QGGPLYVLVE  YAAKGNLREF  LRARRPPGMD
 551  YSFDACRLPE  EQLTCKDLVS  CAYQVARGME  YLASQKCIHR  DLAARNVLVT
 601  EDNVMKIADF  GLARDVHNLD  YYKKTTNGRL  PVKWMAPEAL  FDRVYTHQSD
 651  VWSFGVLLWE  IFTPGGPSPY  PGIPVEELFK  LLKEGHRMDK  PASCTHDLYM
 701  IMRECWHAVP  SQRPTFKQLV  EDLDRILTVT  STDEYLDLSV  PFEQYSPGGQ
 751  DTPSSSSSGD  DSVFTHDLLP  PGPPSNGGPR  T
```

Tyr621 is a potential site of autophosphorylation by similarity.

Amino acid sequence for mouse FGFR-4 [42]

Accession code: GenEMBL X59927

```
 -18  MWLLLALLSI  FQGTPALS
   1  LEASEEMEQE  PCLAPILEQQ  EQVLTVALGQ  PVRLCCGRTE  RGRHWYKEGS
  51  RLASAGRVRG  WRGRLEIASF  LPEDAGRYLC  LARGSMTVVH  NLTLLMDDSL
 101  TSISNDEDPK  TLSSSSSGHV  YPQQAPYWTH  PQRMEKKLHA  VPAGNTVKFR
 151  CPACRNPMPT  IHWLKDGQAF  HGENRIGGIR  LRHQHWSLVM  ESVVPSDRGT
 201  YTCLVENSLG  SIRYSYLLDV  LERSPHRPIL  QAGLPANTTA  VVGSDVELLC
 251  KVYSDAQPHI  QWLKHVVING  SSFGADGFPY  VQVLKTTDIN  ISEVQVLYLR
 301  NVSAEDAGEY  TCLAGNSIGL  SYQSAWLTVL  PEEDLTWTTA  TPEARYTDII
 351  LYVSGSLVLL  VLLLLAGVYH  RQVIRGHYSR  QPVTIQKLSR  FPLARQFSLE
 401  SRSSGKSSLS  LVRGVRLSSS  GPPLLTGLVN  LDLPLDPLWE  FPRDRLVLGK
 451  PLGEGCFGQV  VRAEAFGQVV  RAEAFGMDPS  RPDQTSTVAV  KMLKDNASDK
 501  DLADLVSEME  VMKLIGRHKN  IINLLGVCTQ  EGPLYVIVEC  AAKGNLREFL
 551  RARRPPGPDL  SPDGPRSSEG  PLSFPALVSC  AYQVARGMQY  LESRKCIHRD
 601  LAARNVLVTE  DDVMKIADFG  LARGVHHIDY  YKKTSNGRLP  VKWMAPEALF
 651  DRVYTHQSDV  WSFEILLWEI  FTLGGSPYPG  IPVEELFSLL  REGHRMERPP
 701  NCPSELYGLM  RECWHAAPSQ  RPTFKQLVEA  LDKVLLAVSE  EYLDLRLTFG
 751  PFSPSNGDAS  STCSSSDSVF  SHDPLPLEPS  PFPFSDSQTT
```

Tyr630 is a potential site of autophosphorylation by similarity.

References

1 Basilico, C. and Moscatelli, D. (1992) Adv. Cancer Res. 59, 115–165.
2 Baird, A., and Bohlen, P. (1990) In Peptide Growth Factors and their Receptors I, Sporn, M.B. and Roberts, A.B., eds., Springer–Verlag, New York, pp. 369–418.
3 Gospodarowicz, D. (1990) Clin. Orth. Rel. Res. 257, 231–248.
4 Klagsbrun, M. (1989) Prog. Growth Factor Res. 1, 207–235.
5 Benharroch, D. and Birnbaum, D. (1990) Israel J. Med. Sci. 26, 212–219.
6 Hebert, J.M. et al. (1990) Dev. Biol. 138, 454–463.
7 Yu, Y.-L. et al. (1992) J. Exp. Med. 175, 1073–1080.
8 Eriksson, A.E. et al. (1991) Proc. Natl. Acad. Sci. USA 88, 3441–3445.
9 Zhang, J. et al. (1991) Proc. Natl. Acad. Sci. USA 88, 3446–3450.
10 Mergia, A. et al. (1989) Biochem. Biophys. Res. Commum. 164, 1121–1129.
11 Jaye, M. et al. (1986) Science 233, 541–545.
12 Wang, W.-P. et al. (1989) Mol. Cell. Biol. 9, 2387–2395.
13 Crumley, G. et al. (1990) Biochem. Biophys. Res. Commum. 171, 7–13.
14 Myers, R.L. et al. (1993) Oncogene 8, 341–349.
15 Abraham, J.A. et al. (1986) Cold Spring Harbor Symp. Quant. Biol. LI, 657–668.
16 Abraham, J.A. et al. (1986) EMBO J. 5, 2523–2528.
17 Prats, H. et al. (1989) Proc. Natl. Acad. Sci. USA 86, 1836–1840.
18 Florkiewicz, R.Z. and Sommer, A. (1989) Proc. Natl. Acad. Sci. USA 86, 3978–3981.
19 Goodrich, S.P. et al. (1989) Nucl. Acids Res. 17, 2867.
20 Johnson, D.E. and Williams, L.T. (1993) Adv. Cancer. Res. 60, 1–41.
21 Klagsbrun, M. and Baird, A. (1991) Cell 67, 229–231.
22 Dionne, C.A. et al. (1991) Ann. N.Y. Acad. Sci. 638, 161–166.
23 Robinson, C.J. (1991) Trends Pharmacol. Sci 12, 123–124.
24 Kaner, R.J. et al. (1990) Science 248, 1410–1413.
25 Partanen, J. et al. (1991) EMBO J. 10, 1347–1354.
26 Korhonen, J. et al. (1991) Ann. N.Y. Acad. Sci. 638, 403–405.
27 Bellot, F. et al. (1991) EMBO J. 10, 2849–2854.
28 Isacchi, A. et al. (1990) Nucl. Acids Res. 18, 1906.
29 Dionne, C.A. et al. (1990) EMBO J. 9, 2685–2692.
30 Itoh, N. et al. (1990) Biochem. Biophys. Res. Commum. 169, 680–685.
31 Wennstrom, S. et al. (1991) Growth Factors 4, 197–208.
32 Miki, T. et al. (1992) Proc. Natl. Acad. Sci. USA 89, 246–250.
33 Hattori, Y. et al. (1990) Proc. Natl. Acad. Sci. USA 87, 5983–5987.
34 Keegan, K. et al. (1991) Proc. Natl. Acad. Sci. USA 88, 1095–1099.
35 Partanen, J. et al. (1990) Proc. Natl. Acad. Sci. USA 87, 8913–8917.
36 Reid, H.H. et al. (1990) Proc. Natl. Acad. Sci. USA 87, 1596–1600.
37 Safran, A. et al. (1990) Oncogene 5, 635–643 .
38 Mansukhani, A. et al. (1990) Proc. Natl. Acad. Sci. USA 87, 4378–4382.
39 Werner, S. et al. (1992) Mol. Cell. Biol. 12, 82–88.
40 Raz, V. et al. (1991) Oncogene 6, 753–760.
41 Ornitz, D.M. and Leder, P. (1992) J. Biol. Chem. 267, 16305–16311.
42 Stark, K.L. et al. (1991) Development 113, 641–651.

G-CSF

Other names
Human G-CSF has been known as CSFβ and pluripoietin.

THE MOLECULE

Granulocyte colony stimulating factor is a growth, differentiation and activating factor for neutrophils and their precursors. It also synergizes with IL-3 to stimulate growth of haematopoietic progenitors, and causes proliferation and migration of endothelial cells [1-3].

Crossreactivity
There is about 73% homology between human and mouse G-CSF, which both act across species [5-8].

Sources
Macrophages, fibroblasts, endothelial cells, bone marrow stroma [1].

Bioassays
Bone marrow colony formation in soft agar, proliferation of NFS60 cell line [9].

Physicochemical properties of G-CSF

Property	Human	Mouse
Amino acids – precursor	207	208
– mature	177(174)[a]	178
M_r (K) – predicted	19	19
– expressed	21	21
Potential N-linked glycosylation sites[b]	0	0
Disulphide bonds[c]	2	2

[a] The 177 and 174 amino acid forms are alternatively spliced variants, the 174 amino acid form is predominant. The 177 amino acid form is 20-fold less biologically active.

[b] Human G-CSF has one O-linked site.

[c] Disulphide bonds between Cys39–45 and 67–77(hG-CSF).

3-D structure
G-CSF forms a four α-helical bundle structure similar to growth hormone, GM-CSF, IFNβ, IL-4 and IL-2 [10,11].

Gene structure [8,12]

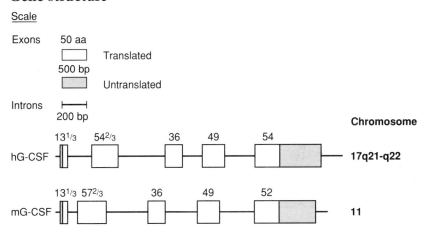

Scale

Exons   50 aa
         ☐ Translated
         500 bp
         ▨ Untranslated

Introns ├──┤
         200 bp

Note: The gene for human G-CSF is located on chromosome 17q21–22. This position corresponds to a translocation found in acute promyelocytic leukaemias [12].

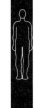

Amino acid sequence for human G-CSF [4,5,6]

Accession code: Swissprot P09919

```
-30   MAGPATQSPM KLMALQLLLW HSALWTVQEA
  1   TPLGPASSLP QSFLLKCLEQ VRKIQGDGAA LQEKLVSECA TYKLCHPEEL
 51   VLLGHSLGIP WAPLSSCPSQ ALQLAGCLSQ LHSGLFLYQG LLQALEGISP
101   ELGPTLDTLQ LDVADFATTI WQQMEELGMA PALQPTQGAM PAFASAFQRR
151   AGGVLVASHL QSFLEVSYRV LRHLAQP
```

Note that the sequence (VSE) in italics (amino acids 36–38) is spliced out in the 174 amino acid variant.

Amino acid sequence for mouse G-CSF [7,8]

Accession code: Swissprot P09920

```
-30   MAQLSAQRRM KLMALQLLLW QSALWSGREA
  1   VPLVTVSALP PSLPLPRSFL LKSLEQVRKI QASGSVLLEQ LCATYKLCHP
 51   EELVLLGHSL GIPKASLSGC SSQALQQTQC LSQLHSGLCL YQGLLQALSG
101   ISPALAPTLD LLQLDVANFA TTIWQQMENL GVAPTVQPTQ SAMPAFTSAF
151   QRRAGGVLAI SYLQGFLETA RLALHHLA
```

135

THE G-CSF RECEPTOR

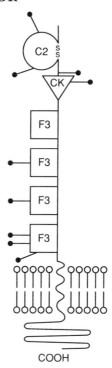

The G-CSF receptor is a hybrid structure containing an immunoglobulin domain, a haematopoietin domain and three FNIII domains [13,14]. The human receptor exists as two forms varying in their intracytoplasmic domains [13]. One form, 25.1, carries a C kinase phosphorylation site. A potential soluble form of the human receptor has been reported which has deleted the transmembrane region [15]. The only murine receptor reported resembles the 25.1 form [16]. Human and mouse receptors share 62.5% homology. The human receptor shares 46.3% sequence homology to the gp130 chain of the IL-6 receptor. Binding specificity for G-CSF resides in the haematopoietin domain, whereas the membrane proximal 57 amino acids are necessary for proliferative signal transduction and residues 57–96 are involved in G-CSF-mediated acute phase protein induction [14,17]. The receptor appears to confer high affinity binding in transfected cells, possibly as a dimeric structure. A G-CSF receptor is present on platelets [19].

Distribution

Neutrophils, myeloid leukaemias, endothelium, platelets, placenta.

Physicochemical properties of the G-CSF receptor

Properties		Human	Mouse
Amino acids	– precursor	836 (783)[a]	837
	– mature	812 (759)[a]	812
M_r (K)	– predicted	90	90
	– expressed	150	95–125
Potential N-linked glycosylation sites		9	11
Affinity K_d (M)		$1–5 \times 10^{-10}$	$2–3 \times 10^{-10}$

[a] Truncated soluble form.

Signal transduction

G-CSF stimulation results in tyrosine phosphorylation of an M_r 56 000 protein in NFS60 cells, and tyrosine and serine phosphorylation of an M_r 75 000 protein. The receptor is thought to bind and mediate auto-phosphorylation of the JAK2 kinase [20].

Chromosomal location
The human receptor is on chromosome 1p35–p34.3

Amino acid sequence for human G-CSF receptor [13]

Accession code: EMBL M59820, M38027, X55720, X55721

```
 -24   MARLGNCSLT WAALIILLLP GSLE
   1   ECGHISVSAP IVHLGDPITA SCIIKQNCSH LDPEPQILWR LGAELQPGGR
  51   QQRLSDGTQE SIITLPHLNH TQAFLSCCLN WGNSLQILDQ VELRAGYPPA
 101   IPHNLSCLMN LTTSSLICQW EPGPETHLPT SFTLKSFKSR GNCQTQGDSI
 151   LDCVPKDGQS HCCIPRKHLL LYQNMGIWVQ AENALGTSMS PQLCLDPMDV
 201   VKLEPPMLRT MDPSPEAAPP QAGCLQLCWE PWQPGLHINQ KCELRHKPQR
 251   GEASWALVGP LPLEALQYEL CGLLPATAYT LQIRCIRWPL PGHWSDWSPS
 301   LELRTTERAP TVRLDTWWRQ RQLDPRTVQL FWKPVPLEED SGRIQGYVVS
 351   WRPSGQAGAI LPLCNTTELS CTFHLPSEAQ EVALVAYNSA GTSRPTPVVF
 401   SESRGPALTR LHAMARDPHS LWVGWEPPNP WPQGYVIEWG LGPPSASNSN
 451   KTWRMEQNGR ATGFLLKENI RPFQLYEIIV TPLYQDTMGP SQHVYAYSQE
 501   MAPSHAPELH LKHIGKTWAQ LEWVPEPPEL GKSPLTHYTI FWTNAQNQSF
 551   SAILNASSRG FVLHGLEPAS LYHIHLMAAS QAGATNSTVL TLMTLTPEGS
 601   ELHIILGLFG LLLLLTCLCG TAWLCCSPNR KNPLWPSVPD PAHSSLGSWV
 651   PTIMEEDAFQ LPGLGTPPIT KLTVLEEDEK KPVPWESHNS SETCGLPTLV
 701   QTYVLQGDPR AVSTQPQSQS GTSDQVLYGQ LLGSPTSPGP GHYLRCDSTQ
 751   PLLAGLTPSP KSYENLWFQA SPLGTLVTPA PSQEDDCVFG PLLNFPLLQG
 801   IRVHGMEALG SF
```

Alternative C-terminus clone D7:

```
 721   AGPPRRSAYF KDQIMLHPAP PNGLLCLFPI TSVL
```

Amino acid sequence for mouse G-CSF receptor [16]

Accession code: EMBL M32699

```
 -25  MVGLGACTLT  GVTLIFLLLP  RSLES
   1  CGHIEISPPV  VRLGDPVLAS  CTISPNCSKL  DQQAKILWRL  QDEPIQPGDR
  51  QHHLPDGTQE  SLITLPHLNY  TQAFLFCLVP  WEDSVQLLDQ  AELHAGYPPA
 101  SPSNLSCLMH  LTTNSLVCQW  EPGPETHLPT  SFILKSFRSR  ADCQYQGDTI
 151  PDCVAKKRQN  NCSIPRKNLL  LYQYMAIWVQ  AENMLGSSES  PKLCLDPMDV
 201  VKLEPPMLQA  LDIGPDVVSH  QPGCLWLSWK  PWKPSEYMEQ  ECELRYQPQL
 251  KGANWTLVFH  LPSSKDQFEL  CGLHQAPVYT  LQMRCIRSSL  PGFWSPWSPG
 301  LQLRPTMKAP  TIRLDTWCQK  KQLDPGTVSV  QLFWKPTPLQ  EDSGQIQGYL
 351  LSWNSPDHQG  QDIHLCNTTQ  LSCIFLLPSE  AQNVTLVAYN  KAGTSSPTTV
 401  VFLENEGPAV  TGLHAMAQDL  NTIWVDWEAP  SLLPQGYLIE  WEMSSPSYNN
 451  SYKSWMIEPN  GNITGILLKD  NINPFQLYRI  TVAPLYPGIV  GPPVNVYTFA
 501  GERAPPHAPA  LHLKHVGTTW  AQLEWVPEAP  RLGMIPLTHY  TIFWADAGDH
 551  SFSVTLNISL  HDFVLKHLEP  ASLYHVYLMA  TSRAGSTNST  GLTLRTLDPS
 601  DLNIFLGILC  LVLLSTTCVV  TWLCCKRRGK  TSFWSDVPDP  AHSSLSSWLP
 651  TIMTEETFQL  PSFWDSSVPS  ITKITELEED  KKPTHWDSES  SGNGSLPALV
 701  QAYVLQGDPR  EISNQSQPPS  RTGDQVLYGQ  VLESPTSPGV  MQYIRSDSTQ
 751  PLLGGPTPSP  KSYENIWFHS  RPQETFVPQP  PNQEDDCVFG  PPFDFPLFQG
 801  LQVHGVEEQG  GF
```

References

[1] Nagata, S. (1990) In Peptide Growth Factors and their Receptors, Sporn, M.B. and Roberts, A.B., eds, Springer-Verlag, Heidelberg.
[2] Gabrilove, J.L. et al. (1988) N. Engl. J. Med. 318, 1414–1422.
[3] Bussolino, F. et al. (1989) Nature 337, 471–473.
[4] Souza, L.M. et al. (1986) Science 232, 61–65.
[5] Nagata, S. et al. (1986) Nature 319, 415–418.
[6] Nagata, S. et al. (1986) EMBO J. 5, 575–581.
[7] Tsuchiya, M. et al. (1986) Proc. Natl. Acad. Sci USA. 83, 7633–7637.
[8] Tsuchiya, M. et al. (1987) Eur. J. Biochem. 165, 7–12.
[9] Testa, N.G. et al. (1991) In Cytokines: A Practical Approach, Balkwill, F.A., ed., IRL Press Oxford, pp. 229–244.
[10] Hill, C.P. et al. (1993) Proc. Natl. Acad. Sci. USA 90, 5167–5171.
[11] Diederichs, K. et al. (1991) Science 254, 1779–1782.
[12] Simmers, R.N. et al. (1987) Blood 70, 330–332.
[13] Larsen, A. et al. (1990) J. Exp. Med. 172, 1559–1570.
[14] Fukunaga, R. et al. (1991) . EMBO J. 10, 2855–2865.
[15] Fukunaga, R. et al. (1990) Proc. Natl Acad. Sci USA 87, 8702–8706.
[16] Fukunaga, R. et al. (1990) Cell 61, 341–350.
[17] Ziegler, S.F. et al. (1993) Mol. Cell. Biol. 13, 2384–2390.
[18] Tweardy, D.J. et al. (1992) Blood 79, 1148–1154.
[19] Shimoda, K. et al. (1993) J. Clin. Invest. 91, 1310–1313.
[20] Witthuhn, B.A. et al. (1993) Cell 74, 227–236.

Other names
Human and mouse GM-CSF have been known as CSFα or pluripoietin-α.

THE MOLECULE

Granulocyte/macrophage colony stimulating factor is a survival and growth factor for haematopoietic progenitor cells, a differentiation and activating factor for granulocytic and monocytic cells, and a growth factor for endothelial cells, erythroid cells, megakaryocytes and T cells [1-4].

Crossreactivity
There is about 56 % homology between human and mouse GM-CSF and no cross species activity.

Sources
T Cells, macrophages, fibroblasts and endothelial cells.

Bioassays
There are no specific bioassays for GM-CSF. Bone marrow colony formation in agar, or the AML-193 cell line can provide sensitive estimates of human GM-CSF activity. Mouse GM-CSF can be measured in bone marrow colony assays or using the DA-1 or FDC-P1 cell lines [5,6].

Physicochemical properties of GM-CSF

Property	Human	Mouse
pI	3.4–4.5	?
Amino acids – precursor	144	141
– mature	127	124
M_r (K) – predicted	16.3	16
– expressed	22	22
Potential N-linked glycosylation sites	2	2
Disulphide bonds[a]	2	2

[a] Disulphide bonds between Cys54–96 and 88–121 in human GM-CSF and 51–93 and 85–118 in mouse GM-CSF [7].

3-D structure
An X-ray crystal structure of human GM-CSF has been determined to 2.4 Å resolution. The molecule comprises a two-stranded antiparallel β-sheet with an open bundle of four α helices, similar to IL-2, IL-4, G-CSF, M-CSF, IFNβ and growth hormone [8,9].

Gene structure [10,11]

Scale

Exons   50 aa

☐ Translated

500 bp

▨ Untranslated

Introns   ⊢——⊣

500 bp

Chromosome

| | 53 | 14 | | 42 | | 35 | |
hGM-CSF ———▢▯——▢———▢▨— **5q21-q32**

| | 50 | 14 | | 42 | | 35 | |
mGM-CSF ——▢▯——▢———▢▨— **11**

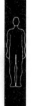

Amino acid sequence for human GM-CSF [12,13]

Accession code: Swissprot P04141

```
-17    MWLQSLLLLG TVACSIS
  1    APARSPSPST QPWEHVNAIQ EARRLLNLSR DTAAEMNETV EVISEMFDLQ
 51    EPTCLQTRLE LYKQGLRGSL TKLKGPLTMM ASHYKQHCPP TPETSCATQI
101    ITFESFKENL KDFLLVIPFD CWEPVQE
```

Conflicting sequence I->T at position 100.

Amino acid sequence for mouse GM-CSF [2,11,14]

Accession code: Swissprot P01587

```
-17    MWLQNLLFLG IVVYSLS
  1    APTRSPITVT RPWKHVEAIK EALNLLDDMP VTLNEEVEVV SNEFSFKKLT
 51    CVQTRLKIFE QGLRGNFTKL KGALNMTASY YQTYCPPTPE TDCETQVTTY
101    ADFIDSLKTF LTDIPFECKK PGQK
```

Conflicting sequence T->I at position 8, T->A at position 91, and Q->V/S at position 123.

THE GM-CSF RECEPTOR

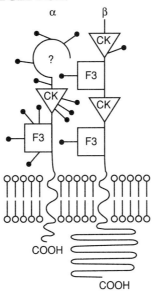

The high affinity GM-CSF receptor is a complex of a low affinity α-chain (CDw116) with a second affinity converting β-chain (human KH97 and murine AIC2B) which is also shared with the IL-3 and IL-5 receptor α-chains [15-18]. (see IL-3 entry). Both the α- and β-chains are members of the haematopoietin family of receptors [19]. A potentially soluble form of the α-chain [20], and a splice variant with an altered intracytoplasmic domain of the α-chain have been described [21]. The intracytoplasmic domain of the β-chain is not required to form a high affinity receptor [16].

Distribution

Granulocytes and monocytes and their precursors, endothelial cells, fibroblasts, Langerhans cells.

Physicochemical properties of the GM-CSF receptors

Properties	Human α-chain	Human β-chain[a]
Amino acids – precursor	400	897
– mature	378	882
M_r (K) – predicted	46	95
– expressed	80	130
Potential N-linked glycosylation sites	11	3
Affinity K_d (M)[b]	3.2×10^{-9}	0
	1.20×10^{-10}	

[a] The β–chain is the same as the human IL-3 receptor KH97 and the murine IL-3 receptor AIC2B [17,18] (see IL-3 entry).

[b] Low and high affinity sites.

Signal transduction

Ligand binding results in tyrosine phosphorylation of several intracellular proteins [19].The receptor is thought to bind and mediate phosphorylation of the JAK2 kinase [22].

Chromosomal location

The human α-chain is located on chromosome Xp22.3, Yp13.3 [23] and the β chain on chromosome 22.

Amino acid sequence for the human GM-CSF receptor α-chain [15]

Accession code: Swissprot P15509

```
-22   MLLLVTSLLL CELPHPAFLL IP
  1   EKSDLRTVAP ASSLNVRFDS RTMNLSWDCQ ENTTFSKCFL TDKKNRVVEP
 51   RLSNNECSCT FREICLHEGV TFEVHVNTSQ RGFQQKLLYP NSGREGTAAQ
101   NFSCFIYNAD LMNCTWARGP TAPRDVQYFL YIRNSKRRRE IRCPYYIQDS
151   GTHVGCHLDN LSGLTSRNYF LVNGTSREIG IQFFDSLLDT KKIERFNPPS
201   NVTVRCNTTH CLVRWKQPRT YQKLSYLDFQ YQLDVHRKNT QPGTENLLIN
251   VSGDLENRYN FPSSEPRAKH SVKIRAADVR ILNWSSWSEA IEFGSDDGNL
301   GSVYIYVLLI VGTLVCGIVL GFLFKRFLRI QRLFPPVPQI KDKLNDNHEV
351   EDEIIWEEFT PEEGKGYREE VLTVKEIT
```

Amino acid sequence for the human GM-CSF receptor β-chain

See IL-3 entry

References
1 Wong, G.C. et al. (1985) Science 228, 810–815.
2 Gough, N.M. et al. (1985) EMBO. J. 4, 645–653.
3 Clarke, S. and Kamen, R. (1987) Science 236, 1229–1237.
4 Groopman, J.E. et al. (1989) New Eng. J. Med. 321, 1449–1459.
5 Testa, N.G. et al. (1991) In Cytokines: A Practical Approach, Balkwill, F.A. ed., IRL Press, Oxford, pp. 229–234.
6 Wadhwa, M. et al. (1991) In Cytokines: A Practical Approach, Balkwill, F.A. ed., IRL Press, Oxford, pp. 309–329.
7 Schrimser, J.L. et al. (1987) Biochem. J. 247, 195–201.
8 Reichert, P. et al. (1990) . J. Biol. Chem. 265, 452–453.
9 Diederichs, K. et al. (1991) Science 254, 1779–1782.
10 Huebner, K. et al. (1985) Science 230, 1282–1285.
11 Mitayake, S. et al. (1985) EMBO. J. 4, 2561–2568.
12 Lee, F. et al. (1985) Proc. Natl. Acad. Sci. USA 82, 4360–4364.
13 Kaushansky, K. et al. (1986) Proc. Natl. Acad. Sci. USA 83, 3101–3105.
14 Delamater, J.F. et al. (1985) EMBO J. 4, 2575–2581.
15 Gearing, D.P. et al. (1989) EMBO J. 8, 3667–3676.

16 Hayashida, K. et al. (1990) Proc. Natl. Acad. Sci. USA. 87, 9655–9659.

17 Kitamura, T. et al. (1991) Cell 66, 1165–1174.

18 Gorman, D.M. et al. (1990) Proc. Natl. Acad. Sci. USA 87, 5459–5463.

19 Cosman, D. (1993) Cytokine 5, 95–106.

20 Raines, M.S. et al. (1991) Proc. Natl. Acad. Sci. USA 88, 8203–8207.

21 Crosier, K.E. et al. (1991) Proc. Natl. Acad. Sci. USA 88, 7744–7748.

22 Witthuhn, B.A. et al. (1993) Cell 74, 227–236.

23 Ashworth, A. and Kraft, A. (1990) Nucleic Acid Res. 18, 7178.

Other names

A splice variant of TCA-3 is known as P500 [1].

THE MOLECULES

I-309 is the human homologue of the murine TCA-3 gene [2-4]. Both molecules are members of the CC family of chemokine/intercrine cytokines [5]. I-309 is a monocyte chemoattractant [6].

Crossreactivity

There is about 42% homology between human I-309 and mouse TCA-3.

Sources

T lymphocytes and mast cells [7].

Bioassays

Monocyte chemoattraction.

Physicochemical properties of I-309/TCA-3

Property	Human (I-309)	Mouse (TCA-3)
Amino acids – precursor	96	92
– mature	73	69
M_r (K) – predicted	8	8
– expressed	8–16	16
Potential N-linked glycosylation sites[a]	1	1
Disulphide bonds[b]	3	3

[a] The TCA-3 splice variant P500 lacks the N-linked glycosylation site in TCA-3.
[b] Putative.

3-D structure

Could be modelled on MCP-1.

Gene structure [8,9]

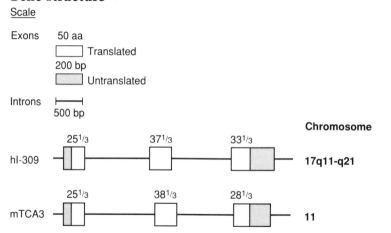

The gene for murine TCA-3 is located on chromosome 11 [9].

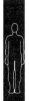

Amino acid sequence for human I-309 [3,9]

Accession code: Swissprot: P22362

```
-23  MQIITTALVC LLLAGMWPED VDS
  1  KSMQVPFSRC CFSFAEQEIP LRAILCYRNT SSICSNEGLI FKLKRGKEAC
 51  ALDTVGWVQR HRKMLRHCPS KRK
```

Amino acid sequence for mouse TCA-3 [4]

Accession code: Swissprot: P10146

```
-23  MKPTAMALMC LLLAAVWIQD VDS
  1  KSMLTVSNSC CLNTLKKELP LKFIQCYRKM GSSCPDPPAV VFRLNKGRES
 51  CASTNKTWVQ NHLKKVNPC
```

In the TCA-3 splice variant P500, amino acids 42–69 are replaced with the sequence shown below [1]:

Accession code: Swissprot P14098

```
 42  VRSSGVPGL TEAEKTVTDS SE
```

THE I-309/TCA-3 RECEPTORS

No information.

References
1 Brown, K.D. et al. (1989) J. Immunol. 142, 679–687.
2 Wilson, S.D. et al. (1990) J. Immunol. 145, 2745–2744.
3 Miller, M.D. et al. (1989) J. Immunol. 143, 2907–2916.
4 Burd, P.R. et al. (1987) J. Immunol. 139, 3126–3131.
5 Schall, T.J. (1991) Cytokine 3, 165–183.
6 Miller, M.D. et al. (1992) Proc. Natl. Acad. Sci. USA 89, 2950–2954.
7 Burd, P.R. et al. (1989) J. Exp. Med. 170, 245–257.
8 Wilson, S.D. et al. (1990) J. Exp. Med. 171, 1301–1314.
9 Miller, M.D. et al. (1990) J. Immunol. 145, 2737–2744.

Other names

Murine γIP-10 has been known as CRG-2 or C7 [1,2].

THE MOLECULE

γIP-10 is a member of the CXC family of chemokine/intercrine cytokines [3-5]. It is a monocyte and T lymphocyte chemoattractant, and promotes lymphocyte adhesion to activated endothelial cells [6]. γIP-10 has been detected in delayed type reactions and leprosy lesions [7].

Crossreactivity

Human γIP-10 shares 67% identity with murine γIP-10 and is active on mouse cells [8].

Sources

Keratinocytes, monocytes, T lymphocytes, endothelial cells, fibroblasts. Induced by IFNγ stimulation (potentiated by IL-2), LPS and IFNβ [9,10].

Bioassays

Monocyte chemoattraction.

Physicochemical properties of γIP-10

Property	Human	Mouse
pI	>8	>8
Amino acids – precursor	98	98
– mature	77	77
M_r (K) – predicted	10.9	10.8
– expressed	6 & 7	?
Potential N-linked glycosylation sites[a]	0	0
Disulphide bonds	2	2

[a] One in signal sequence.

3-D structure

Could be modelled on IL-8.

Gene structure [11]

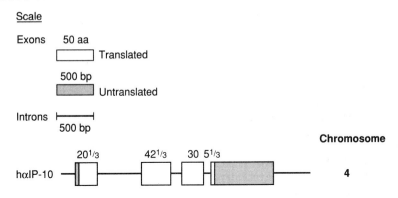

Scale

Exons   50 aa

[ ] Translated

500 bp

[▒▒▒] Untranslated

Introns ├───┤
500 bp

Chromosome

$20^{1/3}$ $42^{1/3}$ 30 $5^{1/3}$

hαIP-10

4

Amino acid sequence for human γIP-10 [3]

Accession code: Swissprot P02778

```
-21  MNQTAILICC LIFLTLSGIQ G
  1  VPLSRTVRCT CISISNQPVN PRSLEKLEII PASQFCPRVE IIATMKKKGE
 51  KRCLNPESKA IKNLLKAVSK EMSKRSP
```

Amino acid sequence for mouse γIP-10 [1,2]

Accession code: Swissprot P17515

```
-21  MNPSAAVIFC LILLGLSGTQ G
  1  IPLARTVRCN CIHDDGPVR MRAIGKLEII PASLSCPRVE IIATMKKNDE
 51  QRCLNPESKT IKNLMKAFSQ KRSKRAP
```

THE RECEPTORS

No information.

References
1 Ohmori, Y. et al. (1990) Biochem. Biophys. Res. Comm. 168, 1261–1267.
2 Vanguri, P. and Farber, J.M. (1990) J. Biol. Chem. 265, 15047–15049.
3 Luster, A.D. et al. (1985) Nature 315, 672–676.
4 Luster, A.D. and Ravetch, J.V. (1987) J. Exp. Med. 166, 1084–1097.
5 Luster, A.D. and Ravetch, J.V. (1987) Mol. Cell. Biol. 7, 3723–3731.
6 Taub, D.D. et al. (1993) J. Exp. Med. 177, 1809–1814.
7 Kaplan, G. et al. (1987) J. Exp. Med. 166, 1098–1108.
8 Luster, A.D. and Peder, P. (1993) J. Cell. Biol. 17B (suppl):E547.
9 Narumi, S. and Hamilton, T.A. (1991) J. Immunol. 146, 3038–3044.
10 Narumi, S. et al. (1992) J. Leucocyte Biol. 52, 27–33.
11 Luster, A.D. et al. (1987) Proc. Natl. Acad. Sci. USA 84, 2868–2871.

IFNα

Other names

Type I interferon, leukocyte interferon, acid stable interferon, B cell interferon, lymphoblast interferon, Namalwa interferon, buffy coat interferon.

THE MOLECULE

The α interferons are a family of inducible secreted proteins which confer resistance to viruses on target cells, inhibit cell proliferation and regulate expression of MHC class I antigens [1-3]. The IFNα family consists of 24 or more genes or pseudo-genes. There are two distinct families (I and II) of human (and bovine) IFNα. Mature IFNα(I) are 166 amino acids long (one is 165 amino acids) whereas IFNα(II) have 172 amino acids. The IFNα genes probably diverged 100 million years ago, prior to mammalian radiation and have about 30% homology with IFNβ.

Crossreactivity

There is about 40% homology between human and mouse IFNα subtypes and there is some species preference in their biological activities depending on the particular IFNα molecule [4].

Sources

Major producers of IFNα are lymphocytes, monocytes, macrophages and cell lines such as Namalwa and KG1.

Bioassays

Inhibition of cytopathic effect of EMCV (encephalomyocarditis virus), VSV (vesicular stomatitis virus) or SFV (Semliki forest virus) on HEP2/C (human epithelial) cell line for human IFN or L929 for mouse IFN. Inhibition of proliferation of DAUDI human lymphoblastoid B cell line.

Physicochemical properties IFN-α

Property	Human		Mouse
	IFNα(I)	IFNα(II)	IFNα
Number of isoforms	≥15	≥1	≥11
pI	5 – 6.5 for most subtypes		
Amino acids – precursor	188/189	195	189/190
– mature[a]	165/166	172	166/167
M_r (K) – predicted	19.2–19.7	20.1	19.1
– expressed[b]	16–27	?	16–27
Potential N-linked glycosylation sites[c]	0	1	1
Disulphide bonds[d]	2	2	2

[a] All human and murine IFNα have a signal peptide of 23 amino acids except for murine IFNα4 which has 24 amino acids.

[b] Apparent M_r on acrylamide gels. Some variation may be due to O-linked glycosylation.

[c] N-glycosylation site at position 78 is present on most murine IFNα sequences. The majority of human IFNα type I molecules are not glycosylated (IFNαH has one potential N-linked site and at least three species have O-linked polysaccharides).

[d] Disulphide bonds between Cys1–99 and 29–139 are present in most human and murine IFNα, and are required for biological activity.

3-D structure

The 3-D structure for IFNα has not yet been reported. From sequence and polypetide folding considerations it is similar to IFNβ.

Gene structure [5-7]

Scale

Exons   50 aa

Introns   NONE

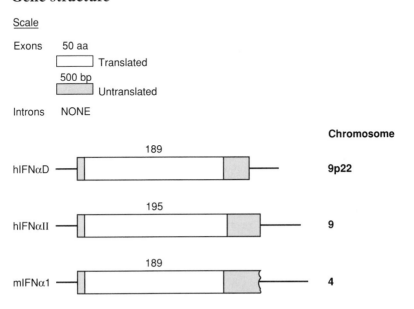

Chromosome

189
hIFNαD — 9p22

195
hIFNαII — 9

189
mIFNα1 — 4

The 3' untranslated sequence is variable in length. It has not been determined for mouse IFNα.

Human IFNα

More than 24 non-allelic genes or pseudo-genes for human IFNα have been identified. Eighteen of these including at least four pseudo-genes are for IFNα(I), and six, of which at least five are pseudo-genes, are for IFNα(II) also known as IFNω. The mature IFNα(I) proteins are mostly 166 amino acids in length, although IFNαA has 165 amino acids. Mature IFNα(II) has 172 amino acids. All have signal peptides of 23 amino acids. Sequences are given here for IFNαD (also called IFNα1) as a typical IFNα(I), and for IFNα(II). For a comparison of human IFNα sequences see the table of Swissprot accession numbers below. An IFNα consensus sequence is given in reference 8.

Amino acid sequence for human IFNαD (IFNα1) [7,8]

Accession code: Swissprot P01562

```
-23   MASPFALLMV LVVLSCKSSC SLG
  1   CDLPETHSLD NRRTLMLLAQ MSRISPSSCL MDRHDFGFPQ EEFDGNQFQK
 51   APAISVLHEL IQQIFNLFTT KDSSAAWDED LLDKFCTELY QQLNDLEACV
101   MQEERVGETP LMNADSILAV KKYFRRITLY LTEKKYSPCA WEVVRAEIMR
151   SLSLSTNLQE RLRRKE
```

Conflicting sequence A->V at position 114 [9]. Disulphide bonds between Cys1–99 and 29–139.

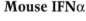

Amino acid sequence for human IFNα(II) (IFNω) [6]

Accession code: Swissprot P05000

```
-23   MALLFPLLAA LVMTSYSPVG SLG
  1   CDLPQNHGLL SRNTLVLLHQ MRRISPFLCL KDRRDFRFPQ EMVKGSQLQK
 51   AHVMSVLHEM LQQIFSLFHT ERSSAAWNMT LLDQLHTELH QQLQHLETCL
101   LQVVGEGESA GAISSPALTL RRYFQGIRVY LKEKKYSDCA WEVVRMEIMK
151   SLFLSTNMQE RLRSKDRDLG SS
```

Disulphide bonds between Cys1–99 and 29–139.

Mouse IFNα

At least 12 non allelic genes or pseudo-genes for mouse IFNα have been identified, 11 of which have been cloned and expressed as biologically active proteins. The mature proteins have 166 or 167 amino acids except for mouse IFNα4 which has a five codon deletion between codons 102 and 108. The example given here is of mouse IFNα1.

Amino acid sequence for mouse IFNα1 [5]

Accession code: Swissprot P01572

```
-23   MARLCAFLMV LAVMSYWPTC SLG
  1   CDLPQTHNLR NKRALTLLVQ MRRLSPLSCL KDRKDFGFPQ EKVDAQQIKK
 51   AQAIPVLSEL TQQILNIFTS KDSSAAWNAT LLDSFCNDLH QQLNDLQGCL
101   MQQVGVQEFP LTQEDALLAV RKYFHRITVY LREKKHSPCA WEVVRAEVWR
151   ALSSSANVLG RLREEK
```

Disulphide bonds between Cys1–99 and 29–139.

Human and mouse IFNα molecules with Swissprot accession numbers

IFNα (alternative name)	Accession code
Human	
IFNα4B	P05014
IFNα7 (IFNαJ1)	P01567
IFNα8 (IFNαB2)	P01565
IFNαA (IFNα2)	P01563/4
IFNαB	P09236, P01565
IFNαC	P01566
IFNαD (IFNα1)	P01562
IFNαF	P01568
IFNαG (IFNα5)	P01569
IFNαH (IFNα14)	P01570
IFNαI	P01571
IFNαK (IFNα6)	P05013
IFNαM1	P13358
IFNaWA (IFN—1-I6)	P05015
IFNα(II)-1 (IFNω)	P05000
Mouse	
IFNα1	P01572
IFNα2	P01573
IFNα4	P07351
IFNα5	P07349
IFNα6	P07350
IFNα7	P06799
IFNα8	P17660
IFNα9	P09235

THE IFNα RECEPTORS

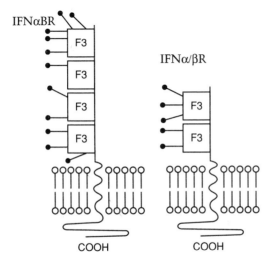

To date, two IFNα receptors have been cloned [10,11]. One of these is apparently specific for IFNαB (IFN-α8) and is called the IFNαB receptor [10]. The other binds both IFNα and IFNβ and is called the IFNα/β receptor [11]. The IFNαB receptor protein is a member of the class II cytokine receptor family which also includes the IFNγ receptor, IL-10 receptor, and tissue factor [12–14]. The extracellular region of 409 amino acids is composed of two homologous regions of about 200 amino acids each of which contains two FNIII domains. The first of these has two conserved tryptophans and a pair of conserved cysteines whereas the second has a unique disulphide loop formed from the second pair of conserved cysteines, but no WSXWS motif characteristic of class I cytokine receptors [15]. Crosslinking studies with ^{125}I IFNαA have shown that the receptor for the IFNαA isoform is a multichain structure [16]. The IFNα/β receptor is also a class II cytokine receptor with two FNIII domains. It is not known if these two receptors are expressed independently on the cell surface or are associated with each other in an IFN receptor complex. A soluble form of the IFNα/β receptor has been identified in human serum and urine [17]. A mouse IFNα receptor cDNA has also been cloned [18].

Distribution

The receptors are present on most cell types.

Physicochemical properties of the IFNα receptors

Properties	IFNαBR Human	IFNα/βR Human	IFNαR Mouse
Amino acids – precursor	557	331	590
– mature[a]	530	305 (239)[b]	564
M_r (K) – predicted	60.9	34.5	63.4
– expressed	95–110	102[c]	?
Potential N-linked glycosylation sites	11	5	8
Affinity K_d (M)	10^{-9}–10^{-11}	?	?

[a] After removal of predicted signal peptide.
[b] Soluble form.
[c] Probably dimer of two disulphide linked M_r 51 000 subunits.

Signal transduction

IFN-α binding to its receptor results in phosphorylation and activation of protein tyrosine kinases TYK2 and JAK1 but not JAK2 [19-21] which directly or indirectly tyrosine phosphorylate the cytoplasmic STAT (signal transducers and activators of transcription) proteins p84/91 and p113 which combine with p48 to form the transcription factor ISGF3 in the cytoplasm [22-27]. Activated ISGF3 moves to the nucleus and binds to the ISRE responsive element on IFNα responsive genes [28]. IFNα has also been shown to activate PLC-A2 releasing arachidonic acid and diacylglycerol

(DAG) [29,30]. Activation of PKC_ϵ (but not $PKC_{\alpha/\beta}$) in the absence of phospholipid turnover or elevation of intracellular calcium has also been described [30]. The IFNα/β receptor is physically associated with JAK1 [11].

Chromosomal location

The human IFNαB receptor is on chromosome 21q22.1

Amino acid sequence for human IFNαB receptor [10]

Accession code: Swissprot P17181

```
-27  MMVVLLGATT  LVLVAVGPWV  LSAAAGG
  1  KNLKSPQKVE  VDIIDDNFIL  RWNRSDESVG  NVTFSFDYQK  TGMDNWIKLS
 51  GCQNITSTKC  NFSSLKLNVY  EEIKLRIRAE  KENTSSWYEV  DSFTPFRKAQ
101  IGPPEVHLEA  EDKAIVIHIS  PGTKDSVMWA  LDGLSFTYSL  LIWKNSSGVE
151  ERIENIYSRH  KIYKLSPETT  YCLKVKAALL  TSWKIGVYSP  VHCIKTTVEN
201  ELPPPENIEV  SVQNQNYVLK  WDYTYANMTF  QVQWLHAFLK  RNPGNHLYKW
251  KQIPDCENVK  TTQCVFPQNV  FQKGIYLLRV  QASDGNNTSF  WSEEIKFDTE
301  IQAFLLPPVF  NIRSLSDSFH  IYIGAPKQSG  NTPVIQDYPL  IYEIIFWENT
351  SNAERKIIEK  KTDVTVPNLK  PLTVYCVKAR  AHTMDEKLNK  SSVFSDAVCE
401  KTKPGNTSKI  WLIVGICIAL  FALPFVIYAA  KVFLRCINYV  FFPSLKPSSS
451  IDEYFSEQPL  KNLLLSTSEE  QIEKCFIIEN  ISTIATVEET  NQTDEDHKKY
501  SSQTSQDSGN  YSNEDESESK  TSEELQQDFV
```

The four pairs of Cys residues at positions 52,60; 172,193; 256,264; and 376,399 are conserved in the class II cytokine receptor family.

Amino acid sequence for human IFNα/β receptor [11]

Accession code: GenEMBL X77722

```
-26  MLLSQNAFIV  RSLNLVLMVY  ISLVFG
  1  ISYDSPDYTD  ESCTFKISLR  NFRSILSWEL  KNHSIVPTHY  TLLYTIMSKP
 51  EDLKVVKNCA  NTTRSFCDLT  DEWRSTHEAY  VTVLEGFSGN  TTLFSCSHNF
101  WLAIDMSFEP  PEFEIVGFTN  HINVMVKFPS  IVEEELQFDL  SLVIEEQSEG
151  IVKKHKPEIK  GNMSGNFTYI  IDKLIPNTNY  CVSVYLEHSD  EQAVIKSPLK
201  CTLLPPGQES  ESAESAKIGG  IITVFLIALV  LTSTIVTLKW  IGYICLRNSL
251  PKVLRQGLTK  GWNAVAIHRC  SHNALQSETP  ELKQSSCLSF  PSSWDYKRAS
301  LCPSD
```

an alternative 4.5kb mRNA transcript gives rise to a truncated soluble form with the same sequence from 1 to 211 plus two additional amino acids followed by a stop codon.

Amino acid sequence for mouse IFNα receptor [18]

Accession code: GenEMBL M89641

```
-26  MLAVVGAAAL  VLVAGAPWVL  PSAAGG
  1  ENLKPPENID  VYIIDDNYTL  KWSSHGESMG  SVTFSAEYRT  KDEAKWLKVP
 51  ECQHTTTTKC  EFSLLDTNVY  IKTQFRVRAE  EGNSTSSWNE  VDPFIPFYTA
```

153

```
101  HMSPPEVRLE  AEDKAILVHI  SPPGQDGNMW  ALEKPSFSYT  IRIWQKSSSD
151  KKTINSTYYV  EKIPELLPET  TYCLEVKAIH  PSLKKHSNYS  TVQCISTTVA
201  NKMPVPGNLQ  VDAQGKSYVL  KWDYIASADV  LFRAQWLPGY  SKSSSGSHSD
251  KWKPIPTCAN  VQTTHCVFSQ  DTVYTGTFFL  HVQASEGNHT  SFWSEEKFID
301  SQKHILPPPP  VITVTAMSDT  LLVYVNCQDS  TCDGLNYEII  FWENTSNTKI
351  SMEKDGPEFT  LKNLQPLTVY  CVQARVLFRA  LLNKTSNFSE  KLCEKTRPGS
401  FSTIWIITGL  GVVFFSVMVL  YALRSVWKYL  CHVCFPPLKP  PRSIDEFFSE
451  PPSKNLVLLT  AEEHTERCFI  IENTDTVAVE  VKHAPEEDLR  KYSSQTSQDS
501  GNYSNEEEES  VGTESGQAVL  SKAPCGGPCS  VPSPPGTLED  GTCFLGNEKY
551  LQSPALRTEP  ALLC
```

The four pairs of Cys residues at positions 52,60; 173,194; 258,266; and 371,393 are conserved in the class II cytokine receptor family.

References

1 Pestka, S. and Langer, J.A. (1987) Annu. Rev. Biochem. 56, 727–777.
2 Balkwill, F.R. (1989) Cytokines in Cancer Therapy. Oxford University Press, Oxford.
3 Sen, G.C. and Lengyel, P. (1992) J. Biol. Chem. 267, 5017–5020.
4 Meager, A. (1990) Cytokines. Open University Press, Milton Keynes.
5 Shaw, G.D. et al. (1983) Nucl. Acids Res. 11, 555–573.
6 Capon, D.J. et al. (1985) Mol. Cell. Biol. 5, 768–779.
7 Mantei, N. et al. (1980) Gene 10, 1–10.
8 Zoon, K.C. (1987) Interferon 9, 1–12.
9 Goeddel, D.V. et al. (1981) Nature 290, 20–26.
10 Uze, G. et al. (1990) Cell 60, 225–234.
11 Novick, D. et al. (1994) Cell 77, 391–400.
12 Bazan, J.F. (1990) Proc. Natl Acad. Sci. USA 87, 6934–6938.
13 Aguet, M. (1991) Br. J. Haematol. 79 , 6–8.
14 Lutfalla, G. et al. (1992) J. Biol. Chem. 267, 2802–2809.
15 Bazan, J.F. (1990) Cell 61, 753–754.
16 Colamonici, O.R. et al. (1992) J. Immunol. 148, 2126–2132.
17 Novick, D. et al. (1992) FEBS Lett. 314, 445–448.
18 Uze, G. et al. (1992) Proc. Natl Acad. Sci. USA 89, 4774–4778.
19 Velazquez, L. et al. (1992) Cell 70, 313–322.
20 Muller, M. et al. (1993) Nature 366, 129–135.
21 Hunter, T. (1993) Nature 366, 114–116.
22 Pellegrini, S. and Schindler, C. (1993) Trends Biochem. Sci. 18, 338–342.
23 David, M. et al. (1993) J. Biol. Chem. 268, 6593–6599.
24 Gutch, M.J. et al. (1992) Proc. Natl. Acad. Sci. USA 89, 11411–11415.
25 Marx, J. (1992) Science 257, 744–745.
26 David, M. and Larner, A.C. (1992) Science 257, 813–815 .
27 Schindler, C. et al. (1992) Science 257, 809–813.
28 Decker, T. et al. (1991) Mol. Cell. Biol. 11, 5147–5153.
29 Hannigan, G.E. and Williams, B.R. (1991) Science 251, 204–207.
30 Pfeffer, L.M. et al. (1991) Proc. Natl. Acad. Sci. USA 88, 7988–7992.

IFNβ

Other names
Type I interferon, fibroblast interferon, acid stable interferon, interferon-β 1.

THE MOLECULE

Interferon-β is related to IFNα with about 30% amino acid sequence homology. IFNα and IFNβ seem to share the same receptor and have very similar biological activities. Both confer resistance to viral infections on target cells, inhibit cell proliferation and regulate expression of MHC class I. Unlike IFNα, there is only one IFNβ gene in humans and in mice. The so called IFNβ2 is now known to be IL-6 [1,2]

Crossreactivity
There is 48% homology between human and mouse IFNβ and no cross-species activity.

Sources
Fibroblasts and some epithelial cells.

Bioassays
See IFNα entry.

Physicochemical properties of IFNβ

Property	Human	Mouse
pI	7.8–8.9	?
Amino acids – precursor	187	182
– mature[a]	166	161
M_r (K) – predicted	20	19.7
– expressed	20	26/35[b]
Potential N-linked glycosylation sites[b]	1	3
Disulphide bonds	1	0

[a] After removal of predicted signal peptide
[b] Two forms of natural murine IFNβ with M_r of 26 000 and 35 000 due to differential glycosylation of the same protein have been reported.

3-D structure
IFNβ conisists of five helices. Three of these are parallel to each other and the other two are antiparallel to the first three. The structure is a variant of the α-helix bundle, but with a new chain folding topology, common to all type I interferons [3].

Gene structure [4-6]

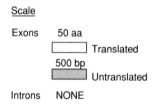

Introns   NONE

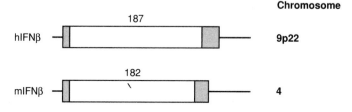

Amino acid sequence for human IFNβ [4,7]

Accession code: Swissprot P01574

```
-21  MTNKCLLQIA LLLCFSTTAL S
  1  MSYNLLGFLQ RSSNFQCQKL LWQLNGRLEY CLKDRMNFDI PEEIKQLQQF
 51  QKEDAALTIY EMLQNIFAIF RQDSSSTGWN ETIVENLLAN VYHQINHLKT
101  VLEEKLEKED FTRGKLMSSL HLKRYYGRIL HYLKAKEYSH CAWTIVRVEI
151  LRNFYFINRL TGYLRN
```

Disulphide bonds betwen Cys31–141. Variant C->Y at position 141 results in loss of disulphide bond and loss of antiviral activity.

Amino acid sequence for mouse IFNβ [8]

Accession code: Swissprot P01575

```
-21  MNNRWILHAA FLLCFSTTAL S
  1  INYKQLQLQE RTNIRKCQEL LEQLNGKINL TYRADFKIPM EMTEKMQKSY
 51  TAFAIQEMLQ NVFLVFRNNF SSTGWNETIV VRLLDELHQQ TVFLKTVLEE
101  KQEERLTWEM SSTALHLKSY YWRVQRYLKL MKYNSYAWMV VRAEIFRNFL
151  IIRRLTRNFQ N
```

THE IFNβ RECEPTOR

See IFN α/β receptor in IFNα entry.

References
1 Pestka, S. and Langer, J. A. (1987) Annu. Rev. Biochem. 56, 727–777.
2 de Maeyer, E. and de Maeyer-Guignard, J. (1991) In The Cytokine Handbook, Thomson, A.W., ed., Academic Press, London, pp. 215–239.
3 Senda, T. et al. (1992) EMBO J. 11, 3193–3201.
4 Derynck, R. et al. (1980) Nature 285, 542–547.
5 Ohno, S. and Taniguchi, T. (1981) Proc. Natl. Acad. Sci. USA 78, 5305–5309.
6 Kuga, T. et al. (1989) Nucl. Acids Res. 17, 3291–3291.
7 Taniguchi, T. et al. (1980) Gene 10, 11–15.
8 Higashi, Y. et al. (1983) J. Biol. Chem. 258, 9522–9529.

IFNγ

Other names

Immune interferon, type II interferon, T cell interferon.

THE MOLECULE

Interferon-γ is a pleiotropic cytokine involved in the regulation of nearly all phases of immune and inflammatory responses, including the activation, growth and differentiation of T cells, B cells, macrophages, NK cells and other cell types such as endothelial cells and fibroblasts. It has weak antiviral and antiproliferative activity, and potentiates the antiviral and anti-tumour effects of IFNα/β [1,2].

Crossreactivity

There is only 40% homology between human and mouse IFNγ and no significant cross-species activity.

Sources

CD8+ and CD4+ T cells, NK cells.

Bioassays

See entry for IFNα.

Physicochemical properties of IFNγ

Property	Human	Mouse
pI	?	5.5–6.0
Amino acids – precursor	166	155
– mature[a]	143	133
M_r (K) – predicted	17.1	15.9
– expressed[b]	40–70 (20, 25)	40–80
Potential N-linked glycosylation sites[c]	2	2
Disulphide bonds	0	0

[a] The predicted sequence after removal of a signal peptide of 20 amino acids for human IFNγ and 19 amino acids for murine IFNγ gives mature proteins of 146 and 136 amino acids respectively. However, sequencing of natural IFNγ has shown that the three N-terminal residues (Cys–Tyr–Cys) are removed during post translational modification yielding mature proteins of 143 and 133 amino acids [3].

[b] Two species (M_r 25 000 and 20 000) of monomeric human IFNγ have been identified on SDS–PAGE which differ only in the degree and sites of N-linked glycosylation. The higher molecular weight forms observed on gel filtration are due to dimerization and some multimerization.

[c] Glycosylation of human IFNγ at position 100 occurs only in the dimer.

3-D structure [4]

IFNγ is a homodimer formed by antiparallel association of two subunits. Each subunit has six α-helices held together by short non-helical sequences. There are no β-sheets. The subunits have a flattened elliptical shape, whereas the overall structure of the dimer is globular.

Gene structure [5,6]

Scale

Exons   50 aa

☐ Translated

500 bp

▨ Untranslated

Introns   ├──┤
500 bp

Chromosome

```
          38          23 61              44
hIFNγ  ──┤│├──      ─┤│├┤ ├──────────┤ │▨├──      12q24.1

          37          22 61              35
mIFNγ  ──┤│├──      ─┤│├┤├──────────┤ │▨├──      10
```

Amino acid sequence for human IFNγ [7]

Accession code: Swissprot P01579

```
-20   MKYTSYILAF QLCIVLGSLG
  1   CYCQDPYVKE AENLKKYFNA GHSDVADNGT LFLGILKNWK EESDRKIMQS
 51   QIVSFYFKLF KNFKDDQSIQ KSVETIKEDM NVKFFNSNKK KRDDFEKLTN
101   YSVTDLNVQR KAIHELIQVM AELSPAAKTG KRKRSQMLFR GRRASQ
```

Variant sequences K->Q at position 9 and R->Q at position 140. The N-glycosylation at position 100 occurs only in the dimer. N-Terminal amino acids Cys–Tyr–Cys are removed during post-translational modification.

Amino acid sequence for mouse IFNγ [6]

Accession code: Swissprot P01580

```
-19   MNATHCILAL QLFLMAVSG
  1   CYCHGTVIES LESLNNYFNS SGIDVEEKSL FLDIWRNWQK DGDMKILQSQ
 51   IISFYLRLFE VLKDNQAISN NISVIESHLI TTFFSNSKAK KDAFMSIAKF
101   EVNNPQVQRQ AFNELIRVVH QLLPESSLRK RKRSRC
```

N-Terminal amino acids Cys–Tyr–Cys are removed during post-translational modification.

THE IFNγ RECEPTOR

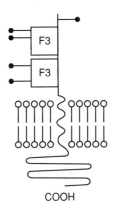

COOH

The IFNγ receptor is a complex of a high affinity IFNγ binding chain (CDw 119) and a second accessory protein required for signal transduction. The IFNγ binding subunit is a single chain transmembrane glycoprotein with a high content of serine and threonine in the intracytoplasmic domain. There is at least one disulphide bond which is essential for function. The receptor is a member of the class II cytokine receptor family which also includes the IFN-α/β receptor, IL10 receptor, and tissue factor [8-10], and is characterised by an extracellular region of about 200 amino acids consisting of two homologous FNIII domains. The first of these has two conserved tryptophans and a pair of conserved cysteines whereas the second has a unique disulphide loop formed from the second pair of conserved cysteines, but no WSXWS motif characteristic of class I cytokine receptors [11]. Although the receptor binds IFNγ with high affinity, signal transduction requires a species specific accessory protein [12,13,14] which associates with the extracellular domain of the receptor [15]. The accessory subunit is encoded by a gene on chromosome 21 and has been called accessory factor 1 (AF-1) [13] and the IFNγ receptor β-chain [14]. It also is a type I membrane spanning glycoprotein and a member of the class II cytokine receptor family with two FNIII domains. Although chromosome 21 encodes the accessory factors required to restore IFNγ induced MHC class I induction and resistance to EMCV infection by cells transfected with the IFNγ receptor, the cloned human accessory protein restores only MHC class I induction and not EMCV resistance suggesting that the accessory subunit belongs to a family of similar proteins [13].

Distribution

The IFNγ receptor is expressed on a wide variety of haematopoietic cells including T cells, B cells, macrophages, polymorphonuclear leukocytes, platelets, but not erythrocytes. The receptor is also on many somatic cells such as epithelial and endothelial cells and on many tumour cells [16].

Physicochemical properties of the IFNγ receptor

Property	IFNγ Receptor		Accessory Chain	
	Human	Mouse	Human	Mouse
Amino acids – precursor	489	477	337	332
– mature[a]	472	455	310	314
M_r (K) – predicted	52.6	50.0	35.0	35.5
– expressed	90	90	?	?
Potential N-linked glycosylation sites	5	5	6	6
Affinity K_d (M)	10^{-9}–10^{-10}	10^{-9}–10^{-10}	?	?

[a] After removal of predicted signal peptide.

Signal transduction

IFN-γ induces receptor dimerisation and internalisation. Receptor mediated ligand internalisation is not sufficient to induce a biological response. Signal transduction is mediated by phosphorylation and activation of JAK1 and JAK2 protein tyrosine kinases [17-19], and involves phosphorylation of the receptor [12,20,21]. The IFNγ and IFNα/β receptors share common signal transduction components including p91 which binds directly to the GAS response element after translocation to the nucleus [19,20,22].

Chromosomal location

The human receptor is on chromosome 6q12-q22 and the receptor accessory protein is on chromosome 21q22. The mouse receptor is on chromosome 10, and the accessory protein is on chromosome 16.

Amino acid sequence for the human IFNγ receptor [23]

Accession code: Swissprot P15260

```
 -17  MALLFLLPLV  MQGVSRA
   1  EMGTADLGPS  SVPTPTNVTI  ESYNMNPIVY  WEYQIMPQVP  VFTVEVKNYG
  51  VKNSEWIDAC  INISHHYCNI  SDHVGDPSNS  LWVRVKARVG  QKESAYAKSE
 101  EFAVCRDGKI  GPPKLDIRKE  EKQIMIDIFH  PSVFVNGDEQ  EVDYDPETTC
 151  YIRVYNVYVR  MNGSEIQYKI  LTQKEDDCDE  IQCQLAIPVS  SLNSQYCVSA
 201  EGVLHVWGVT  TEKSKEVCIT  IFNSSIKGSL  WIPVVAALLL  FLVLSLVFIC
 251  FYIKKINPLK  EKSIILPKSL  ISVVRSATLE  TKPESKYVSL  ITSYQPFSLE
 301  KEVVCEEPLS  PATVPGMHTE  DNPGKVEHTE  ELSSITEVVT  TEENIPDVVP
 351  GSHLTPIERE  SSSPLSSNQS  EPGSIALNSY  HSRNCSESDH  SRNGFDTDSS
 401  CLESHSSLSD  SEFPPNNKGE  IKTEGQELIT  VIKAPTSFGY  DKPHVLVDLL
 451  VDDSGKESLI  GYRPTEDSKE  FS
```

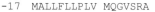

The two pairs of Cys residues at positions 60,68 and 197,218 are conserved in the class II cytokine receptor family.

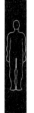

Amino acid sequence of the human IFNγR accessory protein [13]

Accession code: GenEMBL U05875 U05877

```
-27  MRPTLLWSLL LLLGVFAAAA AAPPDPL
  1  SQLPAPQHPK IRLYNAEQVL SWEPVALSNS TRPVVYRVQF KYTDSKWFTA
 51  DIMSIGVNCT QITATECDFT AASPSAGFPM DFNVTLRLRA ELGALHSAWV
101  TMPWFQHYRN VTVGPPENIE VTPGEGSLII RFSSPFDIAD TSTAFFCYYV
151  HYWEKGGIQQ VKGPFRSNSI SLDNLKPSRV YCLQVQAQLL WNKSNIFRVG
201  HLSNISCYET MADASTELQQ VILISVGTFS LLSVLAGACF FLVLKYRGLI
251  KYWFHTPPSI PLQIEEYLKD PTQPILEALD KDSSPKDDVW DSVSIISFPE
301  KEQEDVLQTL
```

Cys59, 67, 147 and 207 are conserved in the IFNR family

Amino acid sequence for the mouse IFNγ receptor [24]

Accession code: Swissprot P15261

```
-22  MGPQAAAGRM ILLVVLMLSA KV
  1  GSGALTSTED PEPPSVPVPT NVLIKSYNLN PVVCWEYQNM SQTPIFTVQV
 51  KVYSGSWTDS CTNISDHCCN IYGQIMYPDV SAWARVKAKV GQKESDYARS
101  KEFLMCLKGK VGPPGLEIRR KKEEQLSVLV FHPEVVVNGE SQGTMFGDGS
151  TCYTFDYTVY VEHNRSGEIL HTKHTVEKEE CNETLCELNI SVSTLDSRYC
201  ISVDGISSFW QVRTEKSKDV CIPPFHDDRK DSIWILVVAP LTVFTVVILV
251  FAYWYTKKNS FKRKSIMLPK SLLSVVKSAT LETKPESKYS LVTPHQPAVL
301  ESETVICEEP LSTVTAPDSP EAAEQEELSK ETKALEAGGS TSAMTPDSPP
351  TPTQRRSFSL LSSNQSGPCS LTAYHSRNGS DSGLVGSGSS ISDLESLPNN
401  NSETKMAEHD PPPVRKAPMA SGYDKPHMLV DVLVDVGGKE SLMGYRLTGE
451  AQELS
```

The two pairs of Cys residues at positions 61,69 and 199,221 are conserved in the class II cytokine receptor family.

Amino acid sequence of the mouse IFNγR accessory protein [14]

Acession code: none yet

```
-18  MRPLPLWLPS LLLCGLGA
  1  AASSPDSFSQ LAAPLNPRLH LYNDEQILTW EPSPSSNDPR PVVYQVEYSF
 51  IDGSWHRLLE PNCTDITETK CDLTGGGRLK LFPHPFTVFL RVRAKRGNLT
101  SKWVGLEPFQ HYENVTVGPP KNISVTPGKG SLVIHFSPPF DVFHGATFQY
151  LVHYWEKSET QQEQVEGPFK SNSIVLGNLK PYRVYCLQTE AQLILKNKKI
201  RPHGLLSNVS CHETTANASA PLQQVILIPL GIFALLLGLT GACFTLFLKY
251  QSRVKYWFQA PPNIPEQIEE YLKDPDQFIL EVLDKDGSPK EDSWDSVSII
301  SSPEKERDDV LQTP
```

References

1 Vilcek, J. et al. (1985) Lymphokines 11, 1–32.

2 Farrar, M.A. and Schreiber, R.D. (1993) Annu. Rev. Immunol. 11, 571–611.

3 Rinderknecht, E. et al. (1984) J. Biol. Chem. 259, 6790–6797.

4 Ealick, S.E. et al. (1991) Science 252, 698–252.

5 Gray, P.W. and Goeddel, D.V. (1982) Nature 298, 859–863.

6 Gray, P.W. and Goeddel, D.V. (1983) Proc. Natl Acad. Sci. USA 80, 5842–5846.

7 Gray, P.W. et al. (1982) Nature 295, 503–508.

8 Bazan, J.F. (1990) Proc. Natl Acad. Sci. USA 87, 6934–6938.

9 Aguet, M. (1991) Br. J. Haematol. 79 , 6–8.

10 Lutfalla, G. et al. (1992) J. Biol. Chem. 267, 2802–2809.

11 Bazan, J.F. (1990) Cell 61, 753–754.

12 Schreiber, R.D. et al. (1992) Int. J. Immunopharmacol. 14, 413–419.

13 Soh, J. et al. (1994) Cell 76, 793–802.

14 Hemmi, S. et al. (1994) Cell 76, 803–810.

15 Gibbs, V.C. et al. (1991) Mol. Cell. Biol. 11, 5860–5866.

16 Valente, G. et al. (1992) Eur. J. Immunol. 22, 2403–2412.

17 Hunter, T. (1993) Nature 366, 114–116.

18 Watling, D. et al. (1993) Nature 366, 166–170.

19 Muller, M. et al. (1993) Nature 366, 129–135.

20 Pellegrini, S. and Schindler, C. (1993) Trends Biochem. Sci. 18, 338–342.

21 Kalina, U. et al. (1993) J. Virol. 67, 1702–1706.

22 Loh, J.E. et al. (1992) EMBO J. 11, 1351–1363.

23 Aguet, M. et al. (1988) Cell 55, 273–280.

24 Gray, P.W. et al. (1989) Proc. Natl Acad. Sci. USA 86, 8497–8501.

Other names

Human LIF has been known as human interleukin for DA cells (HILDA), melanoma-derived lipoprotein lipase inhibitor (MLPLI) and hepatocyte stimulating factor III (HSF III). Mouse LIF has been known as differentiation inhibiting factor (DIA), differentiation retarding factor (DRF) and cholinergic nerve differentiation factor (CNDF).

THE MOLECULE

Leukaemia inhibitory factor is produced by many different cell types and has pleiotropic actions [1]. LIF stimulates the differentiation of the macrophage cell line M1, and the proliferation of haematopoietic stem cells [2-4]. *In vivo*, it has profound effects on haematopoiesis, particularly in combination with other cytokines such as IL-3, causing increased platelet formation [5]. LIF allows embryonic stem cells to remain in an undifferentiated state and can maintain their proliferation in culture [6]. LIF stimulates synthesis of acute phase proteins by liver cells, increases bone resorption, stimulates differentiation of cholinergic nerves and loss of body fat [7-10].

Crossreactivity

There is 78% homology between human and mouse LIF [2,3]. Human LIF is active on mouse cells, mouse LIF is not active on human cells.

Sources

Multiple, including T cells, myelomonocytic lineages, fibroblasts, liver, heart and melanoma.

Bioassays

Human and murine LIF can be measured using the M1 murine leukaemia cell line assay [2].

Physicochemical properties of LIF

Property		Human	Mouse
pI		9	>9
Amino acids	– precursor	202	203[a]
	– mature	180	180
M_r (K)	– predicted	20	20
	– expressed	45	58
Potential N-linked glycosylation sites[b]		6	6
Disulphide bonds		3	3

[a] A second form of murine LIF has an alternative leader peptide which targets LIF to matrix [11].
[b] Disulphide bonds link Cys12–134, 18–131 and 60–163[12].

3-D structure

Predicted to be a four alpha helical bundle structure similar to other hematopoietin cytokines [13]

Gene structure [14,15]

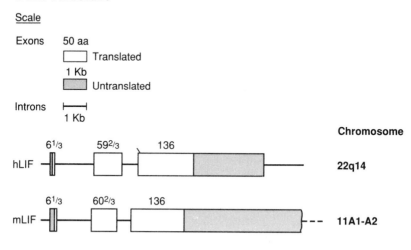

Scale

Exons   50 aa
         ☐ Translated
         1 Kb
         ▨ Untranslated

Introns ├──┤
         1 Kb

                                                    Chromosome

hLIF $6^{1/3}$ $59^{2/3}$ 136   **22q14**

mLIF $6^{1/3}$ $60^{2/3}$ 136   **11A1-A2**

The gene for murine LIF is located on chromosome 11A1-A2 [15].

Amino acid sequence for human LIF [3,7,9]

Accession code: Swissprot P15018

```
-22  MKVLAAGVVP LLLVLHWKHG AG
  1  SPLPITPVNA TCAIRHPCHN NLMNQIRSQL AQLNGSANAL FILYYTAQGE
 51  PFPNNLDKLC GPNVTDFPPF HANGTEKAKL VELYRIVVYL GTSLGNITRD
101  QKILNPSALS LHSKLNATAD ILRGLLSNVL CRLCSKYHVG HVDVTYGPDT
151  SGKDVFQKKK LGCQLLGKYK QIIAVLAQAF
```

Amino acid sequence for mouse LIF [2]

Accession code: Swissprot P09056

```
-23  MKVLAAGIVP LLLLVLHWKH GAG
  1  SPLPITPVNA TCAIRHPCHG NLMNQIKNQL AQLNGSANAL FISYYTAQGE
 51  PFPNNVEKLC APNMTDFPSF HGNGTEKTKL VELYRMVAYL SASLTNITRD
101  QKVLNPTAVS LQVKLNATID VMRGLLSNVL CRLCNKYRVG HVDVPPVPDH
151  SDKEAFQRKK LGCQLLGTYK QVISVVVQAF
```

THE LIF RECEPTOR

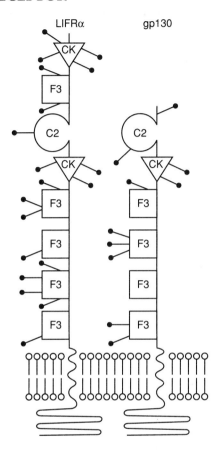

The high affinity (K_d 10–200×10^{-12}M) LIF receptor is a complex of a low affinity (K_d 1–3nM) receptor (LIFRα-chain) belonging to the cytokine receptor superfamily, and a second affinity conversion chain (gp130) (CDw 130) which also forms part of the IL-6R complex [16] (see IL-6 entry). The high affinity LIF receptor is also a high affinity receptor for oncostatin M. The LIF receptor and gp130 also form part of the CNTF receptor complex [17]. Antibodies to gp130 block responses to LIF, IL-6, OSM and CNTF [18]. A soluble murine receptor has been described which shares 76% identity with the human receptor [16]. A membrane-bound murine LIFR also exists [19].

Distribution

Monocytes, liver, placenta, embryonic stem cells.

Physicochemical properties of the LIF receptorα-chain

Properties		Human	Mouse
Amino acids	– precursor	1097	719
	– mature	1053	676
M_r (K)	– predicted	111	76.2
	– expressed	190	130
Potential N-linked glycosylation sites		19	13
Affinity K_d (M)	– low	10^{-9}	$1–3\times10^{-9}$
	– high	0.15×10^{-10}	$0.1–2.0\times10^{-10}$

Signal transduction

There is no evidence that the low affinity receptor (LIFRα-chain) can transduce a signal. The C-terminal 110 amino acids can be removed from the receptor and it can still associate with the affinity converter. By analogy with the IL-6 receptor, the affinity converter is likely to be the signalling chain.

Chromosomal location

The human LIFRα-chain is on chromosome 5p12–13 and the mouse LIFRα-chain is on chromosome 15.

Amino acid sequence for human low affinity LIF receptor [16]

Accession code: Genbank X61615

```
 -44 MMDIYVCLKR PSWMVDNKRM RTASNFQWLL STFILLYLMN QVNS
   1 QKKGAPHDLK CVTNNLQVWN CSWKAPSGTG RGTDYEVCIE NRSRSCYQLE
  51 KTSIKIPALS HGDYEITINS LHDFGSSTSK FTLNEQNVSL IPDTPEILNL
 101 SADFSTSTLY LKWNDRGSVF PHRSNVIWEI KVLRKESMEL VKLVTHNTTL
 151 NGKDTLHHWS WASDMPLECA IHFVEIRCYI DNLHFSGLEE WSDWSPVKNN
 201 SWIPDSQTKV FPQDKVILVG SDITFCCVSQ EKVLSALIGH TNCPLIHLDG
 251 ENVAIKIRNI SVSASSGTNV VFTTEDNIFG TVIFAGYPPD TPQQLNCETH
 301 DLKEIICSWN PGRVTALVGP RATSYTLVES FSGKYVRLKR AEAPTNESYQ
 351 LLFQMLPNQE IYNFTLNAHN PLGRSQSTIL VNITEKVYPH TPTSFKVKDI
 401 NSTAVKLSWH LPGNFAKINF LCEIEIKKSN SVQEQRNVTI QGVENSSYLV
 451 ALDKLNPYTL YTFRIRCSTE TFWKWSKWSN KKQHLTTEAS PSKGPDTWRE
 501 WSSDGKNLII YWKPLPINEA NGKILSYNVS CSSDEETQSL SEIPDPQHKA
 551 EIRLDKNDYI ISVVAKNSVG SSPPSKIASM EIPNDDLKIE QVVGMGKGIL
 601 LTWHYDPNMT CDYVIKWCNS SRSEPCLMDW RKVPSNSTET VIESDEFRPG
 651 IRYNFFLYGC RNQGYQLLRS MIGYIEELAP IVAPNFTVED TSADSILVKW
 701 EDIPVEELRG FLRGYLFYFG KGERDTSKMR VLESGRSDIK VKNITDISQK
 751 TLRIADLQGK TSYHLVLRAY TDGGVGPEKS MYVVTKENSV GLIIAILIPV
 801 AVAVIVGVVT SILCYRKREW IKETFYPDIP NPENCKALQF QKSVCEGSSA
 851 LKTLEMNPCT PNNVEVLETR SAFPKIEDTE IISPVAERPE DRSDAEPENH
 901 VVVSYCPPII EEEIPNPAAD EAGGTAQVIY IDVQSMYQPQ AKPEEEQEND
 951 PVGGAGYKPQ MHLPINSTVE DIAAEEDLDK TAGYRPQANV NTWNLVSPDS
1001 PRSIDSNSEI VSFGSPCSIN SRQFLIPPKD EDSPKSNGGG WSFTNFFQNK
1051 PND
```

Amino acid sequence for mouse low affinity LIF receptor [16]

Accession code: D26177, D17444

```
-43  MAAYSWWRQP  SWMVDNKRSR  MTPNLPWLLS  ALTLLHLTMH  ANG
  1  LKRGVQDLKC  TTNNMRVWDC  TWPAPLGVSP  GTVKDICIKD  RFHSCHPLET
 51  TNVKIPALSP  GDHEVTINYL  NGFQSKFTLN  EKDVSLIPET  PEILDLSADF
101  FTSSLLLKWN  DRGSALPHPS  NATWEIKVLQ  NPRTEPVALV  LLNTMLSGKD
151  TVQHWNWTSD  LPLQCATHSV  SIRWHIDSPH  FSGYKEWSDW  SPLKNISWIR
201  NTETNVFPQD  KVVLAGSNMT  ICCMSPTKVL  SGQIGNTLRP  LIHLYGQTVA
251  IHILNIPVSE  NSGTNIIFIT  DDDVYGTVVF  AGYPPDVPQK  LSCETHDLKE
301  IICSWNPGRI  TGLVGPRNTE  YTLFESISGK  SAVFHRIEGL  TNETYRLGVQ
351  MHPGQEIHNF  TLTGRNPLGQ  AQSAVVINVT  ERVAPHDPTS  LKVKDINSTV
401  VTFSWYLPGN  FTKINLLCQI  EICKANSKKE  VRNATIRGAE  DSTYHVAVDK
451  LNPYTAYTFR  VRCSSKTFWK  WSRWSDEKRH  LTTEATPSKG  PDTWREWSSD
501  GKNLIVYWKP  LPINEANGKI  LSYNVSCSLN  EETQSVLEIF  DPQHRAEIQL
551  SKNDYIISVV  ARNSAGSSPP  SKIASMEIPN  DDITVEQAVG  LGNRIFLTWR
601  HDPNMTCDYV  IKWCNSSRSE  PCLLDWRKVP  SNSTETVIES  DQFQPGVRYN
651  FYLYGCTNQG  YQLLRSIIGY  VEELEA
```

For the affinity converter (gp130) see IL-6 entry.

References

1 Gearing, D.P. (1991) Ann. N.Y. Acad. Sci. 628, 9–18.
2 Gearing, D.P. et al. (1987) EMBO J. 6, 3995–4002.
3 Gough, N.M. et al. (1988) Proc. Natl. Acad. Sci. USA 85, 2623–2627.
4 Escary, J.L. et al. (1993) Nature 363, 361–364.
5 Waring, P. et al. (1993) Br. J. Haematol. 83, 80–87.
6 Williams, R.L. et al. (1988) Nature 336, 684–687.
7 Moreau, J.-F. et al. (1988) Nature 336, 690–692.
8 Yamamori, T. et al. (1989) Science 246, 1412–1416.
9 Baumann, H. and Wong, G.G. (1989) J. Immunol. 143, 1163–1167.
10 Mori, M. et al. (1989) Biochem. Biophys. Res. Commun. 160, 1085–1092.
11 Rathjen, P.D. et al. (1990) Cell 62, 1105–1114.
12 Nicola, N.A. et al. (1993) Biochem. Biophys. Res. Commun. 190, 20–26.
13 Bazan, J.F. (1991) Neuron 7, 197–208.
14 Sutherland, G.R. et al. (1989)Leukemia 3, 9–13.
15 Kola, I. et al. (1989) Growth Factors 2, 235–140.
16 Gearing, D.P. et al. (1991) EMBO J. 10, 2839–2848.
17 Gearing, D.P. et al. (1992) Science 255, 1434–1437.
18 Taga, T. et al. (1993) Proc. Natl. Acad. Sci. USA 89, 10998–11001.
19 Gearing, D.P. et al. (1993) Adv. Immunol. 53, 31–58.

LT (TNFβ)

Other names

Tumour necrosis factor β (TNFβ), cytotoxin, differentiation-inducing factor.

THE MOLECULE

Lymphotoxin has 35% homology with TNFα and binds to the same receptors. Like TNFα, it has a wide range of biological activities from killing of tumour cells *in vitro* to induction of gene expression and stimulation of fibroblast proliferation. It is also an important mediator of inflammation and immune function. Whereas TNFα can be expressed as a membrane protein attached by its long signal sequence, LT has a more conventional signal peptide and is secreted [1-3]. A membrane-bound molecule LTβ has been described. LTβ is a type II integral membrane protein that forms a heteromeric complex with LT on the cell surface [4,5]. The function of this complex is at present unknown.

Crossreactivity

There is 74% homology between human and mouse LT and significant cross-species activity.

Sources

LT is made mostly by activated T and B lymphocytes. There have also been some reports of its production by astrocytes.

Bioassays

The same bioassays for TNFα can be used. Cytotoxicity on murine L929 or WEHI 164 clone 13.

Physicochemical properties of LT

Property	LT (TNFβ) Human	LT (TNFβ) Mouse	LTβ Human
pI	5.8	5.8	?
Amino acids – precursor	205	202	244
– mature[a]	171	169	244/240[b]
M_r (K) – predicted	18.7	18.6	25.4
– expressed[c]	25	25	33
N-linked glycosylation sites[d]	1	1	1
Disulphide bonds	0	0	0

[a] After removal of predicted signal peptide.

[b] LTβ is a type II integral membrane protein. N-Terminal amino acid analysis has shown LTβ to begin with Gly at position 5. There is some evidence that translation is initiated by CTG coding for Leu at position 4 which is subsequently removed.

[c] Corresponds to the subunit secreted by the B lymphoblastoid cell line RPMI 1788. There is also a M_r 20 000 LT secreted by this line which lacks the 23 N-terminal amino acids and may be a breakdown product. The mature molecule is a trimer, except for the membrane-bound complex form [4].

[d] There is N-linked glycosylation and some O-linked glycosylation [6].

3-D structure

The structure of LT has been solved at a resolution of 1.9 Å [7]. It is very similar to TNFα.

Gene structure [5,8–10]

<u>Scale</u>

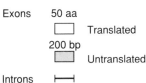

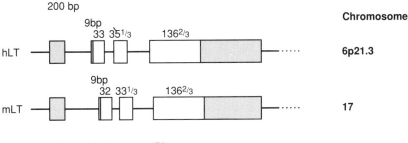

Order on chromosome: centromere - - - - LTβ —— TNFα —— LT
                                         →   ←   ←
                                         2Kb   1.2Kb

Amino acid sequence for human LT [11]

Accession code: Swissprot P01374

```
-34  MTPPERLFLP  RVCGTTLHLL  LLGLLLVLLP  GAQG
  1  LPGVGLTPSA  AQTARQHPKM  HLAHSTLKPA  AHLIGDPSKQ  NSLLWRANTD
 51  RAFLQDGFSL  SNNSLLVPTS  GIYFVYSQVV  FSGKAYSPKA  TSSPLYLAHE
101  VQLFSSQYPF  HVPLLSSQKM  VYPGLQEPWL  HSMYHGAAFQ  LTQGDQLSTH
151  TDGIPHLVLS  PSTVFFGAFA  L
```

Variant sequence T->N at position 26

Amino acid sequence for human LTβ [5]

Accession code: GenEMBL L11015

```
  1  MGALGLEGRG  GRLQGRGSLL  LAVAGATSLV  TLLLAVPITV  LAVLALVPQD
 51  QGGLVTETAD  PGAQAQQGLG  FQKLPEEEPE  TDLSPGLPAA  HLIGAPLKGQ
101  GLGWETTKEQ  AFLTSGTQFS  DAEGLALPQD  GLYYLYCLVG  YRGRAPPGGG
151  DPQGRSVTLR  SSLYRAGGAY  GPGTPELLLE  GAETVTPVLD  PARRQGYGPL
201  WYTSVGFGGL  VQLRRGERVY  VNISHPDMVD  FARGKTFFGA  VMVG
```

Translation may be initiated by CTG coding for Leu at position 4. Removal of the N-terminal amino acid then gives a mature protein begining with Gly at position 5.

169

Amino acid sequence for mouse LT [12]

Accession code: Swissprot P09225

```
-33  MTLLGRLHLL  RVLGTPPVFL  LGLLLALPLG  AQG
  1  LSGVRFSAAR  TAHPLPQKHL  THGILKPAAH  LVGYPSKQNS  LLWRASTDRA
 51  FLRHGFSLSN  NSLLIPTSGL  YFVYSQVVFS  GESCSPRAIP  TPIYLAHEVQ
101  LFSSQYPFHV  PLLSAQKSVY  PGLQGPWVRS  MYQGAVFLLS  KGDQLSTHTD
151  GISHLHFSPS  SVFFGAFAL
```

THE LT RECEPTORS

See under TNFα. TNFα and LT bind the same receptor molecules.

References
1 Paul, N.L. and Ruddle, N. H. (1988) Annu. Rev. Immunol. 6, 407–438.
2 Ruddle, N.H. and Turetskaya, R.L. (1991) In The Cytokine Handbook, Thomson, A.W., ed., Academic Press, London, pp. 257–267.
3 Ruddle, N.H. (1992) Curr. Opin. Immunol. 4, 327–332.
4 Androlewicz, M.J. et al. (1992) J. Biol. Chem. 267, 2542–2547.
5 Browning, J.L. et al. (1993) Cell 72, 847–856.
6 Kofler, G. et al. (1992) Lymphokine Cytokine Res. 11, 9–14.
7 Eck, M.J. et al. (1992) J. Biol. Chem. 267, 2119–2122.
8 Nedwin, G.E. et al. (1985) Nucl. Acids Res. 13, 6361–6373.
9 Semon, D. et al. (1987) Nucl. Acids Res. 15, 9083-9084
10 Gray, P.W. et al. (1987) Nucl. Acids Res. 15, 3937–3937.
11 Gray, P.W. et al. (1984) Nature 312, 721–724.
12 Li, C-B. et al. (1987) J. Immunol. 138, 4496–4501.

Other names

Human MCP-1 has been known as monocyte chemoattractant and activating factor (MCAF), human JE, lymphocyte derived chemotactic factor (LDCF) and glioma derived monocyte chemotactic factor (GDCF). Human MCP-2 has been known as HC14. Mouse MCP-1 has been known as JE, and mouse MCP-3 as MARC [1].

THE MOLECULES

Monocyte chemoattractant protein 1 is a monocyte chemoattractant and activating factor, and an activating factor for basophils [2-6]. MCP-1 is a member of the CC family of chemokine/intercrine cytokines [7]. The related molecules MCP-2 and MCP-3 are also monocyte chemoattractants [8,9].

Crossreactivity
There is about 55% homology between human and mouse MCP-1. Human MCPs are active on rabbit cells [8].

Sources
Monocytes, T lymphocytes, fibroblasts, endothelial cells, smooth muscle cells, keratinocytes and some tumours [10]. IFNγ is a potent stimulus for leucocyte release of MCPs, whilst IL-13 inhibits release.

Bioassays
MCP-1 is measured using Boyden chamber or agarose gel chemotaxis assays. Monocytes and basophils but not neutrophils or lymphocytes are affected. Half maximal responses are seen with 0.5 ng/ml MCP-1. Histamine release from basophils is a sensitive measure of MCP-1 levels.

Physicochemical properties of MCPs

Property	Human (MCP-1, MCP-2, MCP-3)	Mouse (MCP-1)
pI	9.7	10.5
Amino acids – precursor	99/77/100[a]	148
– mature	76	125[b]
M_r (K) – predicted	8.7	12
– expressed	8–18[c]	12–25[c]
Potential N-linked glycosylation sites	1/0/1[a]	1
Disulphide bonds[d]	2	2

[a] For MCP-1, 2 and 3 respectively.

[b] Mature mouse MCP-1 has a C-terminal extension of 49 amino acids.

[c] Variable O-linked glycosylation gives rise to the variation in molecular weight of human MCPs[11]. There is no N-linked glycosylation site in MCP-2.

[d] Disulphide bonds link Cys 11–36 and 12–52 in human and mouse MCP-1, a similar arrangement is predicted for MCP-2 and MCP-3.

3-D structure

A model of MCP-1 has been prepared, based on the solution structure of IL-8, indicating a dimeric structure consisting of two three-stranded Greek keys upon which lie two antiparallel α-helices [12]. Sequence differences between IL-8 and MCP-1 in surface residues suggest that biological specificity is determined by residues in the cleft between the two α-helices.

Gene structure [7,13]

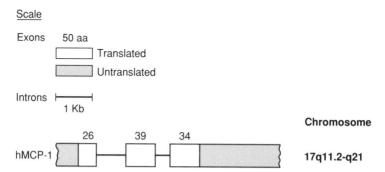

Scale

Exons   50 aa

Translated

Untranslated

Introns

1 Kb

Chromosome

26   39   34

hMCP-1   17q11.2-q21

The gene for murine MCP-1 is located on the distal portion of chromosome 11 [7,13].

Amino acid sequence for human MCP-1 [3-5]

Accession code: Swissprot P13500

```
-23  MKVSAALLCL LLIAATFIPQ GLA
  1  QPDAINAPVT CCYNFTNRKI SVQRLASYRR ITSSKCPKEA VIFKTIVAKE
 51  ICADPKQKWV QDSMDHLDKQ TQTPKT
```

A proteolytically processed variant lacking five amino acids at the N-terminus has been described [14].

Amino acid sequence for mouse MCP-1 [6]

Accession code: NBRF A30209

```
-23  MQVPVMLLGL LFTVAGWSIH VLA
  1  QPDAVNAPLT CCYSFTSKMI PMSRLESYKR ITSSRCPKEA VVFVTKLKRE
 51  VCADPKKEWV QTYIKNLDRN QMRSEPTTLF KTASALRSSA PLNVKLTRKS
101  EANASTTFST TTSSTSVGVT SVTVN
```

Amino acid sequence for human MCP-2 [8]

Accession code: Swissprot P80075

```
-1   A
 1   QPDSVSIPIT CCFNVINRKI PIQRLESYTR ITNIQCPKEA VIFKTKRGKE
51   VCADPKERWV RDSMKHLDQI FQNLKP
```

Amino acid sequence for human MCP-3 [8]

Accession code: GenEMBL X71087

```
-24  MKASAALLCL LLTAAAFSPQ GLA
  1  QPVGINTSTT CCYRFINKKI PKQRLESYRR TTSHSCPREA VIFKTKLDKE
 51  ICADPTQKWV QDFMKHLDKK TQTPKL
```

THE MCP RECEPTOR

There appears to be a specific receptor for MCP-1 on monocytes (IC$_{50}$ 0.5nM, K_d 0.2nM) [15] or (kD 2nM)[16], and at least one other receptor shared with RANTES (IC$_{50}$ 35nM) [15]. MCP-1 has been shown to bind to the cloned MIP-1α receptor with a K_d of 230nM, in a heterologous expression system, but it was a weak stimulus for calcium flux [17]. There is no information on receptors for MCP-2 and 3.

Signal transduction

MCP-1 causes a calcium flux in monocytes and the receptor is G-protein-linked [15,18,19].

References
1 Kulmburg, P.A. et al. (1992) J. Exp. Med. 176, 1773–1778.
2 Leonard, E.J. and Yoshimura, T. (1990) Immunol. Today 11, 97–101.
3 Matsushima, K. et al. (1989) J. Exp. Med. 169, 1485–1490.
4 Yoshimura, T. et al. (1989) FEBS Lett. 244, 487–493.
5 Robinson, E.A. et al. (1989) Proc. Natl. Acad. Sci. USA 86, 1850–1854.
6 Rollins, B.J. et al. (1988) Proc. Natl. Acad. Sci. USA 85, 3738–3742.
7 Schall, T.J. (1991) Cytokine 3, 165–183.
8 Van Damme, J. et al. (1992) J. Exp. Med. 176, 59–65.
9 Minty, A. et al. (1993) Eur. Cyt. Network 4, 99–110.
10 Cushing, S.D. et al. (1990) Proc. Natl. Acad. Sci. USA 87, 5134–5138.
11 Jiang, Y. et al. (1990) J. Biol. Chem. 265, 18318–18321.
12 Gronenborn, A.M. and Clore G.M. (1991) Prot. Eng. 4, 263–269.
13 Wilson, S.D. et al. (1990) J. Exp. Med. 171, 1301–1314.
14 Decock, B. et al. (1990) Biochem. Biophys. Res. Commun. 167, 904–909.
15 Van Riper, B.G. et al. (1993) J. Exp. Med. 177, 851–856.
16 Valente, A.J. et al. (1991) Biochem. Biophys. Res. Commun. 176, 309–314.
17 Neote, K. et al. (1993) Cell 72, 415–425.
18 Rollins, B.J. et al. (1991) Blood 78, 1112–1116.
19 Yoshimura, T. and Leonard, E.J. (1990) J. Immunol. 145, 292–297.

M-CSF

Other names

Human and mouse M-CSF have been known as colony stimulating factor-1 (CSF-1) and macrophage and granulocyte inducer IM (MGI-IM).

THE MOLECULE

Macrophage colony stimulating factor is a survival, growth, differentiation and activating factor for macrophages and their progenitor cells [1,2]. M-CSF is a complex cytokine, which can be produced as integral cell surface or secreted protein variants [3-6].

Crossreactivity

There is about 82% homology between human and mouse M-CSF in the N-terminal 227 amino acid of the mature sequence, falling to 47% in the rest of the molecule[4]. Human M-CSF is active on murine cells but not vice versa [4].

Sources

Multiple, including lymphocytes, monocytes, fibroblasts, epithelial cells, endothelial cells, myoblasts and osteoblasts.

Bioassays

Macrophage colony formation from bone marrow in soft agar, or proliferation of the M-NFS60 murine cell line [7,8].

Physicochemical properties of M-CSF

Property	Human	Mouse
pI	3–5	?
Amino acids – precursor	554	552
– mature	522/406/224[a]	519
M_r (K) – predicted	60	61
– expressed[b]	45–90	45–90
Potential N-linked glycosylation sites	3	3
Disulphide bonds	7–9	7–9

[a] M-CSF is derived from three major mRNA species to yield 522 amino acid (M-CSFb), 406 amino acid (M-CSFg, lacking residues 332–447), and 224 amino acid (M-CSFa, lacking residues 150–447) polypeptides which share the same N- and C-termini.

[b] M-CSF is biologically active as a disulphide-linked homodimer [9]. The active homodimers are made up from N-terminal chains (amino acids 1–221) and are released from the cell membrane by proteolytic cleavage [1]. Residues 1–149 are required for biological activity.

3-D structure

The structure of a recombinant M-CSF residues 4–158 has been determined by X-ray crystallography to 2.5 Å [9]. The molecule is comprised of two bundles of four α-helices laid end to end. The connectivity of the helices is similar to GM-CSF, G-CSF, IL-4, IL-2 and growth hormone.

Gene structure [10,11]

Scale

Exons   50 aa
         ☐ Translated

         500 bp
         ☐ Untranslated

Introns ⊢⊣
         2 Kb

Note: size of exon six can be $341^{2/3}$ or $43^{2/3}$ depending on which splice acceptor site is used (ref 5)
Exon ten gives an alternative 3' untranslated sequence

The mouse M-CSF gene is on chromosome 11 [11].

Amino acid sequence for human M-CSF [2,3,5]

Accession code: Swissprot P09603

```
 -32  MTAPGAAGRC PPTTWLGSLL LLVCLLASRS IT
   1  EEVSEYCSHM IGSGHLQSLQ RLIDSQMETS CQITFEFVDQ EQLKDPVCYL
  51  KKAFLLVQDI MEDTMRFRDN TPNAIAIVQL QELSLRLKSC FTKDYEEHDK
 101  ACVRTFYETP LQLLEKVKNV FNETKNLLDK DWNIFSKNCN NSFAECSSQD
 151  VVTKPDCNCL YPKAIPSSDP ASVSPHQPLA PSMAPVAGLT WEDSEGTEGS
 201  SLLPGEQPLH TVDPGSAKQR PPRSTCQSFE PPETPVVKDS TIGGSPQPRP
 251  SVGAFNPGME DILDSAMGTN WVPEEASGEA SEIPVPQGTE LSPSRPGGGS
 301  MQTEPARPSN FLSASSPLPA SAKGQQPADV TGTALPRVGP VRPTGQDWNH
 351  TPQKTDHPSA LLRDPPEPGS PRISSLRPQG LSNPSTLSAQ PQLSRSHSSG
 401  SVLPLGELEG RRSTRDRRSP AEPEGGPASE GAARPLPRFN SVPLTDTGHE
 451  RQSEGSSSPQ LQESVFHLLV PSVILVLLAV GGLLFYRWRR RSHQEPQRAD
 501  SPLEQPEGSP LTQDDRQVEL PV
```

The biologically active soluble form of M-CSF (residues 1–221) is released by proteolytic cleavage from the membrane-bound propeptide (in italics).

Amino acid sequence for mouse M-CSF [4,12]

Accession code: Swissprot P07141

```
-33   MTARGRAGRC PSSTWLGSRL LLVCLLMSRS IAK
  1   EVSEHCSHMI GNGHLKVLQQ LIDSQMETSC QIAFEFVDQE QLDDPVCYLK
 51   KAFFLVQDII DETMRFKDNT PNANATERLQ ELSNNLNSCF TKDYEEQNKA
101   CVRTFHETPL QLLEKIKNFF NETKNLLEKD WNIFTKNCNN SFAKCSSRDV
151   VTKPDCNCLY PKATPSSDPA SASPHQPPAP SMAPLAGLAW DDSQRTEGSS
201   LLPSELPLRI EDAGSAKQRP PRSTCQTLES TEQPNHGDRL TEDSQPHPSA
251   GGPVPGVEDI LESSLGTNWV LEEASGEASE GFLTQEAKFS PSTPVGGSIQ
301   AETDRPRALS ASPFPKSTED QKPVDITDRP LTEVNPMRPI GQTQNNTPEK
351   TDGTSTLRED HQEPGSPHIA TPNPQRVSNS ATPVAQLLLP KSHSWGIVLP
401   LGELEGKRST RDRRSPAELE GGSASEGAAR PVARFNSIPL TDTGHVEQHE
451   GSSDPQIPES VFHLLVPGII LVLLTVGGLL FYKWKWRSHR DPQTLDSSVG
501   RPEDSSLTQD EDRQVELPV
```

THE M-CSF RECEPTOR

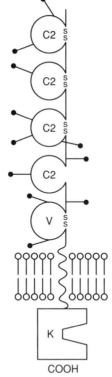

The M-CSF receptor (CD115) is identical to the product of the c-*fms* proto-oncogene and is related to the PDGF receptor, FGFb receptor and c-kit (the stem cell factor receptor) [13-17]. These receptors are all autophosphorylating tyrosine kinases [18]. The intracellular kinase domain contains a 70 amino acid insert which is necessary for association with PI-3′ kinase. The receptor exists in a single affinity form.

Distribution

Macrophages and their progenitors, placental cells.

Physicochemical properties of the M-CSF receptor

Properties	Human	Mouse
Amino acids – precursor	972	976
– mature	953	957
M_r (K) – predicted	106	109
– expressed	150	165
Potential N-linked glycosylation sites	11	9
Affinity K_d (M)	0.4×10^{-10}	$<2 \times 10^{-10}$

Signal transduction

M-CSF binding to its receptor stabilizes dimerisation leading to activation of the kinase which autophosphorylates the receptor, PI-3 kinase, and other cytoplasmic proteins[18]. The M-CSF receptor is also G-protein-linked and stimulates protein kinase C translocation to the cell membrane[19].

Chromosomal location

The human gene is located on chromosome 5q33-q35[16].

Amino acid sequence for human M-CSF receptor [15]

Accession code: Swissprot P07333

```
-19   MGPGVLLLLL  VATAWHGQG
  1   IPVIEPSVPE  LVVKPGATVT  LRCVGNGSVE  WDGPASPHWT  LYSDGSSSIL
 51   STNNATFQNT  GTYRCTEPGD  PLGGSAAIHL  YVKDPARPWN  VLAQEVVVFE
101   DQDALLPCLL  TDPVLEAGVS  LVRVRGRPLM  RHTNYSFSPW  HGFTIHRAKF
151   IQSQDYQCSA  LMGGRKVMSI  SIRLKVQKVI  PGPPALTLVP  AELVRIRGEA
201   AQIVCSASSV  DVNFDVFLQH  NNTKLAIPQQ  SDFHNNRYQK  VLTLNLDQVD
251   FQHAGNYSCV  ASNVQGKHST  SMFFRVVESA  YLNLSSEQNL  IQEVTVGEGL
301   NLKVMVEAYP  GLQGFNWTYL  GPFSDHQPEP  KLANATTKDT  YRHTFTLSLP
351   RLKPSEAGRY  SFLARNPGGW  RALTFELTLR  YPPEVSVIWT  FINGSGTLLC
401   AASGYPQPNV  TWLQCSGHTD  RCDEAQVLQV  WDDPYPEVLS  QEPFHKVTVQ
451   SLLTVETLEH  NQTYECRAHN  SVGSGSWAFI  PISAGAHTHP  PDEFLFTPVV
501   VACMSIMALL  LLLLLLLLYK  YKQKPKYQVR  WKIIESYEGN  SYTFIDPTQL
551   PYNEKWEFPR  NNLQFGKTLG  AGAFGKVVEA  TAFGLGKEDA  VLKVAVKMLK
601   STAHADEKEA  LMSELKIMSH  LGQHENIVNL  LGACTHGGPV  LVITEYCCYG
651   DLLNFLRRKA  EAMLGPSLSP  GQDPEGGVDY  KNIHLEKKYV  RRDSGFSSQG
701   VDTYVEMRPV  STSSNDSFSE  QDLDKEDGRP  LELRDLLHFS  SQVAQGMAFL
751   ASKNCIHRDV  AARNVLLTNG  HVAKIGDFGL  ARDIMNDSNY  IVKGNARLPV
801   KWMAPESIFD  CVYTVQSDVW  SYGILLWEIF  SLGLNPYPGI  LVNSKFYKLV
851   KDGYQMAQPA  FAPKNIYSIM  QACWALEPTH  RPTFQQICSF  LQEQAQEDRR
901   ERDYTNLPSS  SRSGGSGSSS  SELEEESSSE  HLTCCEQGDI  AQPLLQPNNY
951   QFC
```

Tyr680, 689 and 790 are autophosphorylated.

Amino acid sequence for mouse M-CSF receptor [17]

Accession code: Swissprot P09581

```
 -19  MELGPPLVLL  LATVWHGQG
   1  APVIEPSGPE  LVVEPGETVT  LRCVSNGSVE  WDGPISPIWT  LDPESPGSTL
  51  TTSNATFKNT  GTYRCTELED  PMAGSTTIHL  YVKDPAHSWN  LLAQEVTVVE
 101  GQEAVLPCLI  TDPALKDSVS  LMREGGRQVL  RKTVYFFSPW  RGSIIRKAKV
 151  LDSNTYVCKT  MVNGRESTST  GIWLKVNRVH  PEPPQIKLEP  SKLVRIRGEA
 201  AQIVCSATNA  EVGFNVILKR  GDTKLEIPLN  SDFQDNYYKK  VRALSLNAVD
 251  FQDAGIYSCV  ASNDVGTRTA  TMNFQVVESA  YLNLTSEQSL  LQEVSVGDSL
 301  ILTVHADAYP  SIQHYNWTYL  GPFFEDQRKL  EFITQRAIYR  YTFKLFLNRV
 351  KASEAGQYFL  MAQNKAGWNN  LTFELTLRYP  PEVSVTWMPV  NGSDVLFCDV
 401  SGYPQPSVTW  MECRGHTDRC  DEAQALHLWN  DTHPEVLSQK  PFDKVIIQSQ
 451  LPIGPLKHNM  TYFCKTHNSV  GNSSQYFRAV  SLGQSKQLPD  ESLFTPVVVA
 501  CMSVMSLLVL  LLLLLLYKYK  QKPKYQVRWK  IIERYEGNSY  TFIDPTQLPY
 551  NEKWEFPRNN  LQFGKTLGAG  AFGKVVEATA  FGLGKEDAVL  KVAVKMLKST
 601  AHADEKEALM  SELKIMSHLG  QHENIVNLLG  ACTHGGPVLV  YTEYCCYGDH
 651  LNFLRRKAEA  MLGPSLSPGQ  DSEGDSSYKN  IHLEKKYVRR  DSGFSSQGVD
 701  TYVEMRPVST  SSSDSFFKQD  LDKEHSRPLE  LWDLLHFSSQ  VAQGMAFLAS
 751  KNCIHRDVAA  RNVLLTSGHV  AKIGDFGLAR  DIMNDSNYVV  KGNALPVKWM
 801  APESIFDCVI  TVQSDVWSYG  ILLWEIFSLG  LNPYPGIHVN  NKFYKLVKDG
 851  YQMAQPVFAP  KNIYSIMQSC  WDLEPTRRPT  FQQICFLLQE  QARLERRDQD
 901  YANLPSSGGS  SGSDSGGGSS  GGSSSEPEEE  SSSEHLACCE  PGDIAQPLLQ
 951  PNNYQFC
```

Tyr678, 687 and 788 are autophosphorylated.

References

[1] Sherr, C.J. and Stanley, E.R. (1990) In Growth Factors, Differentiation Factors and Cytokines, Habenicht, A., ed., Springer-Verlag, Berlin.

[2] Kawasaki, E.S. et al. (1985) Science 230, 291–296.

[3] Wong, G.C. et al. (1987) Science 235, 1504–1508.

[4] Ladner, M.B. et al. (1988) Proc. Natl. Acad. Sci. USA 85, 6706–6710.

[5] Ladner, M.B. et al. (1987) EMBO J. 6, 2693–2698.

[6] Cerreti, D.P. et al. (1988) Mol. Immunol. 25, 761–770.

[7] Testa, N.G. et al. (1991) In Cytokines: A Practical Approach, Balkwill, F.A., ed., IRL Press, Oxford, pp. 229–244.

[8] Wadhwa, M. et al. (1991) In Cytokines: A Practical Approach, Balkwill, F.A., ed., IRL Press, Oxford, pp. 309–329.

[9] Pandit, J. et al. (1992) Science 258, 1358–1362.

[10] Ladner, M.B. et al. (1987) EMBO J. 6, 2693–2698.

[11] Pettenati, M.J. et al. (1987) Proc. Natl. Acad. Sci. USA 84, 2970–2974.

[12] Delamater, J.F. et al. (1987) Nucl. Acids Res. 15, 2389–2390.

[13] Sherr, C.J. (1990) Blood 75, 1–12.

[14] Sherr, C. et al. (1985) Cell 41, 665–676.

[15] Coussens, L. et al. (1986) Nature 320, 277–280.

[16] Hampe, A. et al. (1989) Oncogene Res. 4, 9–17.

[17] Rothwell, V.M. and Rohrschneider, L.R. (1987) Oncogene Res. 1, 311–324.

[18] Ullrich, A. and Schlessinger, J. (1990) Cell 61, 203–212.

[19] Vairo, G. and Hamilton, J.A. (1991) Immunol Today 12, 362–369.

Other names
None.

THE MOLECULE

Migration inhibition factor is a cytokine which can activate macrophages and also inhibit their migration [1-3]. MIF can be detected immuno-histochemically in inflamed tissues, and in LPS-stimulated anterior pituitary cells acting as a mediator of lethal endotoxaemia [1,4].

Crossreactivity
Human MIF is active on guinea-pig cells. Murine MIF has 89% homology to human MIF.

Sources
Activated T cells, anterior pituitary cells and possibly monocytes and endothelial cells [4,5].

Bioassays
Inhibition of macrophage migration from agar gel drops, or from capillary tubes [6]. The migration is also inhibited by IL-4 and IFNγ.

Physicochemical properties of MIF

Property	Human	Mouse
Amino acids – precursor	115	114
– mature	?	?
M_r – predicted	12.3	12.3
– expressed[a]	12.5	?
Potential N-linked glycosylation sites	2	2
Disulphide bonds	1	1

[a] MIF produced by leucocytes exists as multimers ranging from M_r 25 000 to 68 000.

3-D structure
Not known.

Gene structure
Not known.

Amino acid sequence for human MIF [5]

Accession code: Swissprot P14174

```
  1   MPMFIVNTNV PRASVPDGFL SELTQQLAQA TGKPPQYIAV HVVPDQLMAF
 51   GGSSEPCALC SLHSIGKIGG AQNRSYSKLL CGLLAERLRI SPDRVYINYY
101   DMNAASVGWN NSTFA
```

There is no obvious signal sequence. Conflicting sequence S->N at position 106.

Amino acid sequence for mouse MIF

Accession code: Swissprot P34884

```
  1   PMFIVNTNVP RASVPEGFLS ELTQQLAQAT GKPAQYIAVH VVPDQLMTFS
 51   GTNDPCALCS LHSIGKIGGA QNRNYSKLLC GLLSDRLHIS PDRVYINYYD
101   MNAANVGWNG STFA
```

THE MIF RECEPTORS

No information available yet.

References
1 Malorny, U. et al. (1988) Clin. Exp. Immunol. 71, 164–170.
2 Cunha, F.Q. et al. (1993) J. Immunol. 150, 1908–1912.
3 Weiser, W.Y. et al. (1991) J. Immunol. 147, 2006–2011.
4 Bernhagen, J. et al. (1993) Nature 365, 756–759.
5 Weiser, W.Y. et al. (1989) Proc. Natl. Acad. Sci. USA 86, 7522–7526.
6 Harrington, J.T. and Stastny, P. (1973) J. Immunol. 110, 752–759.

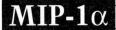

Other names

Human MIP-1α has been known as Hu MIP-1α, pLD78, pAT464 and GOS19. Mouse MIP-1α has been known as MIP-1α, TY5 and stem cell inhibitor.

THE MOLECULE

Macrophage inflammatory protein-1α is a monocyte-, neutrophil- and lymphocyte-derived cytokine [1,2] with activity as an inhibitor of stem cell proliferation [3–5], and as a chemoattractant for B cells, eosinophils and killer T cells. The murine protein may be pyrogenic [6]. MIP-1α is a member of the CC family of chemokine/intercrine cytokines [7].

Crossreactivity

There is about 73% homology between human and mouse MIP-1α. Human and mouse MIP-1α are active on human and murine haematopoietic cells [8].

Sources

T Cells, B cells, Langerhans cells, neutrophils and macrophages [9,10,19].

Bioassays

The only definitive bioassay for MIP-1α is inhibition of the proliferation of haematopoietic stem cells in a CFU-A assay [3]. Chemotaxis for eosinophils.

Physicochemical properties of MIP1α

Property	Human	Mouse
pI	4.6	4.6
Amino acids – precursor	92	92
– mature	70	69
M_r (K) – predicted	8.6	8
– expressed[a]	8–200	8–200
Potential N-linked glycosylation sites	0	0
Disulphide bonds[b]	2	2

[a] MIP-1α probably exists as high molecular weight aggregates under physiological conditions.

[b] By homology with the structures of IL-8 and platelet factor 4, the disulphide bonds should link Cys11–51 and 12–35 (human) and 11–50 and 12–34 (mouse).

3-D structure

Circular dichroism and fluorescence spectroscopy indicate that murine MIP-1α is structurally very similar to other members of the chemokine superfamily of cytokines [5].

Gene structure [11,14]

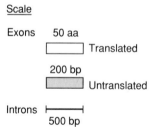

Scale

Exons   50 aa

☐ Translated

200 bp

▨ Untranslated

Introns ├────┤
        500 bp

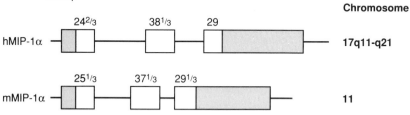

Chromosome

hMIP-1α

$24^{2/3}$ $38^{1/3}$ 29

17q11-q21

mMIP-1α

$25^{1/3}$ $37^{1/3}$ $29^{1/3}$

11

Note: 1. Human MIP-1α is 14 kb from MIP-1β in a head to head configuration.
2. A second non allelic human MIP-1α gene which varies by 5 amino acids has been identified.

Amino acid sequence for human MIP-1α [9,12,13]

Accession code: Swissprot P10147, P16619

```
-22  MQVSTAALAV LLCTMALCNQ FS
  1  ASLAADTPTA CCFSYTSRQI PQNFIADYFE TSSQCSKPGV IFLTKRSRQV
 51  CADPSEEWVQ KYVSDLELSA
```

Conflicting sequence S->P at position 2, G->S at position 39, and S->G at position 47.

Amino acid sequence for mouse MIP-1α [2,14]

Accession code: Swissprot P10855, P14096

```
-23  MKVSTTALAV LLCTMTLCNQ VFS
  1  APYGADTPTA CCFSYSRKIP RQFIVDYFET SSLCSQPGVI FLTKRNRQIC
 51  ADSKETWVQE YITDLELNA
```

Conflicting sequence F->L at position -2, V->A at position 39.

THE MIP-1α RECEPTOR

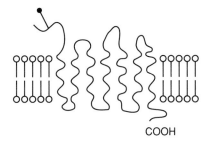

COOH

A MIP-1α receptor has been cloned from human leucocytes [15]. It is a seven membrane spanning receptor and shares 32% homology with the IL-8 receptors. The cloned receptor expressed in human kidney cells binds MIP-1α (K_d 5nM), MCP-1 (K_d 232nM), RANTES (K_d 468nM) and MIP-1β (K_d 122nM). MIP-1α at 10nM and RANTES at 100nM trigger a significant calcium flux via the receptor, MIP-1β at 250nM and MCP-1 at 1000nM give a weak calcium flux. A gene product of cytomegalovirus, hcmv-us28, encodes a functional protein with homology to the MIP-1α receptor [15].

Distribution

A specific receptor for murine MIP-1α has been identified on T cells, macrophages and eosinophils [16,17].

Physicochemical properties of the MIP-1α receptor

Properties	Human
Amino acids – precursor	355
– mature[a]	?
M_r (K) – predicted	41
– expressed	52
Potential N-linked glycosylation sites	1
Affinity K_d (M)	5×10^{-9}

[a] Length of signal sequence is not known.

Signal transduction

Binding of MIP-1α to its receptor triggers a calcium flux.

Chromosomal location

The receptor gene is on human chromosome 3p21 [18].

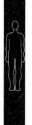

Amino acid sequence for the human MIP-1α receptor [15]

Accession code: Genbank L10918

```
  1  METP**N**TTEDY DTTTEFDYGD ATPCQKVNER AFGAQLLPPL YSLVFVIGLV
 51  GNILVVLVLV QYKRLKNMTS IYLLNLAISD LLFLFTLPFW IDYKLKDDWV
101  FGDAMCKILS GFYYTGLYSE IFFIILLTID RYLAIVHAVF ALRARTVTFG
151  VITSIIIWAL AILASMPGLY FSKTQWEFTH HTCSLHFPHE SLREWKLFQA
201  LKLNLFGLVL PLLVMIICYT GIIKILLRRP NEKKSKAVRL IFVIMIIFFL
251  FWTPYNLTIL ISVFQDFLFT HECEQSRHLD LAVQVTEVIA YTHCCVNPVI
301  YAFVGERFRK YLRQLFHRRV AVHLVKWLPF LSVDRLERVS STSPSTGEHE
351  LSAGF
```

References

 1 Wolpe, S.D. et al. (1988) J. Exp. Med. 167, 570–581.
 2 Davatelis, G. et al. (1988) J. Exp. Med. 167, 1939–1944.
 3 Graham, G.J. et al. (1990) Nature 344, 442–445.
 4 Lord, B.I. et al. (1992) Blood 79, 2605–2609.
 5 Clements, J.C. et al. (1992) Cytokine 4, 76–82.
 6 Davatelis, G. et al. (1989) Science 243, 1066–1068.
 7 Schall, T.J. (1991) Cytokine 3, 165–183.
 8 Broxmeyer, H.E. et al. (1989) J. Exp. Med. 170, 1583–1594.
 9 Obaru, K. et al. (1986) J. Biochem 99, 885–894.
10 Yamamura, Y. et al. (1989) J. Clin. Invest. 84, 1707–1712.
11 Wilson, S.D. et al. (1990) J. Exp. Med. 171, 1301–1314.
12 Irving, S.G. et al. (1990) Nucl. Acids Res. 18, 3261–3270.
13 Nakao, M. et al. (1990) Mol. Cell Biol. 10, 3646–3658.
14 Grove, M. et al. (1990) Nucl. Acids Res. 18, 5561.
15 Neote, K. et al. (1993) Cell 72, 415–425.
16 Oh, K.O. et al. (1991) J. Immunol. 147, 2978–2983.
17 Rot, A. et al. (1992). J. Exp. Med. 176, 1489–1495.
18 Gao, J.-L. et al. (1993) J. Exp. Med. 177, 1421–1427.
19 Kasama, T. et al. (1993) J. Exp. Med 178, 63–72.

Other names

Human MIP-1β has been known as Hu Mip-1β, ACT-2, pAT744, hH400, hSISα, G26 , HC21, MAD-5 and HIMAP. Mouse MIP-1β has been known as MIP-1β, H400 and SISγ.

THE MOLECULE

Macrophage inflammatory protein-1β is a monocyte- and lymphocyte-derived cytokine with stimulatory effects on myelopoietic cell growth and leucocyte chemoattractant activity [1-3]. It is closely related to MIP-1α, and may function in concert with it. MIP-1β is a member of the CC family of chemokine/intercrine cytokines [4].

Crossreactivity

There is about 70% homology between human and mouse MIP-1β [4]. Human and mouse MIP-1β are active on human and murine haematopoietic cells.

Sources

T Cells, B cells and macrophages [5,6].

Bioassays

Human MIP-1β is a chemoattractant for memory T cells. Murine MIP-1β enhances haematopoietic colony formation in the presence of GM-CSF. MIP-1β may antagonize the effects of MIP-1α [7].

Physicochemical properties of MIP-1β

Property	Human	Mouse
pI	4.6	4.6
Amino acids – precursor	92	92
– mature	69	69
M_r (K) – predicted	8.6	8
– expressed	7.8	8–100
Potential N-linked glycosylation sites[a]	0	0
Disulphide bonds[b]	2	2

[a] There may be some O-linked glycosylation.
[b] By homology with the structures of IL-8 and platelet factor 4, the disulphide bonds should link Cys11–35 and 12–51 in human and mouse MIP-1β.

3-D structure

Can be modelled on other chemokine cytokines.

Gene structure [8-10]

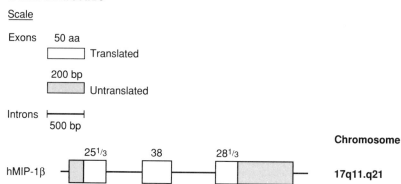

Scale

Exons 50 aa
☐ Translated

200 bp
▨ Untranslated

Introns ├────┤
500 bp

Chromosome

25¹/₃   38   28¹/₃

hMIP-1β

17q11.q21

There are multiple non-allelic genes for human MIP-1β located on chromosome 17 in bands q11–q21. The genes for murine MIP-1β are located on the distal portion of chromosome 11 [8-10]. Both are closely linked to MIP-1α. Human MIP-1β is 14 kb from MIP-1α in a head to head configuration.

Amino acid sequence for human MIP1β [5,6]

Accession code: Swissprot P13236

```
-23  MKLCVTVLSL LMLVAAFCSP ALS
  1  APMGSDPPTA CCFSYTARKL PRNFVVDYYE TSSLCSQPAV VFQTKRSKQV
 51  CADPSESWVQ EYVYDLELN
```

Conflicting sequence L->I at position –14, P->L at position –4, KLPR->EASS/H, at position 19–22, S->I at position 32, S->G at position 47 and S->T at position 57.

Amino acid sequences for mouse MIP-1β [1]

Accession code: Swissprot P14097

```
-23  MKLCVSALSL LLLVAAFCAP GFS
  1  APMGSDPPTS CCFSYTSRQL HRSFVMDYYE TSSLCSKPAV VFLTKRGRQI
 51  CPNPSQPWVT EYMSHLELN
```

Conflicting sequence C->A at position 51, Q->E at position 56, and L->D at position 66.

THE MIP-1β RECEPTOR

MIP-1β binds with low affinity to the cloned MIP-1α receptor. Murine MIP-1α and β compete with human MIP-1β for binding to the human receptor [11].

Distribution

MIP-1β receptors are found on T and B lymphocytes and monocytes, HELA and K562 cells.

References

1 Sherry, B .et al. (1988) J. Exp. Med. 168, 2251–2259.
2 Wolpe, S.D. et al. (1988) J. Exp Med 167, 570–581.
3 Broxmeyer, H.E. et al. (1989) J. Exp. Med. 170, 1583–1594.
4 Schall, T.J. (1991) Cytokine 3, 165–183.
5 Lipes, M.A. et al. (1988) Proc. Natl. Acad. Sci. USA 85, 9704–9708.
6 Zipfel, P.F. et al. (1989) J. Immunol. 142, 1582–1590.
7 Fahey, T.J. et al. (1992) J. Immunol. 148, 2764–2769.
8 Irving, S.G. et al. (1990) Nucl Acids Res. 18, 3261–3270.
9 Wilson, S.D. et al. (1990) J. Exp. Med. 171, 1301–1314.
10 Napolitano, M. et al. (1990) J. Biol. Chem. 266, 17531–17536.
11 Napolitano, M. et al. (1990) J. Exp. Med. 172, 285–289.

The Chemokine Family.

Other names

MIP-2α and MIP-2β have been known as GROβ and GROγ respectively. GRO/MGSA has also been known as NAP-3 [1]. Mouse MIP-2 is also known as KC.

THE MOLECULES

The products of the *MIP-2α, MIP-2β* and *GRO/MGSA* genes [2-4] are the human homologues of the mouse *MIP-2* and *KC* genes [5,6]. They are members of the CXC family of chemokine/intercrine cytokines. The molecules are chemoattractant and activating factors for neutrophils. MIP-2 is also a growth factor for myelopoietic cells and GRO/MGSA for fibroblasts and melanoma cells.

Crossreactivity

There is about 60 % homology between human and mouse MIP2 proteins, 87% homology between the human proteins, and 63% homology between KC and MIP-2. Murine MIP-2 is active on human cells; GRO is active on rodent cells.

Sources

MIP-2 is made by cytokine- or LPS-activated monocytes; GRO/MGSA is made by activated monocytes, fibroblasts, epithelial and endothelial cells and KC by activated monocytes and fibroblasts.

Bioassays

There are no specific assays for these molecules. GRO and MIP-2 are chemotactic and activating factors for neutrophils. GRO is also a growth factor for fibroblasts and melanoma cells.

Physicochemical properties of MIP-2

Property	Human MIP-2α, MIP-2β, GRO/MGSA			Mouse MIP-2	KC
pI	9.7–9.9			?	?
Amino acids – precursor	107	107	107	100	96
– mature	73	73	73	73	72
M_r (K) – predicted	11.4	11.4	11.3	10.6	10.2
– expressed	7.9	7.9	?	7.9	?
Potential N-linked glycosylation sites	0	0	0	0	0
Disulphide bonds[a]	2	2	2	2	2

[a] Disulphide bonds between Cys9–35 and 11–51 in each molecule.

3-D structure

Could be modelled on IL-8.

Gene structure

The genes for human MIP-2α, MIP-2β, and GRO/MGSA are located on chromosome 4q12–21 [1]. The genes for murine MIP-2 and KC are not yet localized .

Amino acid sequence for human MIP-2α [2]

Accession code: Swissprot P19875

```
-34  MARATLSAAP  SNPRLLRVAL  LLLLLVAASR  RAAG
  1  APLATELRCQ  CLQTLQGIHL  KNIQSVKVKS  PGPHCAQTEV  IATLKNGQKA
 51  CLNPASPMVK  KIIEKMLKNG  KSN
```

Amino acid sequence for human MIP-2β [3]

Accession code: Swissprot P19876

```
-34  MAHATLSAAP  SNPRLLRVAL  LLLLLVAASR  RAAG
  1  ASVVTELRCQ  CLQTLQGIHL  KNIQSVNVRS  PGPHCAQTEV  IATLKNGKKA
 51  CLNPASPMVQ  KIIEKILNKG  STN
```

Amino acid sequence for human GRO/MGSA [4]

Accession code: Swissprot P09341

```
-34  MARAALSAAP  SNPRLLRVAL  LLLLLVAAGR  RAAG
  1  ASVATELRCQ  CLQTLQGIHP  KNIQSVNVKS  PGPHCAQTEV  IATLKNGRKA
 51  CLNPASPIVK  KIIEKMLNSD  KSN
```

Amino acid sequence for mouse MIP-2 [5]

Accession code: Swissprot P10889

```
-27  MAPPTCRLLS  AALVLLLLLA  TNHQATG
  1  AVVASELRCQ  CLKTLPRVDF  KNIQSLSVTP  PGPHCAQTEV  IATLKGGQKV
 51  CLDPEAPLVQ  KIIQKILNKG  KAN
```

Amino acid sequence for mouse KC [6]

Accession code: Swissprot P12850

```
-24  MIPATRSLLC  AALLLLATSR  LATG
  1  APIANELRCQ  CLQTMAGIHL  KNIQSLKVIP  SGPHCTQTEV  IATLKNGREA
 51  CLDPEAPLVQ  KIVQKMLKGV  PK
```

THE MIP-2 RECEPTORS

GRO and MIP-2 have been shown to compete with IL-8 for binding to the low affinity IL-8 receptors on neutrophils [7] (see IL-8 entry).

Distribution

MIP-2 receptors are found on neutrophils, monocytes, endothelial cells and melanoma cells.

Signal transduction

MIP-2 causes a calcium flux in both neutrophils and monocytes [8].

References
1 Oppenheim, J.J. et al. (1991) Ann. Rev. Immunol. 9, 617–648.
2 Haskill, S. et al. (1990) Proc. Natl. Acad. Sci. USA 87, 7732–7736.
3 Sager, R. et al. (1991) Adv. Exp. Med. Biol. 305, 73–77.
4 Aniscowicz, A. et al. (1987) Proc. Natl Acad. Sci. USA 84, 7188–7192.
5 Tekamp-Olson, P. et al. (1990) J. Exp. Med. 172, 911–919.
6 Oquendo, P. et al. (1989) J. Biol. Chem. 264, 4133–4137.
7 LaRosa, G.J. et al. (1992) J. Biol. Chem. 267, 25402–25406.
8 Walz, A. et al. (1991) J. Leucocyte Biol. 50, 279–286.

Other names
β-NGF.

THE MOLECULE

Nerve growth factor enhances the survival, growth and neurotransmitter biosynthesis of certain sympathetic and sensory neurons [1-4]. It has also been reported to stimulate the growth and differentiation of B lymphocytes [5].

NGF isolated from mouse submaxillary gland is in the form of a high molecular weight 7S complex (M_r 130 000–140 000) consisting of homodimeric NGF (β-NGF) and two other subunits (α-NGF and γ-NGF) belonging to the kallikrein family of serine proteases. The α– and γ-NGF kallikreins are involved in the processing of the β-NGF precursor to form active NGF by removal of an N-terminal pre-propeptide and a C-terminal dipeptide [2]. The β- and γ-NGF kallikreins are lacking in other species, and processing of human precursor NGF does not include removal of the C-terminal dipeptide.

NGF has about 50% homology with BDNF, NT-3 and NT-4/5.

Crossreactivity
There is 90% sequence homology between human and mouse NGF and complete cross-species reactivity.

Sources
Submaxillary gland of male mice, prostate, brain and nervous system.

Bioassays
Survival and outgrowth of neurites from embryo chicken dorsal root ganglia. Differentiation of PC12 cell line.

Physicochemical properties of NGF

Property	Human	Mouse
pI	~10	~10
Amino acids – precursor	241	241/307/313[a]
– mature[b]	120	118
M_r (K) – predicted	13.5	13.3
– expressed[c]	26	26 (130)
Potential N-linked glycosylation sites[d]	3	3
Disulphide bonds[e]	3	3

[a] There are three forms of murine NGF precursor derived from alternative mRNA splicing. Two high molecular weight forms (M_r 33 900 and 33 800) of 313 and 307 amino acids respectively, and a low molecular weight form (M_r 27 000) of 241 amino acids (see sequence and gene diagram).

[b] After removal of propeptide. The C-terminal dipeptide is also removed from mouse NGF.

[c] Biologically active NGF is a homodimer. Murine NGF is also found in the submaxillary gland as a high molecular weight complex (M_r 130 000) with α- and γ-NGF.

d Includes two sites on propeptide. The one site on mature NGF is not normally glycosylated.

e Disulphide bonds are required for biological activity. All the Cys residues are strictly conserved between species and between NGF, BDNF, NT-3 and NT-4.

3-D structure

Functional NGF is a non-covalently linked parallel homodimer. Crystal structure of the NGF dimer has been resolved at 2.3 Å. It consists of three antiparallel pairs of β-strands together forming a flat surface through which the two subunits associate. There are four loops which contain many of the variable residues between the different NGF-related molecules, and may determine receptor specificity. Clusters of positively charged side-chains may interact with the acidic low affinity NGFR [6].

Gene structure [7]

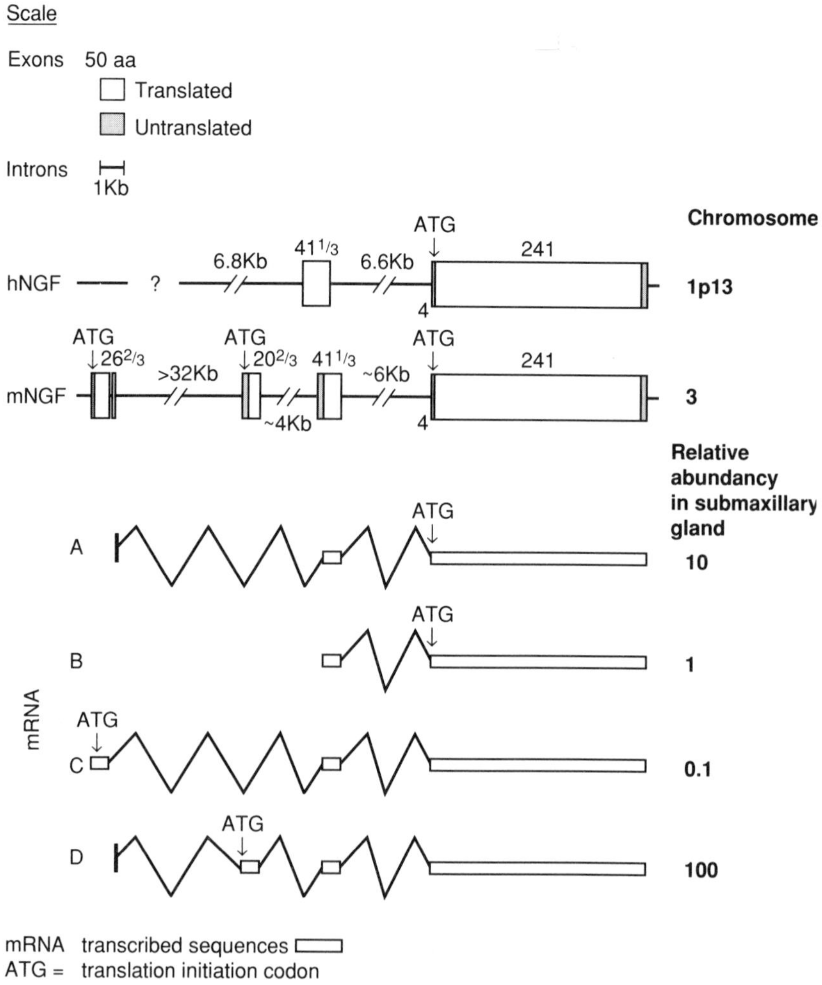

Scale

Exons 50 aa
    ☐ Translated
    ▨ Untranslated

Introns ⊢⊣
    1Kb

mRNA transcribed sequences ⊏⊐
ATG = translation initiation codon

Four species of murine NGF precursor mRNA produced by alternative splicing and independent promoter elements are shown as A–D above [7,8]. These give rise to three different precursor molecules. The abundance of the four mRNA species varies in different sites of production. The A form is the most abundant in submaxillary gland whereas the short forms are more abundant in other sites. The 5' end of the human gene has not yet been sequenced.

Amino acid sequence for human NGF [9]

Accession code: Swissprot P01138

```
-18   MSMLFYTLIT AFLIGIQA
  1   EPHSESNVPA GHTIPQVHWT KLQHSLDTAL RRARSAPAAA IAARVAGQTR
 51   NITVDPRLFK KRRLRSPRVL FSTQPPREAA DTQDLDFEVG GAAPFNRTHR
101   SKRSSSHPIF HRGEFSVCDS VSVWVGDKTT ATDIKGKEVM VLGEVNINNS
151   VFKQYFFETK CRDPNPVDSG CRGIDSKHWN SYCTTTHTFV KALTMDGKQA
201   AWRFIRIDTA CVCVLSRKAV RRA
```

Mature human NGF is formed by removal of a predicted signal peptide and a propeptide (1–103, in italics). Disulphide bonds between Cys118–183, 161–211 and 171–213 by similarity.

Amino acid sequence for mouse NGF [7,10]

Accession code: Swissprot P01139

(A B)
```
-18   MSMLFYTLIT AFLIGVQA
  1   EPYTDSNVPE GDSVPEAHWT KLQHSLDTAL RRARSAPTAP IAARVTGQTR
 51   NITVDPRLFK KRRLHSPRVL FSTQPPPTSS DTLDLDFQAH GTIPFNRTHR
101   SKRSSTHPVF HMGEFSVCDS VSVWVGDKTT ATDIKGKEVT VLAEVNINNS
151   VFRQYFFETK CRASNPVESG CRGIDSKHWN SYCTTTHTFV KALTTDEKQA
201   AWRFIRIDTA CVCVLSRKAT RRG
```

Mature murine NGF is formed by removal of a predicted signal peptide, an N-terminal propeptide (1–103, in italics), and a C-terminal Arg–Gly dipeptide (in italics). Disulphide bonds between Cys118–183, 161–211, and 171–213 by similarity.

Three murine NGF precursors derived from alternative mRNA splicing have been identified. The short form shown above with a total of 241 amino acids is derived from mRNA transcripts A and B shown on the gene diagram. Two other longer forms with additional N-terminal sequences (shown below) are derived from mRNA transcripts C and D. The letters A–D in bold indicate the translated peptides from the four mRNA species.

(C)
```
MSHQLGSYPS LVPRTLTTRT PGSSHSRVLA CGRAVQGAGW HAGPKLTSVS
GPNKGFAKDA AFYTGRSEVH SV
```

(D)
```
MLCLKPVKLG SLEVGHGQHG GVLACGRAVQ GAGWHAGPKL TSVSGPNKGF
AKDAAFYTGR SEVHSV
```

THE NGF RECEPTORS

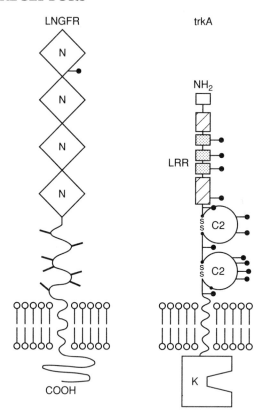

NGF binds to both low affinity (K_d 10^{-9}M) and high affinity (K_d 10^{-11}M) cell surface receptors [11,12]. The low affinity NGF receptor (LNGFR), also known as p75^{LNGF} or fast NGF receptor, belongs to the NGFR/TNFR superfamily with four Cys-rich repeats in the extracellular domain. It is also a low affinity receptor (K_d 10^{-9}M) for the NGF-related neurotrophins, BDNF, NT-3 and NT-4/5. The LNGFR does not mediate the neurotrophic effects of the NGF family [13,14] and it is expressed in non-neuronal cells that do not respond to any of the known members of the NGF family of neurotrophins [15]. Mice lacking the LNGFR gene are viable, and for the most part exhibit normal neuronal development except in certain sensory terminals. Expression of LNGFR has been shown to induce apoptosis which can be inhibited by either NGF or antibody binding to the receptor [16].

The high affinity receptors (K_d 10^{-11}M) mediate NGF neurotrophic activity and are expressed exclusively on NGF responsive cells. Their molecular structure is still a matter of debate. At least one component of the high affinity receptor is the product of the *trk* proto-oncogene gp140^{trk} (trkA). Transfection of trkA into 3T3 cells gives rise to low affinity receptors (Kd 10^{-9}M) and a small proportion of high affinity receptors

$(K_d 10^{-10}M)$. It has been proposed that the high affinity receptors result from receptor dimerization (or oligomerization) [17,18]. On the other hand, high affinity receptors have been shown to depend on co-expression of both trkA and LNGFR on COS cells indicating a role for LNGFR [19]. However, NGF mutants which cannot bind LNGFR can still interact with trkA and retain their full neurotrophic properties [20]. Whatever the structure of the high affinity receptor, trkA can mediate NGF signal transduction in the absence of LNGFR [17,18,21]. TrkA can also mediate NT-3 signal transduction with limited efficiency, at least in some *in vitro* assays [21].

TrkA is a member of the trk family of tyrosine kinases which includes trkB, a receptor for BDNF and NT-3, and trkC, a receptor for NT-3 but not NGF or BDNF [22-24]. This family of receptors is characterized by a novel extracellular domain made up of an N-terminal leucine-rich region (LRR) composed of three tandem leucine rich motifs flanked by two distinct cysteine-rich clusters, followed by two Ig-SF C2 set domains [25]. The LRR region is thought to be involved in cell adhesion and the Ig-SF domains may be important for interaction with other cell surface proteins. Fusion products of trkA with tropomyosin, L7a ribosomal protein, and the EGF receptor signal peptide have been identified as oncogenes [26].

Distribution

NGF receptors are expressed on sensory and sympathetic neurons, non-neuronal cells derived from the neural crest including melanocytes, and Schwann cells, and on mast cells, B lymphocytes, monocytes and the PC12 cell line [4,15,27-29].

Physicochemical properties of the NGF receptors

Properties	LNGF receptor		trkA	
	Human	Rat	Human	Rat
Amino acids – precursor	427	425	790	799
– mature[a]	399	396	758	765
M_r (K) – predicted	42.5	42.5	83.6	84.4
– expressed	70–75	83	140	150
Potential N-linked glycosylation sites[b]	1	2	13	11
Affinity K_d (M)[c]	10^{-9}	10^{-9}–10^{-10}	10^{-9}&10^{-10}	10^{-9}

[a] After removal of predicted signal peptide.

[b] There is some O-linked glycosylation of LNGFR on Ser/Thr-rich region proximal to the transmembrane domain.

[c] Rat and mouse trkA expressed in 3T3 cells have a K_d of approximately $10^{-9}M$ [11,19,30]. Human trkA expressed in 3T3 cells gives rise to two populations of receptors, one with a K_d of about $10^{-9}M$ and a second minor population with a K_d of about $10^{-10}M$ [17]. The higher affinity receptors may be dimers or oligomers [18].

Signal transduction

TrkA has intrinsic protein tyrosine kinase activity [11]. Binding of NGF induces tyrosine phosphorylation of several cellular proteins including PLC-γ1 [31,32], PI3-kinase [33] and autophosphorylation of trkA [31]. Association with the ERK1 Ser/Thr kinase has also been reported [34]. Activation of PLC-γ1 by phosphorylation results in hydrolysis of PIP_2 releasing IP_3 and DAG [32,35]. There is evidence for ligand-induced receptor dimerization [18]. The low affinity receptor is not required for growth and differentiation of neurons in response to NGF [21]. Expression of LNGFR has been shown to induce neuronal cell death by apoptosis which can be prevented by either NGF or monoclonal antibody binding to the receptor [16].

Chromosomal location

LNGFR is on human chromosome 17q21–q22 and trkA is on human chromosome 1q23–q31.

Amino acid sequence for human low affinity NGF receptor (LNGFR) [13]

Accession code: Swissprot P08138

```
-28    MGAGATGRAM  DGPRLLLLLL  LGVSLGGA
  1    KEACPTGLYT  HSGECCKACN  LGEGVAQPCG  ANQTVCEPCL  DSVTFSDVVS
 51    ATEPCKPCTE  CVGLQSMSAP  CVEADDAVCR  CAYGYYQDET  TGRCEACRVC
101    EAGSGLVFSC  QDKQNTVCEE  CPDGTYSDEA  NHVDPCLPCT  VCEDTERQLR
151    ECTRWADAEC  EEIPGRWITR  STPPEGSDST  APSTQEPEAP  PEQDLIASTV
201    AGVVTTVMGS  SQPVVTRGTT  DNLIPVYCSI  LAAVVVGLVA  YIAFKRWNSC
251    KQNKQGANSR  PVNQTPPPEG  EKLHSDSGIS  VDSQSLHDQQ  PHTQTASGQA
301    LKGDGGLYSS  LPPAKREEVE  KLLNGSAGDT  WRHLAGELGY  QPEHIDSFTH
351    EACPVRALLA  SWATQDSATL  DALLAALRRI  QRADLVESLC  SESTATSPV
```

Cys-rich repeats: 3–37, 38–79, 80–119, 120–161. Ser/Thr-rich segment 169–220.

Amino acid sequence for human high affinity NGF receptor (trkA) [26,36]

Accession code: Swissprot P04629, P08119

```
-32    MLRGGRRGQL  GWHSWAAGPG  SLLAWLILAS  AG
  1    AAPCPDACCP  HGSSGLRCTR  DGALDSLHHL  PGAENLTELY  IENQQHLQHL
 51    ELRDLRGLGE  LRNLTIVKSG  LRFVAPDAFH  FTPRLSRLNL  SFNALESLSW
101    KTVQGLSLQE  LVLSGNPLHC  SCALRWLQRW  EEEGLGGVPE  QKLQCHGQGP
151    LAHMPNASCG  VPTLKVQVPN  ASVDVGDDVL  LRCQVEGRGL  EQAGWILTEL
201    EQSATVMKSG  GLPSLGLTLA  NVTSDLNRKN  LTCWAENDVG  RAEVSVQVNV
251    SFPASVQLHT  AVEMHHWCIP  FSVDGQPAPS  LRWLFNGSVL  NETSFIFTEF
301    LEPAANETVR  HGCLRLNQPT  HVNNGNYTLL  AANPFGQASA  SIMAAFMDNP
351    FEFNPEDPIP  DTNSTSGDPV  EKKDETPFGV  SVAVGLAVFA  CLFLSTLLLV
401    LNKCGRRNKF  GINRPAVLAP  EDGLAMSLHF  MTLGGSSLSP  TEGKGSGLQG
451    HIIENPQYFS  DACVHHIKRR  DIVLKWELGE  GAFGKVFLAE  CHNLLPEQDK
```

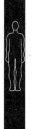

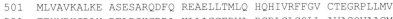

```
501   MLVAVKALKE  ASESARQDFQ  REAELLTMLQ  HQHIVRFFGV  CTEGRPLLMV
551   FEYMRHGDLN  RFLRSHGPDA  KLLAGGEDVA  PGPLGLGQLL  AVASQVAAGM
601   VYLAGLHFVH  RDLATRNCLV  GQGLVVKIGD  FGMSRDIYST  DYYRVGGRTM
651   LPIRWMPPES  ILYRKFTTES  DVWSFGVVLW  EIFTYGKQPW  YQLSNTEAID
701   CITQGRELER  PRACPPEVYA  IMRGCWQREP  QQRHSIKDVH  ARLQALAQAP
751   PVYLDVLG
```

Tyr at position 642 is site of autophosphorylation. Translocation breakpoint forming oncogene between Pro and Asp at position 360–361.

Amino acid sequence for rat low affinity NGF receptor (LNGFR) [14]

(Mouse LNGFR sequence has not been published.)
Accession number: Swissprot P07174

```
-29   MRRAGAACSA  MDRLRLLLLL  ILGVSSGGA
  1   KETCSTGLYT  HSGECCKACN  LGEGVAQPCG  ANQTVCEPCL  DNVTFSDVVS
 51   ATEPCKPCTE  CLGLQSMSAP  CVEADDAVCR  CAYGYYQDEE  TGHCEACSVC
101   EVGSGLVFSC  QDKQNTVCEE  CPEGTYSDEA  NHVDPCLPCT  VCEDTERQLR
151   ECTPWADAEC  EEIPGRWIPR  STPPEGSDST  APSTQEPEVP  PEQDLVPSTV
201   ADMVTTVMGS  SQPVVTRGTT  DNLIPVYCSI  LAAVVGLVA  YIAFKRWNSC
251   KQNKQGANSR  PVNQTPPPEG  EKLHSDSGIS  VDSQSLHDQQ  THTQTASGQA
301   LKGDGNLYSS  LPLTKREEVE  KLLNGDTWRH  LAGELGYQPE  HIDSFTHEAC
351   PVRALLASWG  AQDSATLDAL  LAALRRIQRA  DIVESLCSES  TATSPV
```

Cys-rich repeats: 3–37, 38–79, 80–119, 120–161. Ser/Thr-rich domain 169–220.

Amino acid sequence for rat high affinity NGF receptor (trkA) [37]

(Mouse trkA sequence has not been published.)
Accession code: Swissprot P04629, P08119

```
-34   MLRGQRHGQL  GWHRPAAGLG  GLVTSLMLAC  ACAA
  1   SCRETCCPVG  PSGLRCTRAG  TLNTLRGLRG  AGNLTELYVE  NQRDLQRLEF
 51   EDLQGLGELR  SLTIVKSGLR  FVAPDAFHFT  PRLSHLNLSS  NALESLSWKT
101   VQGLSLQDLT  LSGNPLHCSC  ALLWLQRWEQ  EDLCGVYTQK  LQGSGSGDQF
151   LPLGHNNSCG  VPSVKIQMPN  DSVEVGDDVF  LQCQVEGQAL  QQADWILTEL
201   EGTATMKKSG  DLPSLGLTLV  NVTSDLNKKN  VTCWAENDVG  RAEVSVQVSV
252   SFPASVHLGK  AVEQHHWCIP  FSVDGQPAPS  LRWFFNGSVL  NETSFIFTQF
301   LESALTNETM  RHGCLRLNQP  THVNNGNYTL  LAANPYGQAA  ASIMAAFMDN
351   PFEFNPEDPI  PVSFSPVDTN  STSRDPVEKK  DETPFGVSVA  VGLAVSAALF
400   LSALLLVLNK  CGQRSKFGIN  RPAVLAPEDG  LAMSLHFMTL  GGSSLSPTEG
451   KGSGLQGHIM  ENPQYFSDTC  VHHIKRQDII  LKWELGEGAF  GKVFLAECYN
501   LLNDQDKMLV  AVKALKETSE  NARQDFHREA  ELLTMLQHQH  IVRFFGVCTE
551   GGPLLMVFEY  MRHGDLNRFL  RSHGPDAKLL  AGGEDVAPGP  LGLGQLLAVA
601   SQVAAGMVYL  ASLHFVHRDL  ATRNCLVGQG  LVVKIGDFGM  SRDIYSTDYY
651   RVGGRTMLPI  RWMPPESILY  RKFSTESDVW  SFGVVLWEIF  TYGKQPWYQL
701   SNTEAIECIT  QGRELERPRA  CPPDVYAIMR  GCWQREPQQR  LSMKDVHARL
751   QALAQAPPSY  LDVLG
```

References

1 Levi-Montalcini, R. (1987) Science 237, 1154–1162.

2 Fahnestock, M. (1991) Curr. Topics Microbiol. Immunol. 165, 1–26.

3 Bradshaw, R.A. et al. (1993) Trends Biochem. Sci. 18, 48–52.

4 Ebendal, T. (1992) J. Neurosci. Res. 32, 461–470.

5 Otten, U. et al. (1989) Proc. Natl. Acad. Sci. USA 86, 10059–10063.

6 McDonald, N.Q. et al. (1991) Nature 354, 411– 414 .

7 Selby, M.J. et al. (1987) Mol. Cell. Biol. 7, 3057–3064.

8 Edwards, R.H. et al. (1986) Nature 319, 784–787.

9 Ulrich, A. et al. (1983) Nature 303, 821–825.

10 Scott, J. et al. (1983) Nature 302, 538–540.

11 Meakin, S.O. and Shooter, E.M. (1992) Trends Neurosci. 15, 323–331.

12 Barker, P.A. and Murphy, R.A. (1992) Mol. Cell. Biochem. 110, 1–15.

13 Johnson, D. et al. (1986) Cell 47, 545–554.

14 Radeke, M.J. et al. (1987) Nature 325, 593– 597.

15 Thomson et al. (1988) Exp. Cell Res. 174, 533–539.

16 Rabizadeh, S. et al. (1993) Science 261, 345–348.

17 Klein, R. et al. (1991) Cell 65, 189–197.

18 Jing, S. et al. (1992) Neuron 9, 1067– 1079.

19 Hempstead, B.L. et al. (1991) Nature 350, 678–683.

20 Ibanez, C.F. et al. (1992) Cell 69, 329–341.

21 Cordon-Cardo, C. et al. (1991) Cell 66, 173–183.

22 Soppet, D. et al. (1991) Cell 65, 895–903.

23 Squinto, S.P. et al. (1991) Cell 65, 885–893.

24 Lamballe, F. et al. (1991) Cell 66, 967–979.

25 Schneider, R. and Schweiger, M. (1991) Oncogene 6, 1807–1811.

26 Barbacid, M. et al. (1991) Biochim. Biophys. Acta 1072, 115–127.

27 Brodie, C. and Gelfand, E.W. (1992) J. Immunol. 148, 3492– 3497.

28 Ehrhard, P.B. et al. (1993) Proc. Natl. Acad. Sci. USA 90, 5423–5427.

29 Ernfors, P. et al. (1988) Neuron 1, 983–996.

30 Kaplan, D.R. et al. (1991) Science 252, 554–558.

31 Ohmichi, M. et al. (1991) Biochem. Biophys. Res. Commun. 179, 217–223.

32 Vetter, M.L. et al. (1991) Proc. Natl. Acad. Sci. USA 88, 5650–5654.

33 Ohmichi, M. et al. (1992) Neuron 9, 769–777.

34 Loeb, D.M. et al. (1992) Neuron 9, 1053–1065.

35 Kaplan, D.R. et al. (1991) Nature 350, 158–160.

36 Martin-Zanca, D. et al. (1989) Mol. Cell. Biol. 9, 24–33.

37 Meakin, S.O. et al. (1992) Proc. Natl. Acad. Sci. USA 89, 2374–2378.

Other names
Hippocampus derived neurotrophic factor (HDNF), nerve growth factor 2 (NGF-2).

THE MOLECULE

Neurotrophin-3 is a neurotrophic factor important in the development and maintenance of the vertebrate nervous system. *In vitro*, it promotes the survival and outgrowth of neural crest-derived sensory and sympathetic neurons. It is similar to NGF and NT-3 but with different neuronal specificities [1,2].

Crossreactivity
The amino acid sequences of mature NT-3 from human, mouse and rat are identical. There is complete cross-species reactivity.

Sources
To date, NT-3 protein has not been isolated from natural sources. NT-3 mRNA is present at high levels in the hippocampus and other sites in the foetal brain and at lower levels in adult brain. High levels are also present in the ovary. Transcripts have also been found in all adult tissues tested including skin, spleen, thymus, liver, muscle, lung, intestine and kidney [2].

Bioassays
Survival and outgrowth of neurites from embryo chicken dorsal root ganglia. Survival and differentiation of trkC transfected cell lines.

Physicochemical properties of NT-3

Property	Human	Mouse
pI	9.5	9.5
Amino acids – precursor	257	258
– mature[a]	119	119
M_r (K) – predicted	13.6	13.6
– expressed[b]	27	27
Potential N-linked glycosylation sites[c]	0	0
Disulphide bonds[d]	3	3

[a] After removal of pre-propeptide.
[b] Homodimer.
[c] There is one N-linked glycosylation site in propeptide.
[d] Conserved between NGF, BDNF NT-3 and NT-4.

3-D structure
Has 60% β-sheet. Exists as tightly linked homodimer. Crystal structure not known, but probably very similar to NGF.

Gene structure [3]

Scale

Exons   50 aa

☐ Translated

1 Kb

▨ Untranslated

Chromosome

257

hNT-3   ?——▨[   ]▨—   **12p13**

258

mNT-3   ?——▨[   ]▨—   **6**

There is evidence for more than one RNA species arising by alternative splicing and ATG initiation sites derived from additional upstream exons similar to mouse NGF.

Amino acid sequence for human NT-3 [3,4]

Accession code: Swissprot P20783

```
-16  MSILFYVIFL AYLRGI
  1  QGNNMDQRSL PEDSLNSLII KLIQADILKN KLSKQMVDVK ENYQSTLPKA
 51  EAPREPERGG PAKSAFQPVI AMDTELLRQQ RRYNSPRVLL SDSTPLEPPP
101  LYLMEDYVGS PVVANRTSRR KRYAEHKSHR GEYSVCDSES LWVTDKSSAI
151  DIRGHQVTVL GEIKTGNSPV KQYFYETRCK EARPVKNGCR GIDDKHWNSQ
201  CKTSQTYVRA LTSENNKLVG WRWIRIDTSC VCALSRKIGR T
```

Mature human NT-3 is formed by removal of a predicted signal peptide and a propeptide (1–122, in italics). Other precursor forms with extended N-terminal sequences similar to murine NGF may also exist. Disulphide bonds between Cys136–201, 179–230 and 189–232 by similarity.

Amino acid sequence for mouse NT-3 [5]

Accession code: Swissprot P20181

```
-16  MSILFYVIFL AYLRGI
  1  QGNSMDQRSL PEDSLNSLII KLIQADILKN KLSKQMVDVK ENYQSTLPKA
 51  EAPREPEQGE ATRSEFQPMI ATDTELLRQQ RRYNSPRVLL SDSTPLEPPP
101  LYLMEDYVGN PVVANRTSPR RKRYAEHKSH RGEYSVCDSE SLWVTDKSSA
151  IDIRGHQVTV LGEIKTGNSP VKQYFYETRC KEARPVKNGC RGIDDKHWNS
201  QCKTSQTYVR ALTSENNKLV GWRWIRIDTS CVCALSRKIG RT
```

Mature murine NT-3 is formed by removal of a predicted signal peptide and a propeptide (1–123, in italics). Other precursor forms with extended N-terminal sequences similar to NGF may also exist. Disulphide bonds between Cys137–202, 180–231 and 190–233 by similarity.

THE NT-3 RECEPTORS

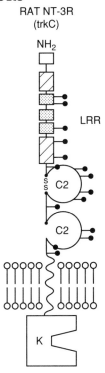

RAT NT-3R
(trkC)

NT-3 binds to both low affinity (K_d 10^{-9}M) and high affinity (K_d 10^{-11}M) cell surface receptors [6,7]. The low affinity receptor is LNGFR which also binds the other members of the NGF neurotrophin family, NGF, BDNF, NT-3 and NT-4 [8] (see NGF entry). Functional high affinity NT-3 receptors (K_d 10^{-11}M) have been identified as gp145^{trkC} (trkC) which is a member of the trk family of protein tyrosine kinases [6,9,10]. The characteristics of this family of receptors is described in the entry for NGF receptors. The rat *trkC* locus is complex and encodes at least four distinct polypeptides of which three are full length receptor tyrosine kinases that differ by novel amino acid insertions in the kinase domain [11,12]. TrkA and trkB are also functional receptors for NT-3 in certain in vitro systems [10,13–16]. In contrast, trkC does not bind NGF, BDNF or NT-4 [9,17]. The LNGFR is not required for high affinity binding of NT-3 nor for signal transduction [14].

Distribution

TrkC mRNA is expressed in pyramidal cells of the hippocampus, dentate gyrus, cortex, and some sites in the cerebellum. *In situ* hybridization experiments have shown it to be present in multiple structures of the peripheral nervous system. Expressed in brain by Nothern blot studies, but not in lung, heart, intestine, kidney, spleen, liver, testes or muscle. Possibly in ovaries.

Physicochemical properties of the NT-3 receptor (trkC)

Properties		Rat
Amino acids	– precursor	825
	– mature[a]	794
M_r (K)	– predicted	89.3
	– expressed	145
Potential N-linked glycosylation sites		14
Affinity K_d (M)		10^{-11}

[a] After removal of predicted signal peptide.

Signal transduction

TrkC has intrinsic protein tyrosine kinase activity. NT-3 binding stimulates receptor autophosphorylation, and phosphorylation of PLC-γl resulting in PIP$_2$ hydrolysis with release of IP$_3$ and DAG [18]. LNGFR is not required for signal transduction [7,10,14].

Chromosomal location
Not known.

Amino acid sequence of rat NT-3 receptor (trkC) [19]
(Human and mouse trkC have not been cloned.)

Accession code: Swissprot P24786

```
 -31   MDVSLCPAKC SFWRIFLLGS VWLDYVGSVL A
   1   CPANCVCSKT EINCRRPDDG NLFPLLEGQD SGNSNGNASI NITDISRNIT
  51   SIHIENWRGL HTLNAVDMEL YTGLQKLTIK NSGLRNIQPR AFAKNPHLRY
 101   INLSSNRLTT LSWQLFQTLS LRELRLEQNF FNCSCDIRWM QLWQEQGEAR
 151   LDSQSLYCIS ADGSQLPLFR MNISQCDLPE ISVSHVNLTV REGDNAVITC
 201   NGSGSPLPDV DWIVTGLQSI NTHQTNLNWT NVHAINLTLV NVTSEDNGFT
 251   LTCIAENVVG MSNASVALTV YYPPRVVSLV EPEVRLEHCI EFVVRGNPTP
 301   TLHWLYNGQP LRESKIIHMD YYQEGEVSEG CLLFNKPTHY NNGNYTLIAK
 351   NALGTANQTI NGHFLKEPFP ESTDFFDFES DASPTPPITV THKPEEDTFG
 401   VSIAVGLAAF ACVLLVVLFI MINKYGRRSK FGMKGPVAVI SGEEDSASPL
 451   HHINHGITTP SSLDAGPDTV VIGMTRIPVI ENPQYFRQGH NCHKPDTYVQ
 501   HIKRRDIVLK RELGEGAFGK VFLAECYNLS PTKDKMLVAV KALKDPTLAA
 551   RKDFQREAEL LTNLQHEHIV KFYGVCGDGD PLIMVFEYMK HGDLNKFLRA
 601   HGPDAMILVD GQPRQAKGEL GLSQMLHIAS QIASGMVYLA SQHFVHRDLA
 651   TRNCLVGANL LVKIGDFGMS RDVYSTDYYR VGGHTMLPIR WMPPESIMYR
 701   KFTTESDVWS FGVILWEIFT YGKQPWFQLS NTEVIECITQ GRVLERPRVC
 751   PKEVYDVMLG CWQREPQQRL NIKEIYKILH ALGKATPIYL DILG
```

Tyr678 is site of autophosphorylation.

References

1 Yancopoulos, G.D. et al. (1990) Cold Spring Harbor Symp. Quant. Biol. LV, 371–379.
2 Maisonpierre, P.C. et al. (1990) Science 247, 1446–1451.
3 Maisonpierre, P.C. et al. (1991) Genomics 10, 558–568.
4 Jones, K.R. and Reichardt, L.F. (1990) Proc. Natl. Acad. Sci. USA 87, 8060–8064.
5 Hohn, A. et al. (1990) Nature 344, 339–341.
6 Meakin, S.O. and Shooter, E.M. (1992) Trends Neurosci. 15, 323–331.
7 Barker, P.A. and Murphy, R.A. (1992) Mol. Cell. Biochem. 110, 1–15.
8 Rodriguez-Tebar, A. et al. (1992) EMBO J. 11, 917–922.
9 Lamballe, F. et al. (1991) Cell 66, 967– 979.
10 Cordon-Cardo, C. et al. (1991) Cell 66, 173–183.
11 Tsoulfas, P. et al. (1993) Neuron 10, 975–990.
12 Valenzuela, D.M. et al. (1993) Neuron 10, 963–974.
13 Klein, R. et al. (1991) Cell 66, 395–403.
14 Glass, D.J. et al. (1991) Cell 66, 405–413.
15 Soppet, D. et al. (1991) Cell 65, 895–903.
16 Squinto, S.P. et al. (1991) Cell 65, 885–893.
17 Klein, R. et al. (1992) Neuron 8, 947–956.
18 Widmer, H.R. et al. (1992) J. Neurochem. 59, 2113–2124.
19 Merlio, J.P. et al. (1992) Neuroscience 51, 513–532.

Other names

Mammalian NT-4 has also been called NT-5 and NT4/5 to distinguish it from *Xenopus* NT-4.

THE MOLECULE

Neurotrophin-4 is a neurotrophic factor which supports the survival and outgrowth of sensory neurons from embryonic chicken dorsal root ganglia, but has no significant effect on embryonic day 8 sympathetic ganglia [1]. It has a strong survival/proliferative action on NIH 3T3 cells expressing trkB but little activity on 3T3 cells expressing trkA. NT-4 was originally identified in *Xenopus* and viper, and was subsequently identified in rat and humans.

Crossreactivity

The mature human and rat NT-4 sequences are 95% identical. Human, rat and *Xenopus* NT-4 are all active on neurites from chicken embryo dorsal root ganglia.

Sources

High levels of NT-4 mRNA have been found in prostate with lower levels in thymus, placenta and skeletal muscle.

Bioassays

Survival and outgrowth of neurites from embryo chicken dorsal root ganglia. Survival and proliferation on NIH 3T3 cells transfected with *trkB*.

Physicochemical properties of NT-4

Property	Human	Rat
Amino acids – precursor	210	209
– mature[a]	130	130
M_r (K) – predicted	13.9	13.9
– expressed[b]	14	14
Potential N-linked glycosylation sites[c]	0	0
Disulphide bonds[d]	3	3

[a] After removal of pre-propeptide.
[b] May also be expressed as a homodimer like the other neurotrophins.
[c] There is one N-linked glycosylation site in the propeptide.
[d] Conserved between NGF, BDNF, NT-3 and NT-4.

3-D structure

Not determined but likely to be very similar to NGF.

Gene structure [1,2]

Scale

Exons   50 aa

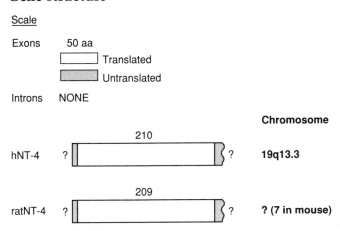

Introns   NONE

Translated

Untranslated

		Chromosome
hNT-4	210	19q13.3
ratNT-4	209	? (7 in mouse)

There may be more than one RNA species arising by alternative splicing and additional ATG initiation sites [1]. Three other partial ORFs that may encode additional members of this acidic protein family have been found on the same region of human chromosome 19 [2].

Amino acid sequence for human NT-4 [1]

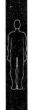

Accession code: GenEMBL M86528

```
-19   MLPLPSCSLP ILLLFLLPS
  1   VPIESQPPPS TLPPFLAPEW DLLSPRVVLS RGAPAGPPLL FLLEAGAFRE
 51   SAGAPANRSR RGVSETAPAS RRGELAVCDA VSGWVTDRRT AVDLRGREVE
101   VLGEVPAAGG SPLRQYFFET RCKADNAEEG GPGAGGGGCR GVDRRHWVSE
151   CKAKQSYVRA LTADAQGRVG WRWIRIDTAC VCTLLSRTGR A
```

Mature human NT-4 is formed by removal of a predicted signal peptide and a propeptide (1–61, in italics). Other precursor forms with extended N-terminal sequences similar to NGF may also exist. Disulphide bonds between Cys78–151, 122–180, and 139–182 by similarity.

Amino acid sequence for rat NT-4 [1]

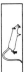

(Mouse NT-4 has not been cloned.)

Accession code: GenEMBL M86742

```
-18   MLPRHSCSLL LFLLLLPS
  1   VPMEPQPPSS TLPPFLAPEW DLLSPRVALS RGTPAGPPLL FLLEAGAYGE
 51   PAGAPANRSR RGVSETAPAS RRGELAVCDA VSGWVTDRRT AVDLRGREVE
101   VLGEVPAAGG SPLRQYFFET RCKAESAGEG GPGVGGGGCR GVDRRHWLSE
151   CKAKQSYVRA LTADSQGRVG WRWIRIDTAC VCTLLSRTGR A
```

Mature rat NT-4 is formed by removal of a predicted signal peptide and a propeptide (1–61, in italics). Other precursor forms with extended N-terminal sequences similar to NGF may also exist. Disulphide bonds between Cys78–151, 122–180 and 139–182 by similarity.

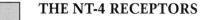

THE NT-4 RECEPTORS

NT-4 binds to LNGFR [3] (see NGF entry), and to trkB [4] (see BDNF entry).

References

[1] Ip, N.Y. et al. (1992) Proc. Natl. Acad. Sci. USA 89, 3060–3064.
[2] Berkemeier, L.R. et al. (1992) Somat. Cell. Mol. Genet. 18, 233–245.
[3] Rodriguez-Tebar, A. et al. (1992) EMBO J. 11, 917–922.
[4] Klein, R. et al. (1992) Neuron 8, 947–956.

Other names
No other names.

THE MOLECULE

Oncostatin M is a cytokine which inhibits the growth of some tumour and normal cell lines, stimulates fibroblast, smooth muscle and Kaposi's sarcoma cell proliferation, cytokine release from endothelial cells and low density lipoprotein receptor expression on hepatoma cells [1-8]. It shares many structural and biological properties with LIF, IL-6 and CNTF [8,9].

Crossreactivity
No rodent OSM has been described.

Sources
Activated T cells and monocytes, Kaposi's sarcoma cells [2,6,10].

Bioassays
Growth inhibition of melanoma cell line A-375 [1,2].

Physicochemical properties of OSM

Property	Human
Amino acids – precursor	252
– mature	227, processed to 196
M_r (K) – predicted	28.5
– expressed[b]	32, 36
Potential N-linked glycosylation sites[c]	2
Disulphide bonds[d]	2

[a] Cys6 and 127, and Cys49 and 167 form disulphide bonds [8].

3-D structure
Predicted four α-helical structure with homology to LIF, CNTF, IL-6, G-CSF and IL-11 [8,11,12].

Gene structure [13]

Scale

Exons   50 aa

☐ Translated

500 bp

▨ Untranslated

Introns ├────┤
        50 bp

Chromosome

11 47¹/₃   193²/₃

hOSM ─║▯──▭─▯─────▭▨▨─────── 22q12

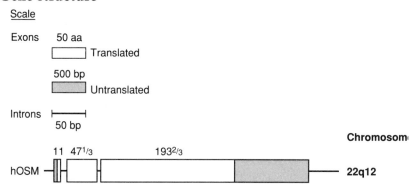

The gene for human OSM on chromosome 22q12 is close to that for LIF [13].

Amino acid sequence for human OSM [1]

Accession code: Genbank M27288, M26966

```
-25 MGVLLTQRTL LSLVLALLFP SMASM
  1 AAIGSCSKEY RVLLGQLQKQ TDLMQDTSRL LDPYIRIQGL DVPKLREHCR
 51 ERPGAFPSEE TLRGLGRRGF LQTLNATLGC VLHRLADLEQ RLPKAQDLER
101 SGLNIEDLEK LQMARPNILG LRNNIYCMAQ LLDNSDTAEP TKAGRGASQP
151 PTPTPASDAF QRKLEGCRFL HGYHRFMHSV GRVFSKWGES PNRSRRHSPH
201 QALRKGVRRT RPSRKGKRLM TRGQLPR
```

The C-terminal 31 amino acids (in italics) are proteolytically removed to release the mature protein.

THE OSM RECEPTOR

The receptor for oncostatin M is composed of a low affinity component which is identical to the gp130 β-chain of the IL-6R and LIFR (see IL-6 entry), and a second affinity-converting α-chain which is identical to the LIF receptor α-chain [14] (see LIF entry). Antibodies to gp130 block responses to OSM, LIF, IL-6 and CNTF [15]. A third oncostatin M-specific binding chain has been suggested [14].

Distribution

See LIF and IL-6 entries.

Signal transduction

Involves a tyrosine kinase in hepatoma, endothelial and smooth muscle cells [8,16].

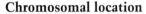
Chromosomal location

See LIF and IL-6 entries.

Amino acid sequence for the human OSM receptors

See IL-6 and LIF entries.

References
1 Malik, N. et al. (1989) Mol. Cell. Biol. 9, 2847–2853.
2 Zarling, J.M. et al. (1986) Proc. Natl. Acad. Sci. USA 83, 9739–9743.
3 Miles, S.A. et al. (1992) Science 255, 1432–1434.
4 Grove, R.I. et al. (1991) J. Biol. Chem. 266, 18194–18199.
5 Grove, R.I. et al. (1993) Proc. Natl. Acad. Sci. USA 90, 823–827.
6 Radka, S.F. et al. (1993) J. Immunol. 150, 5195–5201.
7 Brown, T.J. et al. (1991) J. Immunol. 147, 2175–2180.
8 Bruce, A.G. et al. (1992) Prog. Growth Factor Res. 4, 157–170.
9 Rose, T.M. and Bruce A.G. (1991) Proc. Natl. Acad. Sci. USA 88, 8641–8645.
10 Radka, S.F. et al. (1993) J. Immunol. 150, 5195–5201.
11 Bazan, J.F. (1991) Neuron 7, 197–208.
12 Nicola, N.A. et al. (1993) Biochem. Biophys. Res. Commun. 190, 20–26.
13 Giovannini, M. et al. (1993) Cytogenet. Cell. Genet. 62, 32–34.
14 Gearing, D.P. et al. (1992) Science 255, 1434–1437.
15 Taga, T. et al. (1993) Proc. Natl. Acad. Sci. USA 89, 10998–11001.
16 Grove, R.I. et al. (1993) Proc. Natl. Acad. Sci. USA 90, 823–827.

Other names

CTAP-III is also known as low affinity platelet factor 4 [1].

THE MOLECULES

Platelet basic protein is a CXC chemokine/intercrine cytokine produced by platelets [2] which is sequentially proteolytically processed to form the active mediators CTAP-III (a chondrocyte mitogen [1]), β-thromboglobulin (βTG) [3,4] (a fibroblast chemoattractant), and NAP-2 (a neutrophil chemo-attractant [5,6]). NAP-2 is produced by cleavage with cathepsin G [7].

Crossreactivity

There is no known murine homologue of human PBP.

Sources

Platelets.

Bioassays

CTAP-III, mitogenesis for fibroblasts [8]; βTG, chemotaxis for fibroblasts [9]; NAP2, chemotaxis of neutrophils [10]. PBP has no biological activity [4].

Physicochemical properties of CTAP-III, bTG and NAP-2

Property	Human CTAP-III	Human βTG	Human NAP-2
Amino acids – precursor	128	128	128
– mature	85	81	69
M_r (K) – predicted	9.2	8.8	7.3
– expressed	7.5	7	6
Potential N-linked glycosylation sites	0	0	0
Disulphide bonds	2	2	2

3-D structure

Could be modelled on PF-4. The association state of CTAP-III has been studied by NMR; under physiological conditions the active form is a monomer [11]

Gene structure for human PBP

The gene for PBP is located on chromosome 4q12–21 [12].

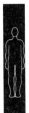

Amino acid sequence for human PBP [1,2]

Accession code: Swissprot P02775

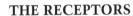

```
-34  MSLRLDTTPS CNSARPLHAL QVLLLLSLLL TALA
  1  SSTKGQTKRN LAKGKEESLD SDLYAELRCM CIKTTSGIHP KNIQSLEVIG
 51  KGTHCNQVEV IATLKDGRKI CLDPDAPRIK KIVQKKLAGD ESAD
```

The N-terminal amino acids for mature CTAP-III, βTG, and NAP-2 are Asn10, Lys15 and Arg28 respectively.

THE RECEPTORS

There is some competition with IL-8 for binding to its receptor.

References

1 Caster, C.W. et al. (1983) Proc. Natl Acad. Sci. USA 80, 765–769.
2 Wenger, R.H. et al. (1989) Blood 73, 1498–1503.
3 Beggs, G.S. et al. (1978) Biochemistry 17, 1739–1744.
4 Holt, J.C. et al. (1986) Biochemistry 25, 1988–1996.
5 Walz, A. et al. (1989) J. Exp. Med. 170, 1745–1750.
6 Walz, A. and Baggiolini, M. (1990) J. Exp. Med. 171, 449–454.
7 Cohen, A.B. et al. (1992) Am. J. Physiol. 263, 1249–1256.
8 Mullenbach, G.T. et al. (1986) J. Biol. Chem. 261, 719–722.
9 Senior, R.M. et al. (1983) J. Cell. Biol. 96, 382–385.
10 Walz, A. et al. (1989) J. Exp. Med. 170, 1745–1750.
11 Mayo, K.H. (1991) Biochemistry 30, 925–934.
12 Modi, W.S. et al. (1990) Hum. Genet. 84, 185–187.

Other names

Murine PBSF is also known as stromal cell-derived factor-1α (SDF-1α) [1].

THE MOLECULES

Pre-B Cell growth stimulating factor is a growth factor for Pre-B cells [1,2]. PBSF is a member of the CXC family of Chemokine cytokines [3].

Crossreactivity

Human PBSF shares 95% identity with murine PBSF [1].

Sources

Fibroblasts, bone marrow stromal cells.

Bioassays

Costimulation with IL-7 of pre-B cell proliferation.

Physicochemical properties of PBSF

Property	Human
Amino acids – precursor	89
– mature	71
M_r (K) – predicted	8.3
– expressed	?
Potential N-linked glycosylation sites	0
Disulphide bonds	2

3-D structure

Could be modelled on MIP-1β [4]

Gene structure

No information.

Amino acid sequence for human PBSF

Not yet reported.

Amino acid sequence for mouse PBSF [1,2]

Accession code: Genbank D21072

```
-18  MDAKVVAVLA LVLAALCI
  1  SDGKPVSLSY RCPCRFFESH IARANVKHLK ILNTPNCALQ VARLKNNNR
 51  QVCIDPKLKW IQEYLEKALN K
```

A variant sequence, SDF-1β, (Genbank L12030) which has a C terminal extension of RLKW has been reported [1].

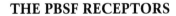
THE PBSF RECEPTORS

No information.

References

1 Tashiro, K. et al. (1993) Science 261, 600–603.
2 Nagasawa, T. et al. (1994) Proc. Natl. Acad. Sci. USA 91, 2305–2309.
3 Schall, T.J. (1991) Cytokine 3, 165–183.
4 Lodi, P.J. et al. (1994) Science 263, 1762–1767.

PDGF

Other names

Osteosarcoma derived growth factor (ODGF), glioma derived growth factor (GDGF).

THE MOLECULES

Platelet derived growth factor is a mitogen for connective tissue cells and glial cells. It plays an important role in wound healing, and may act as an autocrine and/or paracrine growth factor for some malignant cells [1-3]. It is also a chemoattractant for fibroblasts, smooth muscle cells, monocytes and neutrophils. Functional PDGF is secreted as a dimer of disulphide-linked A and B chains (PDGF-AA, PDGF-BB, or PDGF-AB). All three forms are produced naturally. The mature A and B chains have 60% homology and eight conserved Cys residues in each chain. The A chain occurs in two variants arising from alternative splicing in which the three C-terminal amino acids in the short form are replaced by 18 different amino acids derived from exon 6 in the long form [4,5]. The gene coding for human PDGF B chain is the c-sis proto-oncogene [1,6].

Crossreactivity

There is greater than 90% homology between human and mouse mature PDGF-A and complete crossreactivity.

Sources

Platelets (human 70% AB, 20% BB, 10% AA), placental cytotrophoblasts, macrophages, endothelial cells, megakaryocytes, fibroblasts, vascular smooth muscle cells, glial cells, type I astrocytes, myoblasts, kidney epithelial cells mesangial cells and many different tumour cells.

Bioassays

Mitogenic activity on fibroblasts.

Physicochemical properties of PDGF

Property	PDGF-A		PDGF-B	
	Human	Mouse	Human	Mouse
pI	10.2	10	10.2	10
Amino acids – precursor	211/196[b]	196[b]	241	241
– mature[a,b]	125/110[b]	110[b]	109	160
M_r (K) – predicted[b]	14.3/12.5	12.5	12.3	12
– expressed[c]	14–18	16	16	16
Potential N-linked glycosylation sites	1	1	0[d]	0[d]
Disulphide bonds[e]	3	3	3	3

[a] After removal of signal peptide and propeptide (see sequences). Precursors are proteolytically cleaved after dimerization.

214

b Two forms of human PDGF-A derived from alternative mRNA splicing have been identified (see sequence). Long and short forms of murine PDGF-A from alternative splicing have also been found, but mRNA for the short form only has been cloned.

c For monomeric PDGF. M_r of dimers is 30 000–32 000.

d There is one site on the propeptide.

e Dimeric PDGF has two additional interchain disulphide bonds (see sequence).

3-D structure

Biologically active PDGF is an antiparallel disulphide-linked dimer (AA, AB or BB). The crystal structure of the human PDGF BB isoform has been determined to a resolution of 3 Å [7]. The polypeptide chain is folded into two highly twisted antiparallel pairs of β-strands with an unusual knotted arrangement of three intramolecular disulphide bonds. A cluster of three surface loops at each end of the dimer may form the receptor recognition sites.

Gene structure [8,9]

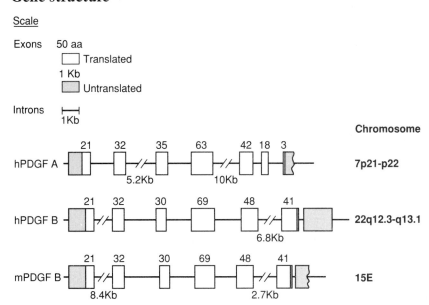

Human chromosome 7p21–p22 is the site of a defined subset of mitogen-induced fragile sites, many of which coincide with well-known oncogenes and the breakpoint in myelodysplastic syndrome.

The gene structure for mouse PDGF-A has not been determined. It is located on chromosome 5. The gene for mouse PDGF-B is closely linked to the gene for the IL-2R β-chain.

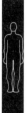

Amino acid sequences for human PDGF-A (long form [10] and short form [4,5,11,12])

Accession code: Swissprot P04085

```
-20  MRTLACLLLL GCGYLAHVLA
  1  EEAEIPREVI ERLARSQIHS IRDLQRLLEI DSVGSEDSLD TSLRAHGVHA
 51  TKHVPEKRPL PIRRKRSIEE AVPAVCKTRT VIYEIPRSQV DPTSANFLIW
101  PPCVEVKRCT GCCNTSSVKC QPSRVHHRSV KVAKVEYVRK KPKLKEVQVR
151  LEEHLECACA TTSLNPDYRE EDTGRPRESG KKRKRKRLKP T
```

Mature PDGF-A is formed by removal of signal peptide and propeptide (1–66, in italics). The short form of human PDGF-A is derived from alternative splicing and terminates with the sequence DVR replacing GRP.. at position 174–176 [4,5]. Intrachain disulphide bonds between Cys76–120, 109–157, 113–159, and interchain disulphide bonds between Cys103–103, 112–112 by similarity.

Amino acid sequence for human PDGF-B (c-*sis* proto-oncogene) [8,13-15]

Accession code: Swissprot P01127

```
-20  MNRCWALFLS LCCYLRLVSA
  1  EGDPIPEELY EMLSDHSIRS FDDLQRLLHG DPGEEDGAEL DLNMTRSHSG
 51  GELESLARGR RSLGSLTIAE PAMIAECKTR TEVFEISRRL IDRTNANFLV
101  WPPCVEVQRC SGCCNNRNVQ CRPTQVQLRP VQVRKIEIVR KKPIFKKATV
151  TLEDHLACKC ETVAAARPVT RSPGGSQEQR AKTPQTRVTI RTVRVRRPPK
201  GKHRKFKHTH DKTALKETLG A
```

Mature PDGF-B is formed by removal of a signal peptide and both N-terminal (1–61) and C-terminal (171–221) propeptides (in italics.) Conflicting sequence E->R at position 1, T->E at position 81, E->C at position 85, and S->C at position 87. Intrachain disulphide bonds between Cys77–121, 110–158, 114–160, and interchain disulphide bonds between Cys104–104, 113–113.

Amino acid sequence for mouse PDGF-A (short form) [16]

Accession code: Swissprot P20033

```
-20  MRTWACLLLL GCGYLAHALA
  1  EEAEIPRELI ERLARSQIHS IRDLQRLLEI DSVGAEDALE TSLRAHGSHA
 51  INHVPEKRPV PIRRKRSIEE AIPAVCKTRT VIYEIPRSQV DPTSANFLIW
101  PPCVEVKRCT GCCNTSSVKC QPSRVHHRSV KVAKVEYVRK KPKLKEVQVR
151  LEEHLECACA TSNLNPDHRE EETDVR
```

Mature PDGF-A is formed by removal of a signal peptide and a propetide (1–66, in italics). Different forms of mouse PDGF-A are produced by alternative splicing. The sequence given here is for the short form. The C-terminal sequence for the long form has not yet been determined. Intrachain disulphide bonds between Cys76–120, 109–157, 113–159, and interchain disulphide bonds between Cys103–103, 112–112 by similarity.

Amino acid sequence for mouse PDGF-B [9]

Accession code: Swissprot P31240

```
-20   MNRCWALFLP  LCCYLRLVSA
  1   EGDPIPEELY  EMLSDHSIRS  FDDLQRLLHR  DSVDEDGAEL  DLNMTRAHSG
 51   VELESSSRGR  RSLGSLAAAE  PAVIAECKTR  TEVFQISRNL  IDRTNANFLV
101   WPPCVEVQRC  SGCCNNRNVQ  CRASQVQMRP  VQVRKIEIVR  KKPIFKKATV
151   TLEDHLACKC  ETIVTPRPVT  RSPGTSREQR  AKTPQARVTI  RTVRIRRPPK
201   GKHRKFKHTH  DKAALKETLG  A
```

Mature mouse PDGF-B is formed by removal of a signal peptide and both N-terminal (1–61) and C-terminal (171–221) propeptides (in italics). Intrachain disulphide bonds between Cys77–121, 110–158, 114–160, and interchain disulphide bonds between Cys104–104, 113–113 by similarity.

THE PDGF RECEPTORS

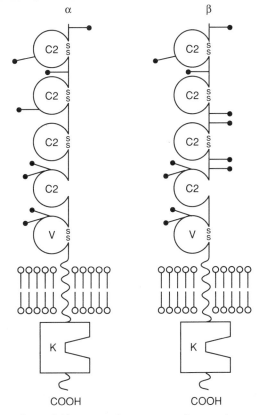

PDGF receptors (α and β) are single transmembrane glycoproteins with an intracellular tyrosine kinase domain split by an inserted sequence of about 100 amino acids [2,3]. They are structurally related to the M-CSF receptor (c-fms) and the SCF receptor (c-kit). Binding of divalent PDGF (AA, AB, or BB)

induces receptor dimerization with three possible configurations (αα, αβ, ββ). The PDGF receptor α-subunit binds both PDGF A and B chains, whereas the receptor β-subunit binds only PDGF B chains. This specificity predicts that PDGF-AA binds only to PDGF receptor αα dimers, PDGF-AB binds to receptor αα and αβ dimers, and PDGF-BB binds to all three possible configurations (PDGF receptor αα, αβ, ββ) [17-19]. Murine and human α- and β-receptors have the same isoform specificity. Both receptors stimulate mitogenic responses, but only the β-receptor can induce chemotaxis and actin reorganization to form circular membrane ruffles. A soluble form of the PDGF-α receptor has been described [20].

Distribution

Widely distributed on cells of mesenchymal origin including fibroblasts, smooth muscle cells, glial cells and chondrocytes. Also on synovia in patients with rheumatoid arthritis and uterine endometrial cells. There are two examples of cells which express one receptor only: O-2A glial progenitor cells of the rat optic nerve express only α-receptors, and capillary endothelial cells of the brain express only β-receptors. PDGF receptors have also been detected on the SMS-SB and NALM6 pre-B cell lines.

Physicochemical properties of the PDGF receptors

	α-receptor		β-receptor	
Properties	Human	Mouse	Human	Mouse
Amino acids – precursor	1089	1089	1106	1098
– mature[a]	1066	1065	1074	1067
M_r (K) – predicted	120 .3	120.1	120.6	119.6
– expressed	170	?	180	180
Potential N-linked glycosylation sites	8	10	11	11
Affinity K_d (M) – PDGF-AB	10^{-10}	?	0	?
– PDGF-AA	2×10^{-10}	?	5×10^{-9}	?
– PDGF-BB	5×10^{-10}	?	5×10^{-10}	?

[a] After removal of predicted signal peptide.

Signal transduction

The PDGF receptor belongs to subclass III of receptor tyrosine kinases which includes SCFR (c-kit) and M-CSFR. PDGF binding induces receptor dimerization and autophosphorylation. Detailed studies of the human β-receptor have identified six autophosphorylation sites (Tyr708, Tyr719 and Tyr739 in the kinase insert, Tyr825 in the second part of the kinase domain, and Tyr977 and Tyr989 in the C-terminal tail) [reviewed in ref. 2].

PLC-γ, PI-3′ kinase, and GTPase activating protein (GAP) bind through their SH2 domains to specific phosphotyrosine-containing motifs on the PDGF receptor and are activated (phosphorylated). Tyr708 and Tyr 719 mediate binding of PI-3′-kinase, and Tyr739 mediates binding of GAP [21,22] whereas Tyr977 and Tyr989 mediate binding of PLC-γ [23]. The PDGF α- and β–receptors activate both common and distinct signal transduction pathways [24].

Chromosomal location

Human PDGFR-α is on chromosome 4q11–q12 and PDGFR-β is on chromosome 5q33–q35. The mouse β-receptor is on chromosome 18, closely linked to the M-CSFR.

Amino acid sequence for human PDGFR-α [15,25]

Accession code: Swissprot P16234

```
 -23  MGTSHPAFLV  LGCLLTGLSL  ILC
   1  QLSLPSILPN  ENEKVVQLNS  SFSLRCFGES  EVSWQYPMSE  EESSDVEIRN
  51  EENNSGLFVT  VLEVSSASAA  HTGLYTCYYN  HTQTEENELE  GRHIYIYVPD
 101  PDVAFVPLGM  TDYLVIVEDD  DSAIIPCRTT  DPETPVTLHN  SEGVVPASYD
 151  SRQGFNGTFT  VGPYICEATV  KGKKFQTIPF  NVYALKATSE  LDLEMEALKT
 201  VYKSGETIVV  TCAVFNNEVV  DLQWTYPGEV  KGKGITMLEE  IKVPSIKLVY
 251  TLTVPEATVK  DSGDYECAAR  QATREVKEMK  KVTISVHEKG  FIEIKPTFSQ
 301  LEAVNLHEVK  HFVVEVRAYP  PPRISWLKNN  LTLIENLTEI  TTDVEKIQEI
 351  RYRSKLKLIR  AKEEDSGHYT  IVAQNEDAVK  SYTFELLTQV  PSSILDLVDD
 401  HHGSTGGQTV  RCTAEGTPLP  DIEWMICKDI  KKCNNETSWT  ILANNVSNII
 451  TEIHSRDRST  VEGRVTFAKV  EETIAVRCLA  KNLLGAENRE  LKLVAPTLRS
 501  ELTVAAAVLV  LLVIVIISLI  VLVVIWKQKP  RYEIRWRVIE  SISPDGHEYI
 551  YVDPMQLPYD  SRWEFPRDGL  VLGRVLGSGA  FGKVVEGTAY  GLSRSQPVMK
 601  VAVKMLKPTA  RSSEKQALMS  ELKIMTHLGP  HLNIVNLLGA  CTKSGPIYII
 651  TEYCFYGDLV  NYLHKNRDSF  LSHHPEKPKK  ELDIFGLNPA  DESTRSYVIL
 701  SFENNGDYMD  MKQADTTQYV  PMLERKEVSK  YSDIQRSLYD  RPASYKKKSM
 751  LDSEVKNLLS  DDNSEGLTLL  DLLSFTYQVA  RGMEFLASKN  CVHRDLAARN
 801  VLLAQGKIVK  ICDFGLARDI  MHDSNYVSKG  STFLPVKWMA  PESIFDNLYT
 851  TLSDVWSYGI  LLWEIFSLGG  TPYPGMMVDS  TFYNKIKSGY  RMAKPDHATS
 901  EVYEIMVKCW  NSEPEKRPSF  YHLSEIVENL  LPGQYKKSYE  KIHLDFLKSD
 951  HPAVARMRVD  SDNAYIGVTY  KNEEDKLKDW  EGGLDEQRLS  ADSGYIIPLP
1001  DIDPVPEEED  LGKRNRHSSQ  TSEESAIETG  SSSSTFIKRE  DETIEDIDMM
1051  DDIGIDSSDL  VEDSFL
```

The extracellular Cys residues form disulphide bonds in Ig-SF domains and are conserved in both PDGF receptors and other members of the split tyrosine kinase family (c-kit, M-CSFR). Tyr708, 719, 739, 826, 970 and 995 are autophosphorylated (by similarity with the β-receptor) and all but Tyr826 have been shown to be involved in binding to SH2 domains of signalling proteins (see above under signal transduction) [2].

Amino acid sequence for human PDGFR-β [26,27]

Accession code: Swissprot P09619

```
 -32  MRLPGAMPAL  ALKGELLLLS  LLLLLEPQIS  QG
   1  LVVTPPGPEL  VLNVSSTFVL  TCSGSAPVVW  ERMSQEPPQE  MAKAQDGTFS
  51  SVLTLTNLTG  LDTGEYFCTH  NDSRGLETDE  RKRLYIFVPD  PTVGFLPNDA
 101  EELFIFLTEI  TEITIPCRVT  DPQLVVTLHE  KKGDVALPVP  YDHQRGFSGI
 151  FEDRSYICKT  TIGDREVDSD  AYYVYRLQVS  SINVSVNAVQ  TVVRQGENIT
 201  LMCIVIGNEV  VNFEWTYPRK  ESGRLVEPVT  DFLLDMPYHI  RSILHIPSAE
 251  LEDSGTYTCN  VTESVNDHQD  EKAINITVVE  SGYVRLLGEV  GTLQFAELHR
 301  SRTLQVVFEA  YPPPTVLWFK  DNRTLGDSSA  GEIALSTRNV  SETRYVSELT
 351  LVRVKVAEAG  HYTMRAFHED  AEVQLSFQLQ  INVPVRVLEL  SESHPDSGEQ
 401  TVRCRGRGMP  QPNIIWSACR  DLKRCPRELP  PTLLGNSSEE  ESQLETNVTY
 451  WEEEQEFEVV  STLRLQHVDR  PLSVRCTLRN  AVGQDTQEVI  VVPHSLPFKV
 501  VVISAILALV  VLTIISLIIL  IMLWQKKPRY  EIRWKVIESV  SSDGHEYIYV
 551  DPMQLPYDST  WELPRDQLVL  GRTLGSGAFG  QVVEATAHGL  SHSQATMKVA
 601  VKMLKSTARS  SEKQALMSEL  KIMSHLGPHL  NVVNLLGACT  KGGPIYIITE
 651  YCRYGDLVDY  LHRNKHTFLQ  HHSDKRRPPS  AELYSNALPV  GLPLPSHVSL
 701  TGESDGGYMD  MSKDESVDYV  PMLDMKGDVK  YADIESSNYM  APYDNYVPSA
 751  PERTCRATLI  NESPVLSYMD  LVGFSYQVAN  GMEFLASKNC  VHRDLAARNV
 801  LICEGKLVKI  CDFGLARDIM  RDSNYISKGS  TFLPLKWMAP  ESIFNSLYTT
 851  LSDVWSFGIL  LWEIFTLGGT  PYPELPMNEQ  FYNAIKRGYR  MAQPAHASDE
 901  IYEIMQKCWE  EKFEIRPPFS  QLVLLLERLL  GEGYKKKYQQ  VDEEFLRSDH
 951  PAILRSQARL  PGFHGLRSPL  DTSSVLYTAV  QPNEGDNDYI  IPLPDPKPEV
1001  ADEGPLEGSP  SLASSTLNEV  NTSSTISCDS  PLEPQDEPEP  EPQLELQVEP
1051  EPELEQLPDS  GCPAPRAEAE  DSFL
```

The extracellular Cys residues form disulphide bonds in Ig-SF domains and are conserved in both PDGF receptors and other members of the split tyrosine kinase family (c-kit, M-CSFR). Tyr708, 719, 739, 825, 977 and 989 are autophosphorylated and all but Tyr825 have been shown to be involved in binding to SH2 domains of signalling proteins (see above under signal transduction) [2]. Conflicting amino acid sequence E->D at position 209.

Amino acid sequence for mouse PDGFR-α

Accession code: Swissprot P26618

```
 -24  MGTSHQVFLV  LSCLLTGPGL  ISCQ
   1  LLLPSILPNE  NEKIVQLNSS  FSLRCVGESE  VSWQHPMSEE  EDPNVEIRSE
  51  ENNSGLFVTV  LEVVNASAAH  TGWYTCYYNH  TQTDESEIEG  RHIYIYVPDP
 101  DMAFVPLGMT  DSLVIVEEDD  SAIIPCRTTD  PETQVTLHNN  GRLVPASYDS
 151  RQGFNGTFSV  GPYICEAAVK  GRTFKTSAFN  VYALKATSEL  NLEMDARQTV
 201  YKAGETIVVT  CAVFNNEVVD  LQWTYPGGVR  NKGITMLEEI  KLPSIKVVYT
 251  LTVPKATVKD  SGEYECAARQ  ATKEVKEMKR  VTISVHEKGF  VEIEPTFSQL
 301  EPVNLHEVRE  FVVEVQAYPT  PRISWLKDNL  TLIENLTEIT  TDVQKSQETR
 351  YQSKLKLIRA  KEEDSGHYTI  IVQNEDDVKS  YTFELSTLVP  ASILDLVDDH
 401  HGSGGGQTVR  CTAEEGPLPE  IDWMICKHIK  KCNNDTSWTV  LASNVSNIIT
 451  ELPRRGRSTV  EGRVSFAKVE  ETIAVRCLAK  NNLSVVAREL  KLVAPTLRSE
 501  LTVAAAVLVL  LVIVIVSLIV  LVVIWKQKPR  YEIRWRVIES  ISPDGHEYIY
 551  VDPMQLPYDS  RWEFPRDGLV  LGRILGSGAF  GKVVEGTAYG  LSRSQPVMKV
```

```
 601  AVKMLKPTAR SSEKQALMSE LKIMTHLGPH LNIVNLLGAC TKSGPIYIIT
 651  EYCFYGDLVN YLHKNRDSFM SQHPEKPKKD LDIFGLNPAD ESTRSYVILS
 701  FENNGDYMDM KQDDTTQYVP MLERKEVSKY SDIQRSLYDR PASYKKKSML
 751  DSEVKNLLSD DDSEGLTLLD LLSFTYQVAR GMEFLASKNC VHRDLAARNV
 801  LLAQGKIVKI CDFGLARDIM HDSNDVSKGS TFLPVKWMAP ESIFDNLYTT
 851  LSDVWSYGIL LWEIFSLGGT PYPGMMVDST FYNKIKSGYR MAKPDHATSE
 901  VYEIMVQCWN SDPEKRPSFY HLSEILENLL PGQYKKSYEK IHLDFLKSDH
 951  PAVARMRVDS DNAYIGVTYK NEEDKLKDWE GGLDEQRLSA DSGYIIPLPD
1001  IDPVPEEEDL GKRNRHSSQT SEESAIETGS SSSTFIKRED ETIEDIDMMD
1051  DIGIDSSDLV EDSFL
```

The extracellular Cys residues form disulphide bonds in Ig-SF domains and are conserved in both PDGF receptors and other members of the split tyrosine kinase family (c-kit, M-CSFR). Tyr707, 718, 738, 969 and 994 are autophosphorylated (by similarity with the human β-receptor) and are involved in binding to SH2 domains of signalling proteins (see above under signal transduction) [2].

Amino acid sequence for mouse PDGFR-β [28]

Accession code: Swissprot P05622

```
 -31  MGLPGVIPAL VLRGQLLLSV LWLLGPQTSR G
   1  LVITPPGPEF VLNISSTFVL TCSGSAPVMW EQMSQVPWQE AAMNQDGTFS
  51  SVLTLTNVTG GDTGEYFCVY NNSLGPELSE RKRIYIFVPD PTMGFLPMDS
 101  EDLFIFVTDV TETTIPCRVT DPQLEVTLHE KKVDIPLHVP YDHQRGFTGT
 151  FEDKTYICKT TIGDREVDSD TYYVYSLQVS SINVSVNAVQ TVVRQGESIT
 201  IRCIVMGNDV VNFQWTYPRM KSGRLVEPVT DYLFGVPSRI GSILHIPTAE
 251  LSDSGTYTCN VSVSVNDHGD EKAINISVIE NGYVRLLETL GDVEIAELHR
 301  SRTLRVVFEA YPMPSVLWLK DNRTLGDSGA GELVLSTRNM SETRYVSELI
 351  LVRVKVSEAG YYTMRAFHED DEVQLSFKLQ VNVPVRVLEL SESHPANGEQ
 401  TIRCRGRGMP QPNVTWSTCR DLKRCPRKLS PTPLGNSSKE ESQLETNVTF
 451  WEEDQEYEVV STLRLRHVDQ PLSVRCMLQN SMGGDSQEVT VVPHSLPFKV
 501  VVISAILALV VLTVISLIIL IMLWQKKPRY EIRWKVIESV SSDGHEYIYV
 551  DPVQLPYDST WELPRDQLVL GRTLGSGAFG QVVEATAHGL SHSQATMKVA
 601  VKMLKSTARS SEKQALMSEL KIMSHLGPHL NVVNLLGACT KGGPIYIITE
 651  YCRYGDLVDY LHRNKHTFLQ RHSNKHCPPS AELYSNALPV GFSLPSHLNL
 701  TGESDGGYMD MSKDESIDYV PMLDMKGDIK YADIESPSYM APYDNYVPSA
 751  PERTYRATLI NDSPVLSYTD LVGFSYQVAN GMDFLASKNC VHRDLAARNV
 801  LICEGKLVKI CDFGLARDIM RDSNYISKGS TYLPLKWMAP ESIFNSLYTT
 851  LSDVWSFGIL LWEIFTLGGT PYPELPMNDQ FYNAIKRGYR MAQPAHASDE
 901  IYEIMQKCWE EKFETRPPFS QLVLLLERLL GEGYKKKYQQ VDEEFLRSDH
 951  PAILRSQARF PGIHSLRSPL DTSSVLYTAV QPNESDNDYI IPLPDPKPDV
1001  ADEGLPEGSP SLASSTLNEV NTSSTISCDS PLELQEEPQQ AEPEAQLEQP
1051  QDSGCPGPLA EAEDSFL
```

The extracellular Cys residues form disulphide bonds in Ig-SF domains and are conserved in both PDGF receptors and other members of the split tyrosine kinase family (c-kit, M-CSFR). Tyr708, 719, 739, 825, 977 and 989 are autophosphorylated (by similarity with the human β-receptor) and all but Tyr825 are involved in binding to SH2 domains of signalling proteins (see abpve under signal transduction) [2].

References

1. Ross, R. et al (1986) Cell 46, 155–169.
2. Heldin, C.-H. (1992) EMBO J. 11, 4251–4259.
3. Raines, E.W. et al (1991) In Peptide Growth Factors and their Receptors I, Sporn, M.B. and Roberts, A.B., eds., Springer-Verlag, New York, pp. 173–262.
4. Collins, T. et al (1987) Nature 328, 621–624.
5. Tong, B.D. et al. (1987) Nature 328, 619–621.
6. Heldin, C.-H. and Westermark, B. (1989) Br. Med. Bull. 45, 453–464.
7. Oefner, C. et al. (1992) EMBO J. 11, 3921–3926.
8. Rao, C.D. et al. (1986) Proc. Natl. Acad. Sci. USA 83, 2392–2396.
9. Bonthron, D.T. et al (1991) Genomics 10, 287–292.
10. Betsholtz, C. et al. (1986) Nature 320, 695–699.
11. Bonthron, D.T. et al. (1988) Proc. Natl. Acad. Sci. USA 85, 1492–1496.
12. Rorsman, F. et al. (1988) Mol. Cell. Biol. 8, 571–577.
13. Chiu, I.-M. et al. (1984) Cell 37, 123–129.
14. Josephs, S.F. et al. (1984) Science 225, 636–639.
15. Collins, T. et al. (1985) Nature 316, 748–750.
16. Mercola, M. et al. (1990) Dev. Biol. 138, 114–122.
17. Seifert, R.A. et al. (1989) J. Biol. Chem. 264, 8771–8778.
18. Hart, C.E. and Bowen-Pope, D.F. (1990) J. Invest. Dermatol. 94, 53S–57S.
19. Westermark, B. et al (1989) Prog. Growth Factor Res. 1, 253–266.
20. Tiesman, J. and Hart, C.E. (1993) J. Biol. Chem. 268, 9621–9628.
21. Fantl, W.J. et al. (1992) Cell 69, 413–423.
22. Kashishian, A. et al (1992) EMBO J. 11, 1373–1382.
23. Ronnstrand, L. et al. (1992) EMBO J. 11, 3911–3919.
24. Eriksson, A. et al. (1992) EMBO J. 11, 543–550.
25. Claesson-Welsh, L. et al. (1989) Proc. Natl. Acad. Sci. USA 86, 4917–4921.
26. Gronwald, R.G.K. et al. (1988) Proc. Natl. Acad. Sci. USA 85, 3435–3439.
27. Claesson-Welsh, L. et al. (1988) Mol. Cell Biol. 8, 3476–3486.
28. Yarden, Y. et al. (1986) Nature 323, 226–232.

Other names

Human PF-4 has been known as oncostatin A [1].

THE MOLECULE

Platelet factor 4 is an inflammatory cytokine [2] released from platelet α-granules [3]. It is a monocyte and neutrophil chemoattractant [4], and binds heparin to act as an anticoagulant [5]. PF-4 also suppresses smooth muscle growth [6], and inhibits megakaryocytopoiesis and angiogenesis [7,8].

Crossreactivity

There is 70% homology between human and rat PF-4 [9,10].

Sources

PF-4 is released during platelet aggregation [11], and from activated T lymphocytes [12].

Bioassays

PF-4 can be measured in neutrophil chemotaxis assays [13].

Physicochemical properties of PF-4

Property	Human	Rat
pI	7.6	?
Amino acids – precursor	101	105
– mature	70	76
M_r (K) – predicted	7.8	11.3
– expressed[a]	32 ?	
Potential N-linked glycosylation sites	0	0
Disulphide bonds[b]	2	2

[a] PF-4 exists in solution as a stable tetramer [14].

[b] Disulphide bonds link the first to third and second to fourth cysteines[15] (see sequence).

3-D structure

The structure of bovine and human PF-4 has been solved by X-ray and NMR spectroscopy [15]. The monomer unit contains a loop, three strands of antiparallel β-sheet in a greek key motif, and an α-helix at the C-terminus. The monomer to dimer and tetramer association pathway has been defined [16].

Gene structure

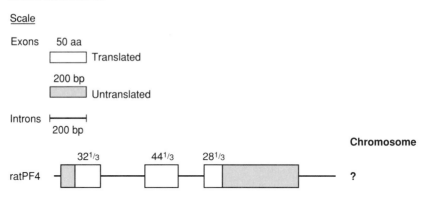

Scale

Exons   50 aa

☐ Translated

200 bp

▨ Untranslated

Introns ⊢———⊣
200 bp

Chromosome

ratPF4

32¹/₃   44¹/₃   28¹/₃

ratPF4   ?

The gene for human PF-4 is located on chromosome 4q12-21 [17].

Amino acid sequence for human PF-4 [2,10]

Accession code: Swissprot P02776

```
-31  MSSAAGFCAS RPGLLFLGLL LLPLVVAFAS A
  1  EAEEDGDLQC LCVKTTSQVR PRHITSLEVI KAGPHCPTAQ LIATLKNGRK
 51  ICLDLQAPLY KKIIKKLLES
```

Amino acid sequence for rat PF-4 [9]

Accession code: Swissprot P06765

```
-29  MSAAAVFRGL RPSPELLLLG LLLLPAVVA
  1  VTRASPEESD GDLSCVCVKT SSSRIHLKRI TSLEVIKAGP HCAVPQLIAT
 51  LKNGSKICLD RQVPLYKKII KKLLES
```

THE PF-4 RECEPTOR

No information is available yet.

References

1 Twardzik, D.R. and Todaro, G.J. (1987) US Patent 4,645,828.
2 Deuel, T.F. et al. (1977) Proc. Natl. Acad. Sci. USA. 74, 2256–2258.
3 Barber, A.J. et al. (1972) Biochim. Biophys. Acta 286, 312–329.
4 Deuel, T.F. et al. (1981) Proc. Natl. Acad. Sci. USA 78, 4584–4587.
5 Loscalzo, J. et al. (1985) Arch. Biochem. Biophys. 240, 446–455.
6 Castellot, J.J. et al. (1982) J. Biol. Chem. 257, 11256–11260.
7 Maione, T.E. et al. (1990) Science 247, 77–79.
8 Han, Z.C. et al. (1990) Blood 75, 1234–1239.
9 Doi, T. et al. (1987) Mol. Cell. Biol. 7, 898–904.
10 Poncz, M. et al. (1987) Blood 69, 219–223.
11 Niewiarowski, S. and Paul, D. (1981) In Platelets in Biology and Pathology, Gordon, J.L,. ed., Elsevier, Amsterdam, pp. 91–106.

12 Zipfel, P.F. et al. (1991) Biochem. Biophys. Res. Commun. 181, 179–183.

13 Van Damme, J. and Conings, R. (1991) In Cytokines: A practical Approach, Balkwill, F.R., ed., IRL Press, London, pp. 187–196.

14 Kurachi, K. (1978) J. Biol. Chem. 253, 8301–8302.

15 St. Charles, R. et al. (1989) J. Biol. Chem. 264, 2092–2099.

16 Mayo, K.H. and Chen, M.-J (1989) Biochemistry 28, 9469–9478.

17 Modi, W.S. et al. (1990) Hum. Genet. 84, 185–187.

RANTES
The chemokine family.

Other names
Human RANTES has been known as human sisδ [1].

THE MOLECULE

RANTES is a member of the CC chemokine/intercrine family of cytokines [2]. It is chemotactic for monocytes and memory T helper cells [3-5], as well as eosinophils [6]. RANTES also causes the release of histamine from human basophils [7], and activates eosinophils [8].

Crossreactivity
There is 85% homology between human and murine RANTES [9]. There is some evidence that the murine protein is active on human cells and vice versa.

Sources
RANTES is produced by T lymphocytes and macrophages, but is unusual in exhibiting a reduction in mRNA levels on activation of T cells [5].

Bioassays
Chemotaxis of monocytes, memory T cells [4], or eosinophils [6]. Release of histamine from mast cells [7].

Physicochemical properties of RANTES

Property	Human	Mouse
pI	9.5	9.0
Amino acids – precursor	91	91
– mature	68	68
M_r (K) – predicted	8	8
– expressed	8	8
Potential N-linked glycosylation sites	0[a]	0
Disulphide bonds	2	2

[a] Possibly some O-linked glycosylation.

3-D structure
Could be modelled on IL-8 structure.

Gene structure

The gene for human RANTES is located on chromosome 17q11–q21 [10].

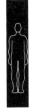

Amino acid sequence for human RANTES [3]

Accession code: Genbank M21121

```
-23  MKVSAARLAV ILIATALCAP ASA
  1  SPYSSDTTPC CFAYIARPLP RAHIKEYFYT SGKCSNPAVV FVTRKNRQVC
 51  ANPEKKWVRE YINSLEMS
```

Amino acid sequence for murine RANTES [9]

Accession code: Genbank M77747

```
-23  MKISAAALTI ILTAAALCTP APA
  1  SPYGSDTTPC CFAYLSLELP RAHVKEYFYT SSKCSNLAVV FVTRRNRQVC
 51  ANPEKKWVQE YINYLEMS
```

THE RANTES RECEPTOR

RANTES has a separate receptor to those for IL-8 and MIP-1α, but can also signal a calcium flux through the cloned MIP-1α receptor at 100nM and can displace MIP-1α from its receptor, with a K_d of 450nM [8,11]. The monocyte receptor for RANTES has an IC_{50} of 7nM, is G-protein linked, and fails to transmit a calcium flux[12].

References

[1] Brown, K.D. et al. (1989). J. Immunol. 142, 679–687.

[2] Oppenheim, J.J. et al. (1991) Annu. Rev. Immunol 9, 617–648.

[3] Schall, T.J. et al. (1988) J. Immunol. 141, 1018–1025.

[4] Schall, T.J. et al. (1990) Nature 347, 669–671.

[5] Schall, T.J. (1991) Cytokine 3, 165–183.

[6] Kamayoshi, Y. et al. (1992) J. Exp. Med. 196, 187–192.

[7] Kuna, P. et al. (1992) J. Immunol. 149, 636–642.

[8] Rot, A. et al. (1992). J. Exp. Med. 176, 1489–1495.

[9] Schall, T.J. et al. (1992) Eur. J. Immunol. 22, 1477–1481.

[10] Donlon, T.A. et al. (1990) Genomics 6, 548–553.

[11] Neote, K. et al. (1993) Cell 72, 415–425.

[12] Van Riper, B.G. et al. (1993) J. Exp. Med. 177, 851–856.

Other names
Mast cell growth factor (MGF), kit ligand (KL), steel factor (SLF).

THE MOLECULE

Stem cell factor is involved in the development of haematopoietic, gonadal and pigment cell lineages. It has a very wide range of activities with direct effects on myeloid and lymphoid cell development and powerful synergistic effects with other growth factors such as GM-CSF, IL-7 and erythropoietin. SCF is encoded by the steel (Sl) locus of the mouse and is the ligand for the c-*kit* proto-oncogene [1,2]. Alternative mRNA splicing gives rise to two forms of SCF both of which have a transmembrane domain and are inserted into the cell membrane. The larger form contains a peptide cleavage site and is processed to yield secreted SCF [3,4]. Both membrane bound and soluble forms are biologically active.

Crossreactivity
There is 81% homology between human and mouse SCF. Human SCF has very little activity on mouse cells whereas rat SCF is active on human cells.

Sources
Bone marrow stromal cells, brain, liver, kidney, lung, placenta, fibroblasts, oocytes, testis.

Bioassays
Synergy with CSFs in progenitor bone marrow colony assay. Proliferation of MO7e cell line.

Physicochemical properties of SCF

Property		Human	Mouse
Amino acids	– precursor	273	273
	– mature[a]	248/220	248/220
M_r (K)	– predicted[b]	27.9/18.5	27.7/18.3
	– expressed[c]	36	28–36
Potential N-linked glycosylation sites[d]		5	4
Disulphide bonds		2	2

[a] Long and short membrane-bound forms after removal of predicted signal peptide.
[b] Long membrane form and mature soluble form.
[c] Mature soluble form.
[d] One site is lost in short form. Also evidence for O-linked glycosylation. Non-glycosylated SCF is biologically active.

3-D structure
Non-covalently linked homodimer. Contains extensive α-helix and β-pleated sheets [5].

Gene structure [6]

Scale

Exons   50 aa
☐ Translated
500 bp
▨ Untranslated

Introns ⊢—⊣
1Kb

Chromosome

```
         5    38   21    57      52     28    37    35
hSCF ─▨┤//┤□┤//┤□┤//┤ □ ┤//┤  □  ┤//┤□┤//┤□┤//┤□▨├─   12q22-q24
```

mouse 10

Amino acid sequence for human SCF [6]

Accession code: Swissprot P21583

```
-25   MKKTQTWILT  CIYLQLLLFN  PLVKT
  1   EGICRNRVTN  NVKDVTKLVA  NLPKDYMITL  KYVPGMDVLP  SHCWISEMVV
 51   QLSDSLTDLL  DKFSNISEGL  SNYSIIDKLV  NIVDDLVECV  KENSSKDLKK
101   SFKSPEPRLF  TPEEFFRIFN  RSIDAFKDFV  VASETSDCVV  SSTLSPEKDS
151   RVSVTKPFML  PPVAASSLRN  DSSSSNRKAK  NPPGDSSLHW  AAMALPALFS
201   LIIGFAFGAL  YWKKRQPSLT  RAVENIQINE  EDNEISMLQE  KEREFQEV
```

Disulphide bonds are formed between Cys4–89 and 43–138. Alternative splicing gives rise to two membrane-bound forms [4]. The longer form contains a cleavage site between Ala164 and Ala165 or Ala165 and Ser166 yielding soluble SCF. The shorter form does not have amino acids 150–177, which contains the cleavage site, and is predominantly membrane bound.

Amino acid sequence for mouse SCF [7–9]

Accession code: Swissprot P20826

```
-25   MKKTQTWIIT  CIYLQLLLFN  PLVKT
  1   KEICGNPVTD  NVKDITKLVA  NLPNDYMITL  NYVAGMDVLP  SHCWLRDMVI
 51   QLSLSLTTLL  DKFSNISEGL  SNYSIIDKLG  KIVDDLVLCM  EENAPKNIKE
101   SPKRPETRSF  TPEEFFSIFN  RSIDAFKDFM  VASDTSDCVL  SSTLGPEKDS
151   RVSVTKPFML  PPVAASSLRN  DSSSSNRKAA  KAPEDSGLQW  TAMALPALIS
201   LVIGFAFGAL  YWKKKQSSLT  RAVENIQINE  EDNEISMLQQ  KEREFQEV
```

Disulphide bonds are formed between Cys4-89 and 43–138. Alternative splicing gives rise to two membrane bound forms [3]. The longer form is shown here. By analogy with rat SCF [10], The longer form contains a cleavage site between Ala164 and Ala165 or Ala165 and Ser166, yielding soluble SCF. The shorter form does not have amino acids 150–177, which contains the cleavage site, and is predominantly membrane-bound. Conflicting sequence A->S at position 182 [9].

THE SCF RECEPTOR

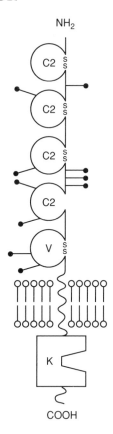

NH₂

The c-*kit* proto-oncogene is the receptor for SCF (CD 117). It is a single transmembrane glycoprotein with five extracellular Ig-SF domains and an intracellular tyrosine kinase domain split by a unique insertion sequence of 77 amino acids which is highly conserved between species. c-kit is structurally closely related to the CSF-1 receptor (c-fms) and the PDGF receptor. The functional receptor is probably a homodimer induced by binding of SCF. In mice, mutations of the W locus which encodes c-kit lead to changes in coat colour, anaemia and defective gonad development. In humans, a mutation resulting in a Gly->Arg substitution at position 642 has been identified in piebaldism.

Distribution

Almost all haematopoietic cell progenitors except B-lineage precursors which form colonies in response to IL-7. Also expressed on mast cells, melanocytes, spermatogonia and oocytes [2].

Physicochemical properties of the SCF receptor (c-kit)

Properties		Human	Mouse
Amino acids	– precursor	976	975
	– mature[a]	954	953
M_r (K)	– predicted	107.4	106.6
	– expressed	145	145–150
Potential N-linked glycosylation sites		10	9
Affinity K_d (M)		?	?

[a] After removal of predicted signal peptide.

Signal transduction

The SCF receptor (c-kit) belongs to the split tyrosine kinase receptor family which includes the PDGF and FGF receptors. The interkinase domain of c-kit contains the binding site for PI-3′ kinase [11]. Ligand binding to the SCF receptor results in auto-tyrosine phosphorylation, and tyrosine phosphorylation of MAP kinase, GAP and PLC-γ, as well as serine phosphorylation of Raf-1 [12].

Chromosomal location

Human chromosome 4q12 and mouse chromosome 5.

Amino acid sequence for human SCF receptor (c-kit) [13]

Accession code: Swissprot P10721

```
 -22  MRGARGAWDF  LCVLLLLLRV  QT
   1  GSSQPSVSPG  EPSPPSIHPG  KSDLIVRVGD  EIRLLCTDPG  FVKWTFEILD
  51  ETNENKQNEW  ITEKAEATNT  GKYTCTNKHG  LSNSIYVFVR  DPAKLFLVDR
 101  SLYGKEDNDT  LVRCPLTDPE  VTNYSLKGCQ  GKPLPKDLRF  IPDPKAGIMI
 151  KSVKRAYHRL  CLHCSVDQEG  KSVLSEKFIL  KVRPAFKAVP  VVSVSKASYL
 201  LREGEEFTVT  CTIKDVSSSV  YSTWKRENSQ  TKLQEKYNSW  HHGDFNYERQ
 251  ATLTISSARV  NDSGVFMCYA  NNTFGSANVT  TTLEVVDKGF  INIFPMINTT
 301  VFVNDGENVD  LIVEYEAFPK  PEHQQWIYMN  RTFTDKWEDY  PKSENESNIR
 351  YVSELHLTRL  KGTEGGTYTF  LVSNSDVNAA  IAFNVYVNTK  PEILTYDRLV
 401  NGMLQCVAAG  FPEPTIDWYF  CPGTEQRCSA  SVLPVDVQTL  NSSGPPFGKL
 451  VVQSSIDSSA  FKHNGTVECK  AYNDVGKTSA  YFNFAFKGNN  KEQIHPHTLF
 501  TPLLIGFVIV  AGMMCIIVMI  LTYKYLQKPM  YEVQWKVVEE  INGNNYVYID
 551  PTQLPYDHKW  EFPRNRLSFG  KTLGAGAFGK  VVEATAYGLI  KSDAAMTVAV
 601  KMLKPSAHLT  EREALMSELK  VLSYLGNHMN  IVNLLGACTI  GGPTLVITEY
 651  CCYGDLLNFL  RRKRDSFICS  KQEDHAEAAL  YKNLLHSKES  SCSDSTNEYM
 701  DMKPGVSYVV  PTKADKRRSV  RIGSYIERDV  TPAIMEDDEL  ALDLEDLLSF
 751  SYQVAKGMAF  LASKNCIHRD  LAARNILLTH  GRITKICDFG  LARDIKNDSN
 801  YVVKGNARLP  VKWMAPESIF  NCVYTFESDV  WSYGIFLWEL  FSLGSSPYPG
 851  MPVDSKFYKM  IKEGFRMLSP  EHAPAEMYDI  MKTCWDADPL  KRPTFKQIVQ
 901  LIEKQISEST  NHIYSNLANC  SPNRQKPVVD  HSVRINSVGS  TASSSQPLLV
 951  HDDV
```

Tyr801 is site of autophosphorylation.

Amino acid sequence for mouse SCF receptor (c-kit) [14]

Accession code: Swissprot P05532

```
 -22  MRGARGAWDL  LCVLLVLLRG  QT
   1  ATSQPSASPG  EPSPPSIHPA  QSELIVEAGD  TLSLTCIDPD  FVRWTFKTYF
  51  NEMVENKKNE  WIQEKAEATR  TGTYTCSNSN  GLTSSIYVFV  RDPAKLFLVG
 101  LPLFGKEDSD  ALVRCPLTDP  QVSNYSLIEC  DGKSLPTDLT  FVPNPKAGIT
 151  IKNVKRAYHR  LCVRCAAQRD  GTWLHSDKFT  LKVREAIKAI  PVVSVPETSH
 201  LLKKGDTFTV  VCTIKDVSTS  VNSMWLKMNP  QPQHIAQVKH  NSWHRGDFNY
 251  ERQETLTISS  ARVDDSGVFM  CYANNTFGSA  NVTTTLKVVE  KGFINISPVK
 301  NTTVFVTDGE  NVDLVVEYEA  YPKPEHQQWI  YMNRTSANKG  KDYVKSDNKS
 351  NIRYVNQLRL  TRLKGTEGGT  YTFLVSNSDA  SASVTFNVYV  NTKPEILTYD
 401  RLINGMLQCV  AEGFPEPTID  WYFCTGAEQR  CTTPVSPVDV  QVQNVSVSPF
 451  GKLVVQSSID  SSVFRHNGTV  ECKASNDVGK  SSAFFNFAFK  EQIQAHTLFT
 501  PLLIGFVVAA  GAMGIIVMVL  TYKYLQKPMY  EVQWKVVEEI  NGNNYVYIDP
 551  TQLPYDHKWE  FPRNRLSFGK  TLGAGAFGKV  VEATAYGLIK  SDAAMTVAVK
 601  MLKPSAHLTE  REALMSELKV  LSYLGNHMNI  VNLLGACTVG  GPTLVITEYC
 651  CYGDLLNFLR  RKRDSFIFSK  QEEQAEAALY  KNLLHSTEPS  CDSSNEYMDM
 701  KPGVSYVVPT  KTDKRRSARI  DSYIERDVTP  AIMEDDELAL  DLDDLLSFSY
 751  QVAKAMAFLA  SKNCIHRDLA  ARNILLTHGR  ITKICDFGLA  RDIRNDSNYV
 801  VKGNARLPVK  WMAPESIFSC  VYTFESDVWS  YGIFLWELFS  LGSSPYPGMP
 851  VDSKFYKMIK  EGFRMVSPEH  APAEMYDVMK  TCWDADPLKR  PTFKQVVQLI
 901  EKQISDSTKH  IYSNLANCNP  NPENPVVVDH  SVRVNSVGSS  ASSTQPLLVH
 951  EDA
```

Tyr799 is site of autophosphorylation.

References

[1] Witte, O.N. (1990) Cell 63, 5–6.

[2] Morrison-Graham, K. and Takahashi, Y. (1993) BioEssays 15, 77–83.

[3] Flanagan, J.G. et al. (1991) Cell 64, 1025–1035.

[4] Anderson, D.M. et al. (1991) Cell Growth Differ. 2, 373–378.

[5] Arakawa, T. et al. (1991) J. Biol. Chem. 266, 18942–18948.

[6] Martin, F.H. et al. (1990) Cell 63, 203–211.

[7] Anderson, D.M. et al. (1990) Cell 63, 235–243.

[8] Zsebo, K.M. et al. (1990) Cell 63, 213–224.

[9] Huang, E. et al. (1990) Cell 63, 225–233.

[10] Lu, H.S. et al. (1991) J. Biol. Chem. 266, 8102–8107.

[11] Lev, S. et al. (1992) Proc. Natl Acad. Sci. USA 89, 678–682.

[12] Miyazawa, K. et al. (1991) Exp. Haematol. 19, 1110–1123.

[13] Yarden, Y. et al. (1987) EMBO J. 6, 3341–3351.

[14] Qiu, F. et al. (1988) EMBO J. 7, 1003–1011.

TGFα

Other names

Sarcoma growth factor.

THE MOLECULE

Transforming growth factor α is a small integral membrane protein which shares biological and structural properties with EGF. The mature 50 amino acid cytokine is released by proteolytic cleavage [1-4]. TGFα can act as an autoinductive growth factor [5].

Crossreactivity

TGFα is active across species. TGFα is closely structurally related to EGF and to vaccinia growth factor, which all bind to the EGF receptor [6,7].

Sources

TGFα is made by monocytes, keratinocytes and many tissues and tumours.

Bioassays

Proliferation of the A431 carcinoma line.

Physicochemical properties of TGFα

Property	Human	Rat
Amino acids – precursor	160	159
– mature[a]	50	50
M_r (K) – predicted	6	6
– expressed	6	6
Potential N-linked glycosylation sites[b]	0	0
Disulphide bonds	3	3

[a] The C-terminal valine in the cytoplasmic tail of proTGFα is required for cleavage to mature TGFα [8].

[b] In mature 50 amino acid TGFα, there is one N-linked glycosylation site in the propeptide.

3-D structure

Similar to EGF [9].

Gene structure

Human TGFα is on chromosome 2.

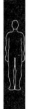

Amino acid sequence for human TGFα[3]

Accession code: Swissprot P01135

```
-23  MVPSAGQLAL FALGIVLAAC QAL
  1  ENSTSPLSAD PPVAAAVVSH FNDCPDSHTQ FCFHGTCRFL VQEDKPACVC
 51  HSGYVGARCE HADLLAVVAA SQKKQAITAL VVVSIVALAV LIITCVLIHC
101  CQVRKHCEWC RALICRHEKP SALLKGRTAC CHSETVV
```

N-terminal and C-terminal sequence in italics are removed during processing to release the active molecule (amino acids 17–66). Disulphide bonds between Cys24–37, 32–48 and 50–59.

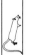

Amino acid sequence for rat TGFα [10]

Accession code: Swissprot P01134

```
-23  MVPAAGQLAL LALGILVAVC QAL
  1  ENSTPPLSDS PVAAAVVSHF NKCPDSHTQY CFHGTCRFLV QEEKPACVCH
 51  SGYVGVRCEH ADLLAVVAAS QKKQAITALV VVSIVALAVL IITCVLIHCC
101  QVRKHCEWCR ALVCRHEKPS ALLKGRTACC HSETVV
```

N-terminal and C-terminal sequence in italics are removed during processing to release the active molecule (amino acids 16–65). Disulphide bonds between Cys23–36, 31–47 and 49–58.

THE TGFα RECEPTOR

The TGF receptor (also known as c-erbB) is a class I receptor tyrosine kinase [11,12]. The receptor is also shared with epidermal growth factor, and with vaccinia virus growth factor. A viral oncogene v-erbB encodes a truncated EGF receptor lacking most of the extracellular domains. See EGF entry for details.

Distribution

See EGF entry.

Chromosomal location

The receptor gene is found on chromosome 7.

References

1 Burgess, A.W. (1989) In Br. Med. Bull. 45, Growth Factors, Waterfeld, M.D., ed, Churchill Livingstone, London, pp. 401–424.
2 DeLarco, J.E. and Todaro, G. (1978) Proc. Natl. Acad. Sci. USA 75, 4001–4005.
3 Dernyck, R. et al. (1984) Cell 38, 287–297.
4 Texido, J. et al. (1987) Nature 326, 883–855.
5 Coffey, R.J. et al. (1987) Nature 328, 817–820.
6 Montelione, G.T. et al. (1986) Proc. Natl. Acad. Sci. USA. 83, 8594–8598.
7 Stroobant, P. et al. (1985) Cell 383–393.
8 Bosenberg, M.W. et al. (1992) Cell 71, 1157–1165.
9 Campbell, I.D. et al. (1989) in Prog. in Growth Factor Res. 1, 13–22.
10 Lee, D.C. et al. (1985) Nature 313, 489–491.
11 Ullrich, A. et al. Nature 309, 418–425.
12 Ullrich, A. and Schlessinger, J. (1990) Cell 61, 203–212.

TGFβ

Other names

Human TGFβ1 has been known as differentiation inhibiting factor and cartilage-inducing factor. Human TGFβ2 has been known as glioblastoma-derived T cell suppressor factor.

THE MOLECULE

Transforming growth factor β is a pleiotropic cytokine involved in tissue remodelling, wound repair, development and haematopoiesis [1]. Its predominant action is to inhibit cell growth. TGFβ is also a switch factor for IgA. TGFβ is comprised of three related dimeric proteins, TGFβ1, 2 and 3, all of which are members of a superfamily including the activins, inhibins and bone morphogenic proteins. The expressed proteins are biologically inactive disulphide-linked dimers which are cleaved to active dimers of 112 amino acid disulphide-linked peptides [2]. Platelet-derived TGFβ1 is covalently associated with an M_r 125 000–160 000 binding protein comprised mainly of 16 EGF domain repeats [3]. (Human sequence in Genbank M34057, rat sequence in Genbank M55431.) A similar protein is found in glioma and fibroblasts. TGFβ binds to proteoglycans such as decorin in the extracellular matrix and α2-macroglobulin in blood [4].

Crossreactivity

There is greater than 98% homology between the functional regions of human and mouse TGFβ species, only the human sequences are given [5-7].

Sources

Platelets contain TGFβ1 and β2. Most nucleated cell types and many tumours also express TGFβ1, β2, β3 or combinations of the three forms.

Bioassays

Inhibition of growth of mink lung cell line MV-1-Lu.

Physicochemical properties of TGFβ1, 2 and 3

Property		TGFβ1	Human TGFβ2	TGFβ3
Amino acids	– precursor	390	414	412
	– mature[a]	112	112	112
M_r (K)	– predicted	44.3	47.8	47.3
	– expressed	25	25	25
Potential N-linked glycosylation sites[b]		0	0	0
Disulphide bonds		1	1	1

[a] Functional TGFβ is a disulphide-linked dimer which must be cleaved from the inactive propeptide. Cleavage of the TGFβ1 propeptide at cell surfaces involves binding of the propeptide to the IGF type II receptor, and requires plasminogen activator and plasmin[8].

[b] There are 2 sites in TGFβ1 propeptide, 3 sites in TGFβ2 propeptide and 4 sites in TGFβ3 propeptide.

3-D structure

The crystal structure of TGFβ2 has been solved and shown to contain an unusual elongated non-globular fold [9]. The structure can be used to model the other TGFβs.

Gene structure [10]

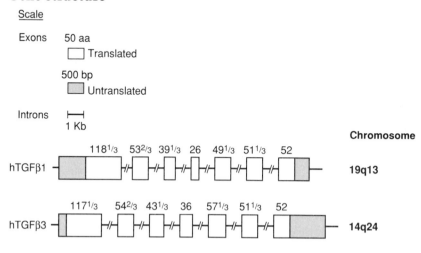

Scale

Exons   50 aa
         ☐ Translated

         500 bp
         ▨ Untranslated

Introns ⊢—⊣
         1 Kb

                                                         Chromosome

         118¹/₃ 53²/₃ 39¹/₃ 26 49¹/₃ 51¹/₃ 52

hTGFβ1   19q13

         117¹/₃ 54²/₃ 43¹/₃ 36 57¹/₃ 51¹/₃ 52

hTGFβ3   14q24

Note: sizes of the introns have not been determined

The gene for human TGFβ1 is located on chromosome19q13, TGFβ2 on 1q41 and TGFβ3 on 14q24. The gene for murine TGFβ1 is located on chromosome 7, β2 on 1 and β3 on 12 .

Amino acid sequence for human TGFβ1 [5]

Accession code: Swissprot P01137

```
-29   MPPSGLRLLL  LLLPLLWLLV  LTPGRPAAG
  1   LSTCKTIDME  LVKRKRIEAI  RGQILSKLRL  ASPPSQGEVP  PGPLPEAVLA
 51   LYNSTRDRVA  GESAEPEPEP  EADYYAKEVT  RVLMVETHNE  IYDKFKQSTH
101   SIYMFFNTSE  LREAVPEPVL  LSRAELRLLR  LKLKVEQHVE  LYQKYSNNSW
151   RYLSNRLLAP  SDSPEWLSFD  VTGVVRQWLS  RGGEIEGFRL  SAHCSCDSRD
201   NTLQVDINGF  TTGRRGDLAT  IHGMNRPFLL  LMATPLERAQ  HLQSSRHRRA
251   LDTNYCFSST  EKNCCVRQLY  IDFRKDLGWK  WIHEPKGYHA  NFCLGPCPYI
301   WSLDTQYSKV  LALYNQHNPG  ASAAPCCVPQ  ALEPLPIVYY  VGRKPKVEQL
351   SNMIVRSCKC  S
```

Propeptide is indicated in italics

Amino acid sequence for human TGFβ2 [6]

Accession code: Swissprot P08112

```
-20   MHYCVLSAFL  ILHLVTVALS
  1   LSTCSTLDMD  QFMRKRIEAI  RGQILSKLKL  TSPPEDYPEP  EEVPPEVISI
 51   YNSTRDLLQE  KASRRAAACE  RERSDEEYYA  KEVYKIDMPP  FFPSENAIPP
101   TFYRPYFRIV  RFDVSAMEKN  ASNLVKAEFR  VFRLQNPKAR  VPEQRIELYQ
```

```
151   ILKSKDLTSP  TQRYIDSKVV  KTRAEGEWLS  FDVTDAVHEW  LHHKDRNLGF
201   KISLHCPCCT  FVPSNNYIIP  NKSEELEARF  AGIDGTSTYT  SGDQKTIKST
251   RKKNSGKTPH  LLLMLLPSYR  LESQQTNRRK  KRALDAAYCF  RNVQDNCCLR
301   PLYIDFKRDL  GWKWIHEPKG  YNANFCAGAC  PYLWSSDTQH  SRVLSLYNTI
351   NPEASASPCC  VSQDLEPLTI  LYYIGKTPKI  EQLSNMIVKS  CKCS
```

Propeptide is indicated in italics.

Amino acid sequence for human TGFβ3 [7]

Accession code: Swissprot P10600

```
-23   MKMHLQRALV  VLALLNFATV  SLS
  1   LSTCTTLDFG  HIKKKRVEAI  RGQILSKLRL  TSPPEPTVMT  HVPYQVLALY
 51   NSTRELLEEM  HGEREEGCTQ  ENTESEYYAK  EIHKFDMIQG  LAEHNELAVC
101   PKGITSKVFR  FNVSSVEKNR  TNLFRAEFRV  LRVPNPSSKR  NEQRIELFQI
151   LRPDEHIAKQ  RYIGGKNLPT  RGTAEWLSFD  VTDTVREWLL  RRESNLGLEI
201   SIHCPCHTFQ  PNGDILENIH  EVMEIKFKGV  DNEDDHGRGD  LGRLKKQKDH
251   HNPHLILMMI  PPHRLDNPGQ  GGQRKKRALD  TNYCFRNLEE  NCCVRPLYID
301   FRQDLGWKWV  HEPKGYYANF  CSGPCPYLRS  ADTTHSTVLG  LYNTLNPEAS
351   ASPCCVPQDL  EPLTILYYVG  RTPKVEQLSN  MVVKSCKCS
```

Propeptide is indicated in italics.

THE TGFβ RECEPTORS

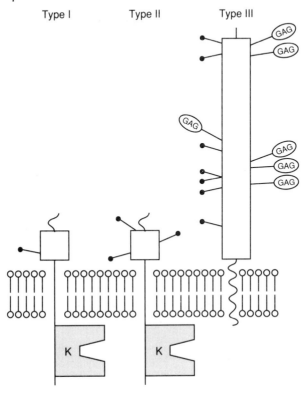

There are three types of TGFβ receptor [11]: high affinity type I (M_r 55 000) [2,12] and II (Mr 80 000) [13], and low affinity type III (M_r 250 000–350 000) [14,15]. The human receptors bind all three TGFβ isoforms. The type I receptor binds β1=β2>β3, type II β1>β2>β3 and type III β1=β2=β3. The human and pig type II receptor and the rat type III receptors have been cloned. The human and murine type I receptors have also been cloned [12,16]. The type I and II receptors are serine/threonine kinases related to the activin receptor. The type III receptors include β-glycan, an integral membrane protein modified by attachment of glycosaminoglycans, and endoglin (CD105) which is a homodimer of two M_r 95 000 disulphide-linked subunits related to β-glycan. Endoglin does not bind TGFβ2 [17]. The type I and II receptors are thought to associate to mediate signal transduction events probably by serine /threonine phosphorylation. It is unclear if the receptors autophosphorylate. There appears to be an emerging family of receptors related to the type I receptor whose role in TGFβ signalling is not yet clear [12,18]. The type III receptors have not been shown to transduce signals, but may function to concentrate TGFβ on the cell surface and present the ligand to its other receptors. Coexpression of type II and III receptors increases the ability of the type II receptor to bind TGFβ. The type III receptor can be released from the cell surface by proteolysis. Two potential cleavage sites exist in the transmembrane region KK and LAVV. The LAVV sequence is also used to release TGFα. The glycosaminoglycan on the type III receptor is not involved in binding TGFβ.

Distribution

Most cell types. The type II receptor is lacking in retinoblastoma cells.

Physicochemical properties of the TGFβ receptors

Properties	Type I human	Type I mouse	Type II human	Type III Rat
Amino acids – precursor	503	509	565	853
– mature	479	492	542	829
M_r (K) – predicted	51	53	60	91.6
– expressed	53	68	65	250–350
Potential N-linked glycosylation sites	1	1	3	7
Affinity K_d (M)	$5–30\times10^{-12}$			$3–30\times10^{-11}$

Signal transduction

Requires the formation of a heteromeric complex of type I and type II receptors (Ser/Thr kinases) for effects, possibly also homodimers [19]. Purified type II receptor can autophosphorylate on Ser and Thr.

Chromosomal location

Not known yet.

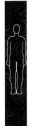

Amino acid sequence for human type I TGFβ receptor ALK-1 [12]

Accession code: Genbank L11695.

```
 -24   MEAAVAAPRP  RLLLLVLAAA  AAAA
   1   AALLPGATAL  QCFCHLCTKD  NFTCVTDGLC  FVSVTETTDK  VIHNSMCIAE
  51   IDLIPRDRPF  VCAPSSKTGS  VTTTYCCNQD  HCNKIELPTT  VKSSPGLGPV
 101   ELAAVIAGPV  CFVCISLMLM  VYICHNRIVI  HHRVPNEEDP  SLDRPFISEG
 151   TTLKDLIYDM  TTSGSGSGLP  LLVQRTIART  IVLQESIGKG  RFGEVWRGKW
 201   RGEEVAVKIF  SSREERSWFR  EAERYQTVML  RHENILGFIA  ADNKDNGTWT
 251   QLWLVSDYHE  HGSLFDYLNR  YTVTVEGMIK  LALSTASGLA  HLHMEIVGTG
 301   GKPAIAHRDL  KSKNILVKKN  GTCCIADLGL  AVRHDSATDT  IDIAPNHRVG
 351   TKRYMAPEVL  DDSINMKHFE  SFKRADIYAM  GLVFWEIARR  CSIGGIAGDY
 401   QLPYYDLVPS  DPSVEEMRKV  VCEQKLRPNI  PNRWQSCEAL  RVMAKIMREC
 451   WYANGAARLT  ALRIKKTLSQ  LSQQEGIKM
```

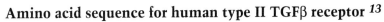

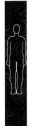

Amino acid sequence for human type II TGFβ receptor [13]

Accession code: Genbank M85079

```
 -23   MGRGLLRGLW  PLHIVLWTRI  AST
   1   IPPHVQKSVN  NDMIVTDNNG  AVKFPQLCKF  CDVRFSTCDN  QKSCMSNCSI
  51   TSICEKPQEV  CVAVWRKNDE  NITLETVCHD  PKLPYHDFIL  EDAASPKCIM
 101   KEKKKPGETF  FMCSCSSDEC  NDNIIFSEEY  NTSNPDLLLV  IFQVTGISLL
 151   PPLGVAISVI  IIFYCYRVNR  QQKLSSTWET  GKTRKLMEFS  EHCAIILEDD
 201   RSDISSTCAN  NINHNTELLP  IELDTLVGKG  RFAEVYKAKL  KQNTSEQFET
 251   VAVKIFPYEE  YASWKDRKDI  FSDINLKHEN  ILQFLTAEER  KTELGKQYWL
 301   ITAFHAKGNL  QEYLTRHVIS  WEDLRNVGSS  LARGLSHLHS  DHTPCGRPKM
 351   PIVHRDLKSS  NILVKNDLTC  CLCDFGLSLR  LGPYSSVDDL  ANSGQVGTAR
 401   YMAPEVLESR  MNLENAESFK  QTDVYSMALV  LWEMTSRCNA  VGEVKDYEPP
 451   FGSKVRDPVV  ESMKDNVLRD  RGTRNSSFWL  NHQGIQMVCE  TLTECWDHDP
 501   EARLTAQCVA  ERFSELEHLD  RLSGRSCSEE  KIPEDGSLNT  TK
```

Potential phosphorylation sites at Ser263, 378, 418, 462 and Thr180, 183, 398, 435 and 540.

Amino acid sequence for murine type I TGFβ receptor [16]

Accession code: Genbank L15436.

```
 -17   MVDGVMILPV  LMMMAFP
   1   SPSVEDEKPK  VNQKLYMCVC  EGLSCGNEDH  CEGQQCFSSL  SIYDGFHVYQ
  51   KGCFQVYEQG  KMTCKTPPSP  GQAVECCQGD  WCNRNITAQL  PTKGKSFPGT
 101   QNFHLEVGLI  ILSVVFAVCL  LACILGVALR  KFKRRNQERL  NPRDVEYGTI
 151   EGLITTNVGD  STLAELLDHS  CTSGSGSGLP  FLVQRTVARQ  ITLLECVGKG
 201   RYGEVWRGSW  QGENVAVKIF  SSRDEKSWFR  ETELYNTVML  RHENILGFIA
 251   SDMTSRHSST  QLWLITHYHE  MGSLYDYLQL  TTLDTVSCLR  IVLSIASGLA
 301   HLHIEIFGTQ  GKSAIAHRDL  KSKNILVKKN  GQCCIADLGL  AVMHSQSTNQ
 351   LDVGNNPRVG  TKRYMAPEVL  DETIQVDCFD  SYKRVDIWAF  GLVLWEVARR
 401   MVSNGIVEDY  KPPFYDVVPN  DPSFEDMRKV  VCVDQQRPNI  PNRWFSDPTL
 451   TSLAKLMKEC  WYQNPSARLT  ALRIKKTLTK  IDNSLDKLKT  DC
```

Potential phosphorylation sites at Ser 222 and 255

Amino acid sequence for rat type III TGFβ receptor (β-glycan) [14,15]

Accession code: Genbank M80784 and M77809

```
-24   MAVTSHHMIP VMVVLMSACL ATAG
  1   PEPSTRCELS PINASHPVQA LMESFTVLSG CASRGTTGLP REVHVLNLBS
 51   TDQGPGQRQR EVTLHLNPIA SVHTHHKPIV FLLNSPQPLV WHLKTERLAA
101   GVPBLFLVSE GSVVQFPSGN FSLTAETEER NFPQENEHLL RWAQKEYGAV
151   TSFTELKIAR NIYIKVGEDQ VFPPTCNIGK NFLSLNYLAE YLQPKAAEGC
201   VLPSQPHEKE VHIIELITPS SNPYSAFQVD IIVDIRPAQE DPEVVKNLVL
251   ILKCKKSVNW VIKSFDVKGN LKVIAPNSIG FGKESERSMT MTKLVRDDIP
301   STQENLMKWA LDNGYRPVTS YTMAPVANRF HLRLENNEEM RDEEVHTIPP
351   ELRILLDPHD PPALDNPLFP GEGSPNGGLP FPFPDIPRRG WKEGEDRIPR
401   PKQPIVPSVQ LLPDHREPEE VQGGVDIALS VKCDHEKMVV AVDKDSFQTN
451   GYSGMELTLL DPSCKAKMNG THFVLESPLN GCGTRHRRST PDGVVYYNSI
501   VVQAPSPGDS SGWPDGYEDL ESGDNGFPGD GDEGETAPLS RAGVVVFNCS
551   LRQLRNPSGF QGQLDGNATF NMELYNTDLF LVPSPGVFSV AENEHVYVEV
601   SVTKADQDLG FAIQTCFLSP YSNPDRMSDY TIIENICPKD DSVKFYSSKR
651   VHFPIPHAEV DKKRFSFLFK SVFNTSLLFL HCELTLCSRK KGSLKLPRCV
701   TPDDACTSLD ATMIWTMMQM KKTFTKPLAV VLQVDYKENV PSTKDSSPIP
751   PPPPQIFHGL DTLTVMGIAF AAFVIGALLT GALWYIYSHT GETARRQQVP
801   TSPPASENSS AAHSIGSTQS TPCSSSSTA
```

Potential glycosaminoglycan sites at Ser29, 118, 511, 522, 558

References
1 Roberts, A.B. and Sporn, M.B. (1990) in Handbook of Experimental Pharmacology, Sporn, M.B. and Roberts, A.B., eds., Vol. 65 Springer-Verlag, Heidelberg, pp. 419–472.
2 Brown, P.D. et al. (1990) Growth Factors 3, 35–43.
3 Kanzaki, T. et al. (1990) Cell 61, 1051–1061.
4 Yamaguchi, Y. et al. (1990) Nature 346, 281–284.
5 Derynck, R. et al. (1985) Nature 316, 701–705.
6 De Martin, R. et al. (1987) EMBO J. 6, 3673–3677.
7 Derynck, R. et al. (1988) EMBO J. 7, 3737–3743.
8 Dennis, P.A. and Rifkin, D.B. (1991) Proc. Natl. Acad. Sci. USA 88, 580–584.
9 Daopin, S. et al. (1992) Science 257, 369–373.
10 Derynck, R. et al. (1987) Nucl. Acids Res. 15, 3188–3189.
11 Massague, J. (1992) Cell 69, 1067–1070.
12 Franzen, P. et al. (1993) Cell 75, 681–692.
13 Lin, H.Y. et al. (1992) Cell 68, 775–785.
14 Lopez-Casillas, F. et al. (1991) Cell 67, 785–795.
15 Wang, X.-F. et al. (1991) Cell 67, 797–805.
16 Ebner, R. et al. (1993) Science 260, 1344–1348.
17 Cheifetz, S. et al. (1992) J. Biol. Chem. 267, 19027–19030.
18 Attisano, L. et al. (1993) Cell 75, 671–680.
19 Wrana, J.L. et al. (1993) Cell 71, 1003–1014.

Other names

Tumour necrosis factor (TNF), cachectin, macrophage cytotoxin, necrosin, cytotoxin, haemorrhagic factor, macrophage cytotoxic factor, differentiation-inducing factor.

THE MOLECULE

Tumour necrosis factor α is a potent paracrine and endocrine mediator of inflammatory and immune functions. It is also known to regulate growth and differentiation of a wide variety of cells types. TNFα is selectively cytotoxic for many transformed cells, especially in combination with IFNγ. In vivo, it leads to necrosis of methylcholanthrene-induced murine sarcomas. Many of the actions of TNFα occur in combination with other cytokines as part of the "cytokine network" [1-3]. TNFα is expressed as a type II membrane protein attached by a signal anchor transmembrane domain in the propeptide, and is processed by a Matrix metalloproteinase [4].

Crossreactivity

There is 79% homology between human and mouse TNFα and significant cross-species reactivity. Human TNF binds to mouse p55 receptor but not to mouse p75 receptor. Mouse TNF binds to both human receptors.

Sources

TNFα is secreted by activated monocytes and macrophages, and many other cells including B cells, T cells and fibroblasts.

Bioassays

Cytotoxicity on murine fibroblast lines L929 or L-M. Assay is faster and more sensitive in the presence of 0.1 μg/ml of actinomycin D. Specific neutralizing antibodies can be used to distinguish between TNFα and TNFβ.

Physicochemical properties of TNFα

Property	Human	Mouse
pI	5.6	5.6
Amino acids – precursor	233	235
– mature[a]	157	156
M_r (K) – predicted	17.4	17.3
– expressed[b]	52	18–150 [c]
Potential N-linked glycosylation sites	0	1
Disulphide bonds[d]	1	1

[a] Processing is by proteolytic cleavage of an atypical signal/propeptide of 76 residues in human TNFα and 79 residues in mouse TNFα. The unprocessed pro-form of TNF-α is expressed as a type II membrane protein by a signal anchor domain in the propeptide.

b TNFα is normally secreted as a homotrimer. Monomeric TNF is not biologically active.

c Differential processing of the murine propeptide and glycosylation results in several higher molecular weight isoforms.

d The disulphide bond is not required for biological activity.

3-D structure

TNFα exists as a homotrimer characterized by edge-to-face association of the antiparallel sandwich structure of the wedge-shaped monomers. The tertiary structure is very similar to the so-called "jelly roll" motif of some plant and animal virus capsids [5].

Gene structure [6,7]

Scale

Exons   50 aa
         ☐ Translated
         200 bp
         ▨ Untranslated

Introns ⊢—⊣
         200 bp

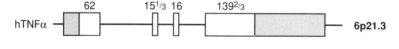

TNFβ is about 1200 bp upstream from TNFα

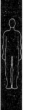

Amino acid sequence for human TNFα [8]

Accession code: Swissprot P01375

```
-76   MSTESMIRDV ELAEEALPKK TGGPQGSRRC LFLSLFSFLI VAGATTLFCL
-26   LHFGVIGPQR EEFPRDLSLI SPLAQA
  1   VRSSSRTPSD KPVAHVVANP QAEGQLQWLN RRANALLANG VELRDNQLVV
 51   PSEGLYLIYS QVLFKGQGCP STHVLLTHTI SRIAVSYQTK VNLLSAIKSP
101   CQRETPEGAE AKPWYEPIYL GGVFQLEKGD RLSAEINRPD YLDFAESGQV
151   YFGIIAL
```

Conflicting sequence F->S at position −14. Disulphide bond between Cys69–101. Signal anchor sequence −41 to −21 (underlined). Myristylation on Lys−58/−57.

Amino acid sequence for mouse TNFα [9]

Accession code: Swissprot P06804

```
-79   MSTESMIRDV ELAEEALPQK MGGFQNSRRC LCLSLFSFLL VAGATTLFCL
-29   LNFGVIGPQR DEKFPNGLPL ISSMAQTLT
  1   LRSSSQNSSD KPVAHVVANH QVEEQLEWLS QRANALLANG MDLKDNQLVV
 51   PADGLYLVYS QVLFKGQGCP DYVLLTHTVS RFAISYQEKV NLLSAVKSPC
101   PKDTPEGAEL KPWYEPIYLG GVFQLEKGDQ LSAEVNLPKY LDFAESGQVY
151   FGVIAL
```

Conflicting sequence G->R at position 152. Disulphide bond between
Cys69–100 (by similarity). Signal membrane anchor sequence –44 to –24
(underlined). Alternative terminus at L-10 reported.

THE TNF RECEPTORS

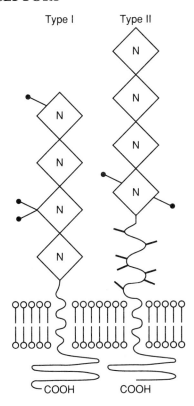

Type I   Type II

There are two receptors for TNF. The type I receptor (CD120a) has an M_r of
55 000 and the type II receptor (CD120b) has an M_r of 75 000. Both
receptors bind TNFα and TNFβ (lymphotoxin). The mouse p75 receptor
does not bind human TNFα which may explain some cases of non-species
crossreactivity. Both receptors are members of the NGFR/TNFR

superfamily with four Cys-rich repeats in the extracellular domain. The two receptors are <25% identical and have no more homology to each other than to other members of the superfamily. There is no significant homology between the intracellular domains of the two TNF receptors, indicating different signalling mechanisms [10]. Soluble forms of both the human p55 and p75 receptors have been found in serum of cancer patients and in urine. The soluble receptors are derived from the extracellular domain of each receptor as indicated on the sequence and are thought to act as inhibitors of TNF action [11]. Myxoma virus encodes a soluble protein related to the TNF receptor [12].

Distribution

TNF receptors are present on nearly all cell types with few exceptions such as erythrocytes and resting T cells. The type I p55 receptor is found on most cell types whereas the type II p75 receptor seems more restricted to haematopoietic cells.

Physicochemical properties of the TNF receptors

Properties	p55 (type I)		p75 (type II)	
	human	mouse	human	Mouse
Amino acids – precursor	455	454	461	474
– mature[a]	426	425	439	452
M_r (K) – predicted	48.3	48	46.1	47.9
– expressed	55	55	75–80	75
Potential N-linked glycosylation sites[b]	3	3	2	2
Affinity K_d (M)	5×10^{-10}	2×10^{-10}	10^{-10}	5×10^{-11}

[a] After removal of predicted signal peptide.
[b] The p75 receptor is also O-glycosylated.

Signal transduction

Receptor crosslinking by the TNF trimer is important for signal transduction. TNF activates a sphingomyelinase resulting in release of ceramide from sphingomyelin [13] which in turn activates a Mg^{2+}-dependent protein kinase [14]. TNF-induced sphingomyelinase activity is secondary to the generation of DAG produced by a phosphorylcholine-specific phospholipase C (PC-PLC) [15,16]. Activation of phospholipase D (PLD) [17] and phospholipase A2 (PLA2) [18] by TNF has also been described. There is some evidence for G protein coupling of the TNF receptor to PLA2 [19]. Type I and type II receptors probably activate different cellular responses [10], and they may be coupled to distinct signal transduction pathways. Mice with the type I receptor gene deleted are resistant to TNF-mediated toxicity and susceptible to infection by *Listeria monocytogenes* [20].

Chromosomal location

The human type I receptor is on chromosome 12p13 and the type II receptor is on chromosome 1p36-p32.

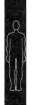

Amino acid sequence for human TNF type I (p55) receptor [21,22]

Accession code: Swissprot P19438

```
-21   MGLSTVPDLL LPLVLLELLV G
  1   IYPSGVIGLV PHLGDREKRD SVCPQGKYIH PQNNSICCTK CHKGTYLYND
 51   CPGPGQDTDC RECESGSFTA SENHLRHCLS CSKCRKEMGQ VEISSCTVDR
101   DTVCGCRKNQ YRHYWSENLF QCFNCSLCLN GTVHLSCQEK QNTVCTCHAG
151   FFLRENECVS CSNCKKSLEC TKLCLPQIEN VKGTEDSGTT VLLPLVIFFG
201   LCLLSLLFIG LMYRYQRWKS KLYSIVCGKS TPEKEGELEG TTTKPLAPNP
251   SFSPTPGFTP TLGFSPVPSS TFTSSSTYTP GDCPNFAAPR REVAPPYQGA
301   DPILATALAS DPIPNPLQKW EDSAHKPQSL DTDDPATLYA VVENVPPLRW
351   KEFVRRLGLS DHEIDRLELQ NGRCLREAQY SMLATWRRRT PRREATLELL
401   GRVLRDMDLL GCLEDIEEAL CGPAALPPAP SLLR
```

Conflicting sequence Pro391 missing, `GPAA->APP` at positions 422–425. Soluble receptor amino acids 20-180.

Amino acid sequence for human TNF type II (p75) receptor [23]

Accession code: GenEMBL M32315

```
-22   MAPVAVWAAL AVGLELWAAA HA
  1   LPAQVAFTPY APEPGSTCRL REYYDQTAQM CCSKCSPGQH AKVFCTKTSD
 51   TVCDSCEDST YTQLWNWVPE CLSCGSRCSS DQVETQACTR EQNRICTCRP
101   GWYCALSKQE GCRLCAPLRK CRPGFGVARP GTETSDVVCK PCAPGTFSNT
151   TSSTDICRPH QICNVVAIPG NASMDAVCTS TSPTRSMAPG AVHLPQPVST
201   RSQHTQPTPE PSTAPSTSFL LPMGPSPPAE GSTGDFALPV GLIVGVTALG
251   LLIIGVVNCV IMTQVKKKPL CLQREAKVPH LPADKARGTQ GPEQQHLLIT
301   APSSSSSSLE SSASALDRRA PTRNQPQAPG VEASGAGEAR ASTGSSDSSP
351   GGHGTQVNVT CIVNVCSSSD HSSQCSSQAS STMGDTDSSP SESPKDEQVP
401   FSKEECAFRS QLETPETLLG STEEKPLPLG VPDAGMKPS
```

Amino acid sequence for mouse TNF type I (p55) receptor [24]

Accession code: Swissprot P25118

```
-21   MGLPTVPGLL LSLVLLALLM G
  1   IHPSGVTGLV PSLGDREKRD SLCPQGKYVH SKNNSICCTK CHKGTYLVSD
 51   CPSPGRDTVC RECEKGTFTA SQNYLRQCLS CKTCRKEMSQ VEISPCQADK
101   DTVCGCKENQ FQRYLSETHF QCVDCSPCFN GTVTIPCKET QNTVCNCHAG
151   FFLRESECVP CSHCKKNEEC MKLCLPPPLA NVTNPQDSGT AVLLPLVILL
201   GLCLLSFIFI SLMCRYPRWR PEVYSIICRD PVPVKEEKAG KPLTPAPSPA
251   FSPTSGFNPT LGFSTPGFSS PVSSTPISPI FGPSNWHFMP PVSEVVPTQG
301   ADPLLYESLC SVPAPTSVQK WEDSAHPQRP DNADLAILYA VVDGVPPARW
351   KEFMRFMGLS EHEIERLEMQ NGRCLREAQY SMLEAWRRRT PRHEDTLEVV
401   GLVLSKMNLA GCLENILEAL RNPAPSSTTR LPR
```

Amino acid sequence for mouse TNF type II (p75) receptor [24]
Accession code: Genbank M60469

```
-22  MAPAALWVAL  VFELQLWATG  HT
  1  VPAQVVLTPY  KPEPGYECQI  SQEYYDRKAQ  MCCAKCPPGQ  YVKHFCNKTS
 51  DTVCADCEAS  MYTQVWNQFR  TCLSCSSSCT  TDQVEIRACT  KQQNRVCACE
101  AGRYCALKTH  SGSCRQCMRL  SKCGPGFGVA  SSRAPNGNVL  CKACAPGTFS
151  DTTSSTDVCR  PHRICSILAI  PGNASTDAVC  APESPTLSAI  PRTLYVSQPE
201  PTRSQPLDQE  PGPSQTPSIL  TSLGSTPIIE  QSTKGGISLP  IGLIVGVTSL
251  GLLMLGLVNC  IILVQRKKKP  SCLQRDAKVP  HVPDEKSQDA  VGLEQQHLLT
301  TAPSSSSSSL  ESSASAGDRR  APPGGHPQAR  VMAEAQGFQE  ARASSRISDS
351  SHGSHGTHVN  VTCIVNVCSS  SDHSSQCSSQ  ASATVGDPDA  KPSASPKDEQ
401  VPFSQEECPS  QSPCETTETL  QSHEKPLPLG  VPDMGMKPSQ  AGWFDQIAVK
451  VA
```

References
1 Manogue, K.R. et al. (1991) In The Cytokine Handbook, Thomson, A.W. ed., Academic Press, London, pp. 241–256.
2 Fiers, W. (1991) FEBS 285, 199–212.
3 Ruddle, N.H. (1992) Curr. Opin. Immunol. 4, 327–332.
4 Gearing, A.J.H. et al. (1994) Nature 370, 555–557.
5 Jones, E.Y. et al. (1989) Nature 338, 225–228.
6 Nedwin, G.E. et al. (1985) Nucl. Acids Res. 13, 6361–6373.
7 Semon, D. et al. (1987) Nucl. Acids Res. 15, 9083–9084.
8 Pennica, D. et al. (1984) Nature 312, 724–729.
9 Pennica, D. et al. (1985) Proc. Natl. Acad. Sci. USA 82, 6060–6064.
10 Tartaglia, L.A. and Goeddel, D.V. (1992) Immunol. Today 13, 151–153.
11 Nophar, Y. et al. (1990) EMBO J. 9, 3269–3278.
12 Upton, C. et al. (1991) Virology 184, 370–382.
13 Dressler, K.A. et al. (1992) Science 255, 1715–1718.
14 Mathias, S. et al. (1991) Proc. Natl Acad. Sci. USA 88, 10009–10013.
15 Schutze, S. et al. (1992) Cell 71, 765–776.
16 Schutze, S. et al. (1991) J. Exp. Med. 174, 975–988.
17 De-Valck, D. et al. (1993) Eur. J. Biochem. 212, 491–497.
18 Wiegmann, K. et al. (1992) J. Biol. Chem. 267, 17997–18001.
19 Yanaga, F. et al. (1992) J. Biol. Chem. 267, 5114– 5121 .
20 Rothe, J. et al. (1993) Nature 364, 798–801.
21 Loetscher, H. et al. (1990) Cell 61, 351–359.
22 Schall, T. J. et al. (1990) Cell 61, 361–370.
23 Smith, C.A. et al. (1990) Science 248, 1019–1023.
24 Lewis, M. et al. (1991) Proc. Natl. Acad. Sci USA 88, 2830–2834.

Tpo

Other names
Megakaryocyte colony stimulating factor, c-MPL ligand

THE MOLECULE

Thrombopoietin is a megakaryocytic lineage specific growth and differentiation factor [1,2,3]. It acts in an analogous fashion to erythropoietin functioning as a circulating regulator of platelet numbers [1,5].

Cross reactivity
Human Tpo is active on murine cells and vice versa [2,3,4]. There is 23% identity between the first 153 amino acids of Tpo and erythropoietin.

Sources
Serum from aplastic individuals, liver, kidney, skeletal muscle.

Bioassays
Generation of megakaryocytes/megakaryocytic colonies from bone marrow cultures[2,3,4,5].

Physicochemical properties of thrombopoietin

Property		Human	Mouse
Amino acids	– precursor	353	356
	– mature[a]	332	335
M_r (K)	– predicted	38	35
	– expressed[b]	60	?
Potential N-linked glycosylation sites		6	7
Disulphide bonds[c]		2	2

[a] The mature protein may be proteolytically processed to give a minimal functional unit corresponding to the N-terminal, epo-like domain. Dibasic (RR) cleavage sites are present in the C-terminal domain. Both mature protein and the epo-like domain are biologically active.

[b] The Mr 60,000 form represents the fully glycosylated mature protein. Other species of human Tpo of Mr 18, 28 and 30k have been described.

[c] By homology to erythropoietin the first and last cysteines may form a critical disulphide bond.

3-D structure
The structure of the N-terminal 156 amino acids could be modelled on erythropoietin.

Gene structure

No information is available.

Amino acid sequence for human thrombopoietin [2]

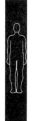

```
-21  MQLTQLLLVV MLLLTARLTL S
  1  SPAPPACDLR VLSKLLRDSH VLHSRLSQCP EVHPLPTPVL LPAVDFLGES
 51  WKTQMEETKA QDILGAVTLL LEGVMAARGQ LGPTCLSSLL GQLSGQVRLL
101  LGALQSLLGT QLPPQGRTTA HKDPMAIFLS FQHLLRGKVR FLMLVGGSTL
151  CVRRAPPTTA VPSRTSLVLT LNELPNRTSG LLETNFTASA RTTGSGLLKW
201  QQGFRAKIPG LLNQTSRSLD QIPGYLNRIH ELLNGTRGLF PGPSRRTLGA
251  PDISSGTSDT GSLPPNLQPG YSPSPTHPPT GQYTLFPLPP TLPTPVVQLH
301  PLLPDPSAPT PTPTSPLLNT SYTHSQNLSQ EG
```

Epo-like domain amino acids 1–156.

Amino acid sequence for murine thrombopoietin [3]

```
-21  MELTDLLLAA MLLAVARLTL S
  1  SPVAPACDPR LLNKLLRDSH LLHSRLSQCP DVDPLSIPVL LPAVDFSLGE
 51  WKTQTEQSKA QDILGAVSLL LEGVMAARGQ LEPSCLSSLL GQLSGQVRLL
101  LGALQGLLGT QLPLQGRTTA HKDPNALFLS LQQLLRGKVR FLLLVEGPTL
151  CVRRTLPTTA VPSSTSQLLT LNKFPNRTSG LLETNFSVTA RTAGPGLLSR
201  LQGFRVKITP GQLNQTSRSP VQISGYLNRT HGPVNGTHGL FAGTSLQTLE
251  ASDISPGAFN KGSLAFNLQG GLPPSPSLAP DGHTPFPPSP ALPTTHGSPP
301  QLHPLFPDPS TTMPNSTAPH PVTMYPHPRN LSQET
```

Epo-like domain amino acids 1–157.

THE THROMBOPOIETIN RECEPTOR (c-mpl)

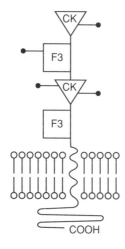

The thrombopoietin receptor also known as c-mpl is a member of the cytokine receptor superfamily with two extracellular segments each with a CKR and a FNIII domain containing a WSXWS (or WGXWS) motif similar to the LIFR and the common β-subunit of the IL-3, IL-5 and GM-CSF receptors. A soluble form of the mouse receptor has been identified [6]. A portion of the c-mpl (thrombopoietin receptor) gene has been found fused to viral sequences encoding the envelope protein of a mutant strain of Friend leukaemia virus called myeloproliferative leukaemia virus (MPLV) [7]. The viral oncogene v-mpl includes the entire cytoplasmic and transmembrane domains of the c-mpl gene and 40 amino acids including the WSXWS motif of the extracellular domain. The remainder of the extracellular domain is replaced by viral envelope sequences.

Distribution

Megakaryocytes and megakaryocyte precursors, platelets. c-mpl mRNA is found in BAF3 and HEL cell lines.

Physicochemical properties of the thrombopoietin receptor (c-mpl)

Properties	Human	Mouse
Amino acids – precursor	635 (579)[a]	625 (457)[a]
– mature[b]	610 (554)	600 (432)
M_r (K) – predicted	68.6 (62.8)	67.1 (48.5)
– expressed	?	78 (55)
Potential N-linked glycosylation sites	4	4

[a] Truncated form in parenthesis.
[b] After removal of predicted signal peptide.

Signal transduction

The mechanism of signal transduction is not known.

Chromosomal location
The human thrombopoietin receptor is on chromosome 1p34, and the mouse receptor is on the D band of chromosome 4.

Amino acid sequence for the human thrombopoietin receptor (c-mpl) [8]

Accession code: GenEMBL M90102

```
-25  MPSWALFMVT  SCLLLAPQNL  AQVSS
  1  QDVSLLASDS  EPLKCFSRTF  EDLTCFWDEE  EAAPSGTYQL  LYAYPREKPR
 51  ACPLSSQSMP  HFGTRYVCQF  PDQEEVRLFF  PLHLWVKNVF  LNQTRTQRVL
101  FVDSVGLPAP  PSIIKAMGGS  QPGELQISWE  EPAPEISDFL  RYELRYGPRD
151  PKNSTGPTVI  QLIATETCCP  ALQRPHSASA  LDQSPCAQPT  MPWQDGPKQT
201  SPSREASALT  AEGGSCLISG  LQPGNSYWLQ  LRSEPDGISL  GGSWGSWSLP
251  VTVDLPGDAV  ALGLQCFTLD  LKNVTCQWQQ  QDHASSQGFF  YHSRARCCPR
301  DRYPIWENCE  EEEKTNPGLQ  TPQFSRCHFK  SRNDSIIHIL  VEVTTAPGTV
351  HSYLGSPFWI  HQAVRLPTPN  LHWREISSGH  LELELEWQHPSS  WAAQETCYQL
401  RYTGEGHQDW  KVLEPPLGAR  GGTLELRPRS  RYRLQLRARL  NGPTYQGPWS
451  SWSDPTRVET  ATETAWISLV  TALHLVLGLS  AVLGLLLLRW  QFPAHYRRLR
501  HALWPSLPDL  HRVLGQYLRD  TAALSPPKAT  VSDTCEEVEP  SLLEILPKSS
551  ERTPLPLCSS  QAQMDYRRLQ  PSCLGTMPLS  VCPPMAESGS  CCTTHIANHS
601  YLPLSYWQQP
```

A second mRNA species (GenBank M90103) predicts a truncated form with a cytoplasmic domain of 66 amino acids compared with 122 amino acids for the full length form. The truncated form is identical to the full length form in the extracellular and transmembrane domains and the first 9 amino acids of the cytoplasmic domain.

Amino acid sequence for the mouse thrombopoietin receptor (c-mpl) [6,9]

Accession code: GenEMBL Z22649

```
-25  MPSWALFMVT  SCLLLALPNQ  AQVTS
  1  QDVFLLALGT  EPLNCFSQTF  EDLTCFWDEE  EAAPSGTYQL  LYAYRGEKPR
 51  ACPLYSQSVP  TFGTRYVCQF  PAQDEVRLFF  PLHLWVKNVS  LNQTLIQRVL
101  FVDSVGLPAP  PRVIKARGGS  QPGELQIHWE  APAPEISDFL  RHELRYGPTD
151  SSNATAPSVI  QLLSTETCCP  TLWMPNPVPV  LDQPPCVHPT  ASQPHGPAPF
201  LTVKGGSCLV  SGLQASKSYW  LQLRSQPDGV  SLRGSWGPWS  FPVTVDLPGD
251  AVTIGLQCFT  LDLKMVTCQW  QQQDRTSSQG  FFRHSRTRCC  PTDRDPTWEK
301  CEEEEPRPGS  QPALVSRCHF  KSRNDSVIHI  LVEVTTAQGA  VHSYLGSPFW
351  IHQAVLLPTP  SLHWREVSSG  RLELEWQHQS  SWAAQETCYQ  LRYTGEGRED
401  WKVLEPSLGA  RGGTLELRPR  ARYSLQLRAR  LNGPTYQGPW  SAWSPPARVS
451  TGSETAWITL  VTALLLVLSL  SALLGLLLLK  WQFPAHYRRL  RHALWPSLPD
501  LHRVLGQYLR  DTAALSPSKA  TVTDSCEEVE  PSLLEILPKS  SESTPLPLCP
551  SQPQMDYRGL  QPCLRTMPLS  VCPPMAETGS  CCTTHIANHS  YLPLSYWQQP
```

A truncated form of murine thrombopoietin with a 257 bp deletion coding for 55 amino acids of the extracellular domain including the WSXWS motif, the transmembrane domain and the first 8 amino acids of the intracellular domain has also been identified (amino acids 402–488). The deletion generates a frame shift and terminates after a further 30 amino acids.

References

1 McDonald, T.P. (1988) Exp. Hematol. 16, 201–205.
2 De Sauvage, F.J. et al. (1994) Nature 369, 533–538.
3 Lok, S. et al. (1994) Nature 369, 565–568.
4 Kaushanksky, K. et al. (1994) Nature 369, 568–571.
5 Wendling, F. et al. (1994) Nature 369, 571–574.
6 Skoda, R.C. et al. (1993) EMBO. J. 12, 2645–2653.
7 Souyri, M. et al. (1990) Cell 63, 1137–1147.
8 Vignon, I. et al. (1992) Proc. Natl. Acad. Sci. USA 89, 5640–5644.
9 Vignon, I. et al. (1993) Oncogene 8, 2607–2615.

Other names

Human VEGF has been known as vascular permeability factor VPF, folliculo-stellate cell-derived growth factor and glioma-derived vascular endothelial cell mitogen.

THE MOLECULE

Vascular endothelial growth factor is a heparin-binding, dimeric protein related to the PDGF/sis family of growth factors [1]. It is a mitogen for endothelial cells, activates and is chemoattractant for monocytes, enhances blood vessel permeability and is a procoagulant [2,3]. A homologue of VEGF is encoded by the orf virus [4].

Crossreactivity

There is about 88% homology between human and rat VEGF, 18% homology with PDGF-B and 15% homology with PDGF-A [1]. Rodent VEGF is active on human cells and vice versa [2].

Sources

Pituitary cells, monocyte/macrophages, smooth muscle, keratinocytes [2,3].

Bioassays

Proliferation of bovine endothelial cells [5].

Physicochemical properties of VEGF

Property		Human	Rat
pI		Basic	Basic
Amino acids	– precursor	215,191,147	190
	– mature	189,165,121[a]	164
M_r (K)	– predicted	25	22.4
	– expressed[b]	45	45
Potential N-linked glycosylation sites		1	1
Disulphide bonds[c]		8?	8?

[a] The 121 and 165 amino acid forms are secreted, the 189 amino acid form is cell associated [6].

[b] The protein forms dimers, it is not known whether these are hetero- or homodimers.

[c] There are 16 Cys residues with eight possible disulphide bonds.

3-D structure

No information, likely to be similar to PDGF.

Gene structure for Human VEGF [7]

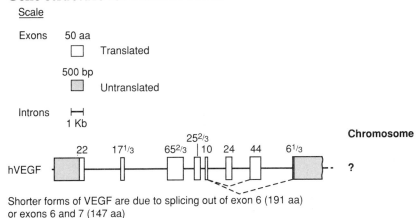

Scale

Exons   50 aa

☐ Translated

500 bp

☐ Untranslated

Introns ⊢⊣
1 Kb

Shorter forms of VEGF are due to splicing out of exon 6 (191 aa)
or exons 6 and 7 (147 aa)

Amino acid sequence for human VEGF [1,3]

Accession code: Swissprot P15692

```
-26   MNFLLSWVHW  SLALLLYLHH  AKWSQA
  1   APMAEGGGQN  HHEVVKFMDV  YQRSYCHPIE  TLVDIFQEYP  DEIEYIFKPS
 51   CVPLMRCGGC  CNDEGLECVP  TEESNITMQI  MRIKPHQGQH  IGEMSFLQHN
101   KCECRPKKDR  ARQEKKSVRG  KGKGQKRKRK  KSRYKSWSVP  CGPCSERRKH
151   LFVQDPQTCK  CSCKNTDSRC  KARQLELNER  TCRCDKPRR
```

Residues encoded by exons 6 and 7 (in italics) may be spliced out.
Conflicting sequence K->N at position 116.

Amino acid sequence for rat VEGF [8]

Accession code: Swissprot P16612

```
-25   MNFLLSWVHW  TLALLLYLHH  AKWSQ
  1   AAPTTEGEQK  AHEVVKFMDV  YQRSYCRPIE  TLVDIFQEYP  DEIEYIFKPS
 51   CVPLMRCAGC  CNDEALECVP  TSESNVTMQI  MRIKPHQSQH  IGEMSFLQHS
101   RCECRPKKDR  TKPENHCEPC  SERRKHLFVQ  DPQTCKCSCK  NTDSRCKARQ
151   LELNERTCRC  DKPRR
```

THE VEGF RECEPTORS

There are three published receptors for VEGF. One is the fms-like tyrosine
kinase flt [9,10], the second receptor is the KDR gene product (the murine
homologue of KDR is the flk-1 gene product) [11,12], and the third receptor is
the flt4 gene product [13]. All are related to the PDGF receptor/M-CSF
receptor/c-kit family of class III tyrosine kinases, but contain seven
extracellular immunoglobulin domains, and an intracellular tyrosine kinase
domain with a kinase insert. The receptors are thought to dimerize in the
presence of ligand to transmit a signal. It is unknown if heterodimers of the
different receptors can form.

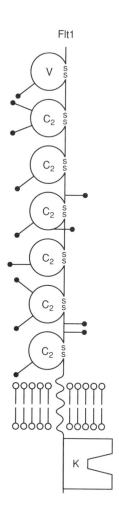

Distribution

The receptors are found on endothelial cells, primitive haematopoietic stem cells, monocytes and erythroleukaemia cells [14].

Physicochemical properties of the VEGF receptors

Properties	Human		
	flt1	flt4	KDR
Amino acids – precursor	1338	1298	1356
– mature	1316	1276	1336
M_r (K) – predicted	150	145	151
– expressed	160	?	195/235
Potential N-linked glycosylation sites	13	12	17
Affinity K_d (M)	0.2×10^{-10}		0.75×10^{-10}

Signal transduction

Ligand binding causes receptor dimerization, tyrosine phosphorylation of a 200 000 Mr protein in endothelial cells, autophosphorylation and a calcium flux [12].

Chromosomal location

Flt1 is located on human chromosome 13q12 [14], kdr is on human chromosome 4, and flt4 is found on chromosome 5q33-qter [13].

Amino acid sequence for human flt1 VEGF receptor [9]

Accession code: Swissprot P17948

```
 -22  MVSYWDTGVL  LCALLSCLLL  TG
   1  SSSGSKLKDP  ELSLKGTQHI  MQAGQTLHLQ  CRGEAAHKWS  LPEMVSKESE
  51  RLSITKSACG  RNGKQFCSTL  TLNTAQANHT  GFYSCKYLAV  PTSKKKETES
 101  AIYIFISDTG  RPFVEMYSEI  PEIIHMTEGR  ELVIPCRVTS  PNITVTLKKF
 151  PLDTLIPDGK  RIIWDSRKGF  IISNATYKEI  GLLTCEATVN  GHLYKTNYLT
 201  HRQTNTIIDV  QISTPRPVKL  LRGHTLVLNC  TATTPLNTRV  QMTWSYPDEK
 251  NKRASVRRRI  DQSNSHANIF  YSVLTIDKMQ  NKDKGLYTCR  VRSGPSFKSV
 301  NTSVHIYDKA  FITVKHRKQQ  VLETVAGKRS  YRLSMKVKAF  PSPEVVWLKD
 351  GLPATEKSAR  YLTRGYSLII  KDVTEEDAGN  YTILLSIKQS  NVFKNLTATL
 401  IVNVKPQIYE  KAVSSFPDPA  LYPLGSRQIL  TCTAYGIPQP  TIKWFWHPCN
 451  HNHSEARCDF  CSNNEESFIL  DADSNMGNRI  ESITQRMAII  EGKNKMASTL
 501  VVADSRISGI  YICIASNKVG  TVGRNISFYI  TDVPNGFHVN  LEKMPTEGED
 551  LKLSCTVNKF  LYRDVTWILL  RTVNNRTMHY  SISKQKMAIT  KEHSITLNLT
 601  IMNVSLQDSG  TYACRARNVY  TGEEILQKKE  ITIRDQEAPY  LLRNLSDHTV
 651  AISSSTTLDC  HANGVPEPQI  TWFKNNHKIQ  QEPGIILGPG  SSTLFIERVT
 701  EEDEGVYHCK  ATNQKGSVES  SAYLTVQGTS  DKSNLELITL  TCTCVAATLF
 751  WLLLTLLIRK  MKRSSSEIKT  DYLSIIMDPD  EVPLDEQCER  LPYDASKWEF
 801  ARERLKLGKS  LGRGAFGKVV  QASAFGIKKS  PTCRTVAVKM  LKEGATASEY
 851  KALMTELKIL  THIGHHLNVV  NLLGACTKQG  GPLMVIVEYC  KYGNLSNYLK
 901  SKRDLFFLNK  DAALHMEPKK  EKMEPGLEQG  KKPRLDSVTS  SESFASSGFQ
 951  EDKSLSDVEE  EEDSDGFYKE  PITMEDLISY  SFQVARGMEF  LSSRKCIHRD
1001  LAARNILLSE  NNVVKICDFG  LARDIYKNPD  YVRKGDTRLP  LKWMAPESIF
1051  DKIYSTKSDV  WSYGVLLWEI  FSLGGSPYPG  VQMDEDFCSR  LREGMRMRAP
1101  EYSTPEIYQI  MLDCWHRDPK  ERPRFAELVE  KLGDLLQANV  QQDGKDYIPI
1151  NAILTGNSGF  TYSTPAFSED  FFKESISAPK  FNSGSSDDVR  YVNAFKFMSL
1201  ERIKTFEELL  PNATSMFDDY  QGDSSTLLAS  PMLKRFTWTD  SKPKASLKID
1251  LRVTSKSKES  GLSDVSRPSF  CHSSCGHVSE  GKRRFTYDHA  ELERKIACCS
1301  PPPDYNSVVL  YSTPPI
```

An alternative terminus of GV at amino acid 1255 has been described. Tyr1031 is phosphorylated. Thr770 can be replaced with Phe.

Amino acid sequence for human flt4 VEGF receptor [13]

Accession code: GenEMBL X69878, X68203

```
 -22  MQRGAALCLR  LWLCLGLLDG  LV
   1  SDYSMTPPTL  NITEESHVID  TGDSLSISCR  GQHPLEWAWP  GAQEAPATGD
  51  KDSEDTGVVR  DCEGTDARPY  CKVLLLHEVH  ANDTGSYVCY  YKYIKARIEG
 101  TTAASSYVFV  RDFEQPFINK  PDTLLVNRKD  AMWVPCLVSI  PGLNVTLRSQ
 151  SSVLWPDGQE  VVWDDRRGML  VSTPLLHDAL  YLQCETTWGD  QDFLSNPFLV
 201  HITGNELYDI  QLLPRKSLEL  LVGEKLVLNC  TVWAEFNSGV  TFDWDYPGKQ
 251  AERGKWVPER  RSQQTHTELS  SILTIHNVSQ  HDLGSYVCKA  NNGIQRFRES
 301  TEVIVHENPF  ISVEWLKGPI  LEATAGDELV  KLPVKLAAYP  PPEFQWYKDG
 351  KALSGRHSPH  ALVLKEVTEA  STGTYTLALW  NSAAGLRRNI  SLELVVNVPP
 401  QIHEKEASSP  SIYSRHSRQA  LTCTAYGVPL  PLSIQWHWRP  WTPCKMFAQR
 451  SLRRRQQQDL  MPQCRDWRAV  TTQDAVNPIE  SLDTWTEFVE  GKNKTVSKLV
 501  IQNANVSAMY  KCVVSNKVGQ  DERLIYFYVT  TIPDGFTIES  KPSEELLEGQ
 551  PVLLSCQADS  YKYEHLRWYR  LNLSTLHDAH  GNPLLLDCKN  VHLFATPLAA
 601  SLEEVAPGAR  HATLSLSIPR  VAPEHEGHYV  CEVQDRRSHD  KHCHKKYLSV
 651  QALEAPRLTQ  NLTDLLVNVS  DSLEMQCLVA  GAHAPSIVWY  KDERLLEEKS
 701  GVDLADSNQK  LSIQRVREED  AGPYLCSVCR  PKGCVNSSAS  VAVEGSEDKG
 751  SMEIVILVGT  GVIAVFFWVL  LLLIFCNMRR  PAHADIKTGY  LSIIMDPGEV
 801  PLEEQCEYLS  YDASQWEFPR  ERLHLGRVLG  YGAFGKVVEA  SAFGIHKGSS
 851  CDTVAVKMLK  EGATASEQRA  LMSELKILIH  IGNHLNVVNL  LGACTKPQGP
 901  LMVIVEFCKY  GNLSNFLRAK  RDAFSPCAEK  SPEQRGRFRA  MVELARLDRR
 951  RPGSSDRVLF  ARFSKTEGGA  RRASPDQEAE  DLWLSPLTME  DLVCYSFQVA
1001  RGMEFLASRK  CIHRDLAARN  ILLSESDVVK  ICDFGLARDI  YKDPDYVRKG
1051  SARLPLKWMA  PESIFDKVYT  TQSDVWSFGV  LLWEIFSLGA  SPYPGVQINE
1101  EFCQRVRDGT  RMRAPELATP  AIRHIMLNCW  SGDPKARPAF  SDLVEILGDL
1151  LQGRGLQEEE  EVCMAPRSSQ  SSEEGSFSQV  STMALHIAQA  DAEDSPPSLQ
1201  RHSLAARYYN  WVSFPGCLAR  GAETRGSSRM  KTFEEFPMTP  TTYKGSVDNQ
1251  TDSGMVLASE  EFEQIESRHR  QESGFR
```

Amino acid sequence for human KDR VEGF receptor [12]

Accession code: GenEMBL X61656, L04947

```
 -19  MSKVLLAVAL  WLCVETRAA
   1  SVGLPSVSLD  LPRLSIQKDI  LTIKANTTLQ  ITCRGQRDLD  WLWPNNQSGS
  51  EQRVEVTECS  DGLFCKTLTI  PKVIGNDTGA  YKCFYRETDL  ASVIYVYVQD
 101  YRSPFIASVS  DQHGVVYITE  NKNKTVVIPC  LGSISNLNVS  LCARYPEKRF
 151  VPDGNRISWD  SKKGFTIPSY  MISYAGMVFC  EAKINDESYQ  SIMYIVVVVG
 201  YRIYDVVLSP  SHGIELSVGE  KLVLNCTART  ELNVGIDFNW  EYPSSKHQHK
 251  KLVNRDLKTQ  SGSEMKKFLS  TLTIDGVTRS  DQGLYTCAAS  SGLMTKKNST
 301  FVRVHEKPFV  AFGSGMESLV  EATVGERVRI  PAKYLGYPPP  EIKWYKNGIP
 351  LESNHTIKAG  HVLTIMEVSE  RDTGNYTVIL  TNPISKEKQS  HVVSLVVYVP
 401  PQIGEKSLIS  PVDSYQYGTT  QTLTCTVYAI  PPPHHIHWYW  QLEEECANEP
 451  SQAVSVTNPY  PCEEWRSVED  FQGGNKIEVN  KNQFALIEGK  NKTVSTLVIQ
 501  AANVSALYKC  EAVNKVGRGE  RVISFHVTRG  PEITLQPDMQ  PTEQESVSLW
 551  CTADRSTFEN  LTWYKLGPQP  LPIHVGELPT  PVCKNLDTLW  KLNATMFSNS
 601  TNDILIMELK  NASLQDQGDY  VCLAQDRKTK  KRHCVVRQLT  VLERVAPTIT
```

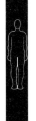

```
 651  GNLENQTTSI  GESIEVSCTA  SGNPPPQIMW  FKDNETLVED  SGIVLKDGNR
 701  NLTIRRVRKE  DEGLYTCQAC  SVLGCAKVEA  FFIIEGAQEK  TNLEIIILVG
 751  TTVIAMFFWL  LLVIILGTVK  RANGGELKTG  YLSIVMDPDE  LPLDEHCERL
 801  PYDASKWEFP  RDRLNLGKPL  GRGAFGQEIE  ADAFGIDKTA  TCRTVAVKML
 851  KEGATHSEHR  ALMSELKILI  HIGHHLNVVN  LLGACTKPGG  PLMVIVEFCK
 901  FGNLSTYLRS  KRNEFVPYKT  KGARFRQGKD  YVGAIPVDLK  RRLDSITSSQ
 951  SSASSGFVEE  KSLSDVEEEE  APEDLYKDFL  TLEHLICYSF  QVAKGMEFLA
1001  SRKCIHRDLA  ARNILLSEKN  VVKICDFGLA  RDIYKDPDYV  RKGDARLPLK
1051  WMAPETIFDR  VYTIQSDVWS  FGVLLWEIFS  LGASPYPGVK  IDEEFCRRLK
1101  EGTRMRAPDY  TTPEMYQTML  DCWHGEPSQR  PTFSELVEHL  GNLLQANAQQ
1151  DGKDYIVLPI  SETLSMEEDS  GLSLPTSPVS  CMEEEEVCDP  KFHYDNTAGI
1201  SQYLQNSKRK  SRPVSVKTFE  DIPLEEPEVK  VIPDDNQTDS  GMVLASEELK
1251  TLEDRTKLSP  SFGGMVPSKS  RESVASEGSN  QTSGYQSGYH  SDDTDTTVYS
1301  SEEAELLKLI  EIGVQTGSTA  QILQPDTGTT  LSSPPV
```

References

[1] Leung, D.W. et al. (1989) Science 246, 1306–1309.

[2] Clauss, M. et al. (1990) J. Exp. Med. 172, 1535–1545.

[3] Keck, P.J. et al. (1989) Science 246, 1309–1312.

[4] Lythe, D.J. et al. (1994) J. Virol. 68, 84–92.

[5] Connolly, D.T. et al. (1989) J. Clin. Invest. 84, 1470.

[6] Houck, K.A. et al. (1992) J. Biol. Chem. 267, 26031–26037.

[7] Tischer, E. et al. (1991) J. Biol. Chem. 266, 11947–11954.

[8] Conn, G. et al. (1990) Proc. Natl. Acad. Sci. USA 87, 20017–20024.

[9] De Vries, C. et al. (1992) Science 255, 989–991.

[10] Shibuya, M. et al. (1990) Oncogene 5, 519–524.

[11] Millauer, B. et al. (1993) Cell 72, 835–846.

[12] Terman, B.I. et al. (1992) Biochem. Biophys. Res. Commun. 187, 1579–1586.

[13] Galland, F. et al. (1993) Oncogene 8, 1233–1240.

[14] Jakeman, L.B. et al. (1992) J. Clin. Invest. 89, 244–253.

[15] Myoken, Y. et al. (1991) Proc. Natl. Acad. Sci. USA 88, 5819–5823.

Appendix: Cytokine standards

The inherent variability of immunoassays, and particularly biological assays, means that cytokine assays should include a standard or reference preparation. Each laboratory should have an aliquoted frozen preparation of its own cytokine standards. Each assay should include at least one standard curve of the lab standard. The lab standard can be assigned an arbitrary potency of x units/ml which can then be compared with the activity of unknown samples by probit analysis. For most human cytokines, and some murine cytokines, an official WHO standard or reference reagent is available from NIBSC, Blanche lane, South Mimms, Potters Bar, Herts, UK or in the USA from BRMP, National Cancer Institutes, Frederick, Maryland 21701. These are listed below. The official standards should be used to calibrate lab standards.

Preparation	Code
Interleukin 1 alpha rDNA (International Standard)	86/632
Interleukin 1 beta rDNA (International Standard)	86/680
Interleukin 2 cell line derived (International Standard)	86/504
Interleukin 2 rDNA	86/564
Interleukin 3 rDNA	88/780
Interleukin 4 rDNA	88/656
Interleukin 5 rDNA	90/586
Interleukin 6 rDNA (International Standard)	89/548
Interleukin 7 rDNA	90/530
Interleukin 8 rDNA	89/520
Interleukin 9 rDNA	91/678
Interleukin 10 rDNA	92/516
Interleukin 11 rDNA	72/788
M-CSF rDNA (International Standard)	89/512
G-CSF rDNA (International Standard)	88/502
GM-CSF rDNA (International Standard)	88/646
Leukaemia inhibitory factor rDNA	91/602
Stem cell factor/MGF rDNA	91/682
Rantes rDNA	92/520
MIP-1 α rDNA	92/518
TGF β 1 rDNA	89/514
TGF β 1 (Natural Bovine)	89/516
TGF β 2 rDNA	90/696
TNF α rDNA (International Standard)	87/650
TNF β rDNA	87/640

General Bibliography

There now follows a list of useful references in Cytokines:

Aggarwal, B.B. and Gutterman, J.U. (1992) Human Cytokines: Handbook for Basic and Clinical Research, Blackwell Scientific, Oxford.

Aggarwal, B.B. and Vilcek, J. (1991) Tumour Necrosis Factors: Structure, Function and Mechanism of Action, Dekker, New York.

Baggiolini, M. and Sorg, C. (1991) Neutrophil-activating Peptides and Other Chemotactic Cytokines. Karger, Basle.

Baird, A. and Klagsbrun, M. (1993) Fibroblast Growth Factor Family. Annals of the New York Academy of Sciences.

Balkwill, Frances R. (1991) Cytokines: A Practical Approach. IRL Press, Oxford.

Baxter, A. and Ross, R. (1991) Cytokine Interactions and Their Control, Wiley, New York.

Bienvenu, J. and Fradelizi, D. (1991) Cytokines and Inflammation. J. Libbey.

Bothwell, M. (1991) Neuronal Growth Factors. Springer-Verlag, Berlin.

Cacciola, E. (1993) Hemopoeitic Growth Factors, Oncogenes and Cytokines in Clinical Hematology: Current Aspects and Future Directions, Karger, Basle.

Callard, R.E. (1990) Cytokines and B-Lymphocytes, Academic Press, London.

Clemens, M.J. (1991) Cytokines. BIOS Scientific Publishers.

Crowther, D.G. (1991) Interferons: Mechanisms of Action and Role in Cancer Therapy. Springer-Verlag, Berlin.

Crumpton, M.J. and Dexter, M.T. (1990) Growth Factors in Differentiation and Development, Royal Society, London.

Cummins, P. (1993) Growth Factors and the Cardiovascular System: Developments in Cardiovascular Medicine, Vol. 147, Kluwer, Dordrecht.

Dawson, M.M. (1991) Lymphokines and Interleukins, Open University, Press, Milton Keynes.

Freund Mathias etc (1990) Cytokines in Haemopoiesis, Oncology and AIDS, Springer-Verlag, Berlin.

Galvani, D. and Cawley, J.C. (1992) Cytokine Therapy, Cambridge University Press, Cambridge.

Gowen, M. (1992) Cytokines and Bone Metabolism, CRC Press Wolfe Pub.

Hamblin, A.S. (1994) Cytokines and Cytokine Receptors: In Focus. In Focus Series. IRL Press, Oxford.

Kimball, E.S. (1991) Cytokines and Inflammation. C.R.C.P.

Kunkel, S.L. and Remmick, D.G. (1992) Cytokines in Health and Disease, Dekker, New York.

Lord, B.A. and Dexter, T.M. (1992) Growth Factors in Haemopoiesis, Baillière Tindall, London.

Luger, T.A. and Scharz, T. (1993) Epidermal Growth Factors and Cytokines: Clinical Dermatology Vol. 10. Dekker, New York.

McKay, I.A. and Leigh, I. (1993) Growth Factors: A Practical Approach, Practical Approach Vol. 119. IRL Press, Oxford

Meager, A. (1990) Cytokines. Open University Press, Milton Keynes

Mertelsmann, R. (1990) Lymphohaematopoietic Growth Factors in Cancer Therapy, Springer-Verlag, Berlin.

Metcalf, D. (1992) Polyfunctional Cytokines; IL-6 and LIF: Ciba Foundation Symposium, Vol. 167 Wiley.

Oppenheim, J.J. (1990) Molecular and Cellular Biology of Cytokines, Wiley.

Oppenheim, J.J. and Shevach, E.M. (1990) Immunophysiology: The Role of Cells and Cytokines in Immunity and Inflammation. Oxford University Press, New York.

Oppenheim, J.J., Rossio, J.L. and Gearing, A.J.H. (1993) Clinical Applications of Cytokines: Role in diagnosis, Pathogenesis and Therapy, Oxford University Press, New York.

Piez, K.A. and Sporn, M.A. (1990) Transforming Growth Factor-betas; Chemistry, Biology and Therapeutics, New York Academy of Sciences.

Pollo, E.E. (1992) Haematopoietic Growth Factors; Biology and Clinical Use. Acta Haematologica, Vol.86, No. 3, Karger, Basle.

Robertson, D.M. and Herington, A. (1991) Growth Factors in Endocrinology. Bailière Tindall, London.

Ross, R.P. (1990) Growth Factors and Their Receptors: Genetic Control and Rational Application, Wiley, New York.

Rothwell, N. and Dantzer, R. (1992) Interleukin-1 in the Brain, Pergamon Press, Oxford.

Schomberg, D.W. (1991) Growth Factors in Reproduction; Symposium Proceedings, Springer-Verlag, Berlin.

Sporn, M.B. (1992) Control of Growth Factors and Prevention of Cancer, ESO Monographs, Springer-Verlag, Berlin.

Sporn, M.B. and Roberts, A.B. (1990) Peptide Growth Factors and Their Receptors, Springer-Verlag, Berlin.

Tache, Y. and Rivier, C. (1993) Corticotropin-releasing Factor and Cytokines Role in the Stress Response: Annals of the New York Academy of Sciences.

Thomson, A.W. (1991) Cytokine Handbook. Academic Press, London.

Waterfield, M.D. (1991) Growth Factors in Cell and Development Biology, Company of Biologists, Portland Press.

Westwick, J. (1991) Chemotactic Cytokines: Biology of the Inflammatory Peptide Supergene Family – International Symposium Proceedings, Plenum Press, New York.

Index